Human Touch in Healthcare

Stephanie Margarete Mueller
Claudia Winkelmann • Martin Grunwald

Human Touch in Healthcare

Textbook for Therapy, Care and Medicine

Springer

Stephanie Margarete Mueller
Haptic Research Lab
Paul-Flechsig-Institute for Brain Research
Leipzig University
Leipzig, Germany

Claudia Winkelmann
Alice Salomon University of Applied Sciences
Berlin, Berlin, Germany

Martin Grunwald
Haptic Research Lab
Paul-Flechsig-Institute for Brain Research
Leipzig University
Leipzig, Germany

ISBN 978-3-662-67859-6 ISBN 978-3-662-67860-2 (eBook)
https://doi.org/10.1007/978-3-662-67860-2

Translation from the German language edition: "Lehrbuch Haptik" by Stephanie Margarete Mueller et al., © Springer-Verlag GmbH Deutschland, ein Teil von Springer Nature 2022. Published by Springer Berlin Heidelberg. All Rights Reserved.

This Springer imprint is published by the registered company Springer-Verlag GmbH, DE, part of Springer Nature.
The registered company address is: Heidelberger Platz 3, 14197 Berlin, Germany

Paper in this product is recyclable.

Preface

Direct physical contact is one of the essential requirements of preventive, curative, rehabilitative, palliative, and nursing activities in all health professions. Despite modern technology and robot-assisted healthcare, physical contact is an elementary part of healing and nursing activities. Physical contact ranges from greeting gestures to painful but unavoidable procedures; from treating premature infants to caring for older adults.

Depending on the occupational field, physical contact with other people is frequent and intensive or sporadic and of low intensity. However, physical contact is not only a professional requirement; most often it is used to transmit sympathy and as a sign of humanity. The physical interactions in the health professions are therefore diverse and an integral part of everyday working life. As natural as the interpersonal contact in the various health professions between patient and specialist is, the precise knowledge of the psychological and physical effects of professional physical contact is not a matter of course.

The diverse effects of human touch are only rarely discussed within the healthcare system, and subject-specific knowledge is seldom implemented in teaching. However, in order to understand how touch affects the patient and what health effects even the smallest touch stimuli can trigger, a basic knowledge of the human haptic system is essential, because touch—socially mediated or professional touch—is not processed and evaluated through visual or acoustic systems, but through the haptic system.

The haptic system is fundamentally different from all other sensory systems in terms of its complexity, and it is also the largest human sensory system due to its multidimensionality. Its complexity and size may have contributed to the fact that the human sense of touch was investigated only marginally in the history of science. However, in the last 30 years, this sensory system has encountered a rapid increase in scientific attention, which is reflected in a growing number of scientific findings and clinical applications.

Studies on the inner workings of the human haptic system were scarce 30 years ago, but today publications on the subject fill entire rows of shelves and many digital folders. The increase in knowledge has thus reached a magnitude for which there is an urgent need to condense the essences in the form of textbooks. Therefore, the authors of this book have compiled both basic scientific and clinically relevant findings on the structure, function, and effects of the haptic system, and prepared a wide spectrum of topics in such a way that it can serve as a teaching tool for various healthcare professions.

With this textbook, the authors hope to support teachers and students in the areas of physical therapy, occupational therapy, health and nursing care, midwifery and obstetrics, speech therapy, geriatric care, and human medicine in developing skills specific to the sense of touch.

Leipzig, Germany — Stephanie Margarete Mueller
Berlin, Germany — Claudia Winkelmann
Leipzig, Germany — Martin Grunwald
Oct. 2023

Acknowledgments

This textbook was only possible thanks to the energetic help of many people. The authors would like to take this opportunity to thank them once again for their support. This thanks goes in particular to Prof. em. Dr. Lothar Beyer, who, due to his expertise in teaching, especially in manual medicine and as editor of the journal *Manual Medicine—European Journal of Manual Medicine*, very urgently pointed out the need for such a textbook a long time ago.

A textbook thrives on illustrations and tables. We would therefore like to thank Julius Ecke, Maria Huettig, Verena Kuehn, and Anna Zender, who supported us in a very creative, committed, and patient manner.

We would like to thank Jente Spille, Alina Mohr, and Sven Martin for the laborious final correction of the manuscript and valuable advice. We would also like to thank the two English-speaking editors, A. St. John Wallis and Dr. K. Barabas, for their invaluable proofreading support.

Last but not least, the book project could not have been completed without the structural support of the Medical Faculty of the University of Leipzig as well as the Alice Salomon Hochschule and the Institute for Applied Research Berlin.

Contents

Perceptual Dimensions of the Haptic System

1

Stephanie Margarete Mueller and Martin Grunwald

Contents

S. M. Mueller (✉) · M. Grunwald
Haptic Research Lab, Paul-Flechsig-Institute for Brain Research, Leipzig University, Leipzig, Germany
e-mail: s.mueller@medizin.uni-leipzig.de; mgrun@medizin.uni-leipzig.de

S. M. Mueller et al., *Human Touch in Healthcare*, https://doi.org/10.1007/978-3-662-67860-2_1

The task of each sensory system is to inform the organism about the properties of the external world and the properties and states of the body.

The outward function of a sensory system is called **exteroception** (Sect. 1.1). All sensory systems—visual, auditory, gustatory, olfactory, and haptic—enable the organism to perceive the physical and chemical properties of the external environment and their changes.

The properties and functions of the organism itself can be perceived via epiphenomena on the body surface through visual, auditory, gustatory, and olfactory receptors. Consequently, secretions can be smelled and tasted, color or shape changes in the skin, eyes, and mucous membranes can be seen, and stomach growls can be heard. In contrast, only the haptic system can perceive information directly inside the body, for example, heartbeat, intestinal peristalsis, and chest expansion. This **interoception** (Sect. 1.2) is possible due to a unique feature of the haptic system: while all other sensory systems consist of specialized biological receptors that are concentrated in a specific region of the body (eye, ear, nose, and mouth), the receptors of the haptic system (mechanoreceptors) exist in varying concentrations throughout the body. Therefore, the interoceptive and exteroceptive functions of the haptic system are not limited to a specific region of the organism.

During all active and passive movement and exploration processes, another class of perceptual qualities of the haptic system is of crucial importance: **Proprioception** (Sect. 1.3) refers to the ability of an organism to adequately detect the position, force, and movement of its limbs at all times in relation to its own body and the external environment. Proprioception forms the basis for all exploratory and motor activities of the body and is crucial for both exteroceptive and interoceptive processes.

To provide exteroceptive, proprioceptive, and interoceptive information, the haptic system relies on highly sensitive and **highly differentiated mechanoreceptors** (Sect. 2.1) that are located around hair follicles, in the skin, connective tissue, organs, musculature, tendons, and joints. The primary function of mechanoreceptors is to register any "deformation" of the organism (mechanosensation). The physical causes of deformations are forces in the form of pressure, stretch, vibration, or shear on the organism or corresponding stimuli inside the body. In addition, there are pain and temperature sensations. These mechanoreceptors form the distal part of a network of neural structures in the body and brain that processes mechanosensory stimuli (i.e., the somatosensory system).

▶ **Definition** The **haptic system** comprises all sensory and psychological aspects associated with the processing of physical stimuli (e.g., pressure, shear, temperature). Physical stimuli are processed by mechanoreceptors to form exteroceptive, proprioceptive, and interoceptive perceptions, as well as pain and temperature sensations. The psychological (e.g., evaluations, expectations, and emotions) and sensory processes of the haptic system influence each other.

In neuroscience and physiology, the neural network in the body and brain that processes physical stimuli is called the **somatosensory system**.

1.1 Sensitivity of the Skin and Perception of Environmental Stimuli (Exteroception)

Exteroception refers to the perception of external stimuli by a living being. To perceive the external environment adequately, signals from all sensory systems—visual, auditory, gustatory, olfactory, and haptic—are processed by the central nervous system (CNS) and complement each other to generate an overall, multisensory impression. The environmental stimuli processed by the haptic system are first detected by the **skin and body hair**. Depending on the intensity and force of the external stimuli, receptors in deeper tissue layers, such as the musculature, connective tissue, and joints, can also be activated. If the external stimulus influences the position of the head or the whole body, the vestibular organ will also respond.

The perceptual dimensions of the skin and mechanoreceptors located deep inside the body are described in separate chapters (Sect. 1.2 Interoception and Sect. 1.3 Proprioception).

The skin is the largest organ in the human body; it covers an area of about 2 m^2 (approx. 21 sqft). The skin is the sensory boundary of the human body, a protective layer, an organ of perception, and a means of communication. The dense network of mechanoreceptors in the skin and the underlying fatty and connective tissue register mechanical, thermal, and chemical changes (Fig. 1.1; Sect. 2.1 Mechanoreceptors). Mechanoreceptors are present in remarkably large numbers. Each square centimeter of body skin is equipped with at least 300 sensitive units, which equates to more than 750 per square inch. (For an estimate of the number of mechanoreceptors in the entire body, see Sect. 2.1.1) The density of receptors varies depending on the body area. Near body orifices that represent potential weak points of the organism, the receptor density is very high (Grunwald 2019). Similarly, the palpatory areas of the extremities (palms and soles), which have frequent contact with the external environment, contain a high density of receptors.

The mechanoreceptors in the skin allow objects to be recognized, roughness, firmness, and temperature to be perceived, interpersonal touch to be felt, and impending tissue damage to be registered. In addition, the skin's highly sensitive signal function protects the body against injuries and penetration from the smallest insects.

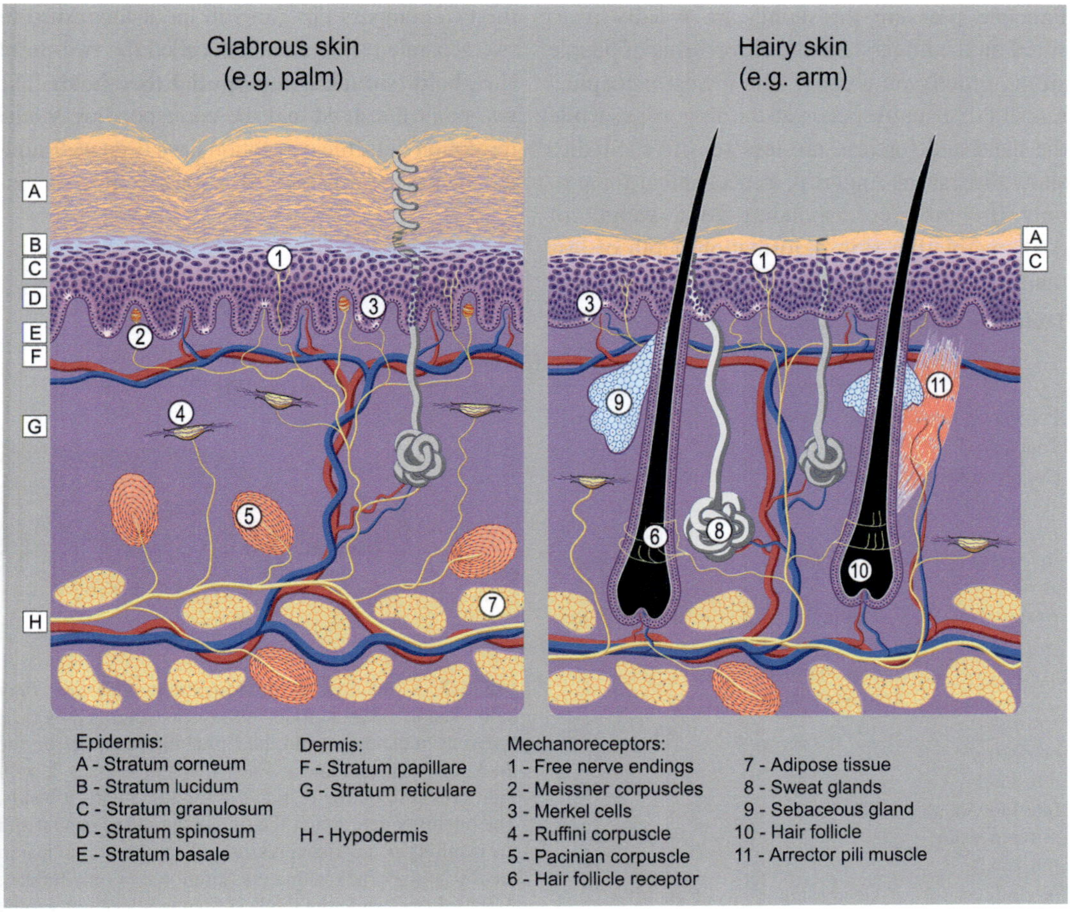

Fig. 1.1 Graphical representation of the skin layers. Localization of mechanoreceptors in hairless (left) and hairy (right) skin. (Illustration from hegasy.de, edited)

1.1.1 Tactile Perception

Exteroceptive functions of the human haptic system are distinguished by whether the perceiving person is exploring and actively moving or whether they are passive, motionless, and being touched. This distinction is important because it determines the complexity of the required perceptual processing and the resulting perceptual thresholds. The sensations that arise in a motionless person who is passively touched are called **tactile perceptions.** However, if the person performs active movements and explorations, **haptic perceptions** arise (Table 1.1). A special type of perception is generated by moving tactile stimuli (Sect. 1.1.2).

1.1.1.1 Sensory Thresholds for Tactile Punctate Pressure Stimuli

Punctate pressure thresholds are usually measured on the fingers, hands, or forearms of people sitting quietly on a chair. The lowest perceptual thresholds usually occur at the fingertips, while the hand and forearm are less sensitive. Studies show that, at the fingertip, a mechanical force of only 0.1 mN (corresponding to a weight of 0.01 mg) with a skin deformation depth of less than 10 μm can be reliably perceived (Johansson et al. 1980). So-called **von Frey hairs (alternative designation: Semmes–Weinstein monofilaments)** are used for this test (Fig. 1.2). This method is one of the oldest tactile threshold tests. Von Frey, the inventor of this method, was one of the first to discover that rapid placement of the stimulus hairs improved the sensation (cf. Sect. 1.1.2 Moving tactile stimuli) (Frey 1896). Like all tactile and haptic perception dimensions, this simple sensation threshold is characterized by large interindividual differences (Sect. 3.2) and a decrease in sensitivity with age (Sect. 3.1).

Table 1.1 Tactile versus haptic perception

	Tactile perception	Haptic perception
Perceiving person	Motionless	Moving
Touch type	Passive	Active
Cognitive demand	Low	High (touch and motion information)
Relevant body areas	Body surface	All body tissues
Example	Resting person feels how another person/object touches them	Person explores an object
Absolute perception threshold	10 μm	1 μm
Interindividual differences in sensitivity	Yes	Yes
Age effects	Decreasing sensitivity	Possibly decreasing sensitivity

1.1.1.2 Spatial Resolution (Two-Point Discrimination)

The accuracy of tactile perception is traditionally measured via two-point discrimination. Two blunted compass tips are simultaneously placed lightly on the skin. The smallest distance at which the two compass tips can still be distinguished as two separate tactile stimuli is called the **two-point threshold (simultaneous spatial threshold).** The two-point threshold and the corresponding spatial resolution of tactile perception have been well studied in various body parts. The tongue, lips, and fin-

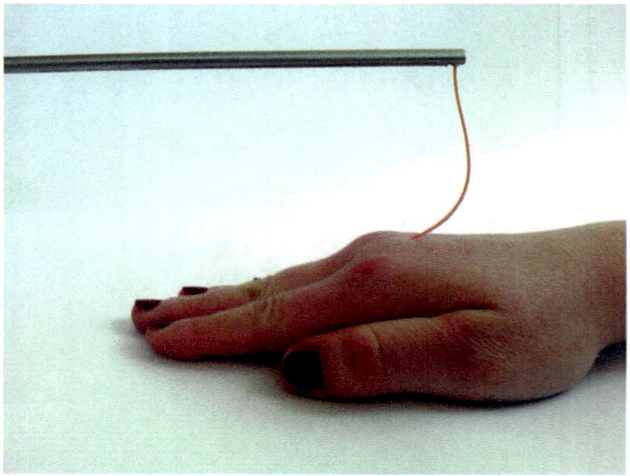

Fig. 1.2 Evaluating tactile sensitivity with von Frey hairs. The nylon monofilaments are characterized by their different thicknesses, and their pliability depends on the thickness of the filament. Each filament is placed, with light pressure, on the skin at a right angle until it bends. The pliability determines the force required to bend it and the resulting perceptible pressure. The thinnest filament in the test series bends with a pressure force of only 0.008 g (0.00028 oz), while the thickest filament bends at a force of 300 g (10.58 oz). (Fig. Haptic Research Laboratory, University of Leipzig)

gertips have the highest spatial resolution. At these sites, a 2–4-mm distance is sufficient to distinguish two simultaneously impinging tactile stimuli (Lederman and Klatzky 2009). The upper arm, thigh, and back have the lowest resolution, and a two-point distance of 50–100 mm is required in these regions (Fig. 1.3). Due to greater objectivity during the application, **grating domes** (stamps with different groove spacings; Sect. 4.2.2) are used in scientific investigations of spatial resolution.

▶ **Important** The higher tactile surface sensitivity in the face, hands, and feet is due to the greater density of mechanoreceptors in these body areas and their larger representational zones (due to frequent use) in the primary somatosensory cortex and thalamus (Birbaumer and Schmidt 2006).

Gridding of human surface sensitivity based on two-point thresholds is easy to illustrate. However, it captures only a small part of the perceptual spectrum and the actual sensitivity of the body surface. Much higher sensitivity can be achieved by haptic stimuli and by touching body hair.

Conclusion

Due to higher receptor density, the tongue, lips, and fingertips have lower two-point thresholds (i.e., a *higher* spatial resolution) than other areas of the body surface. A low threshold indicates that a person has high sensitivity.

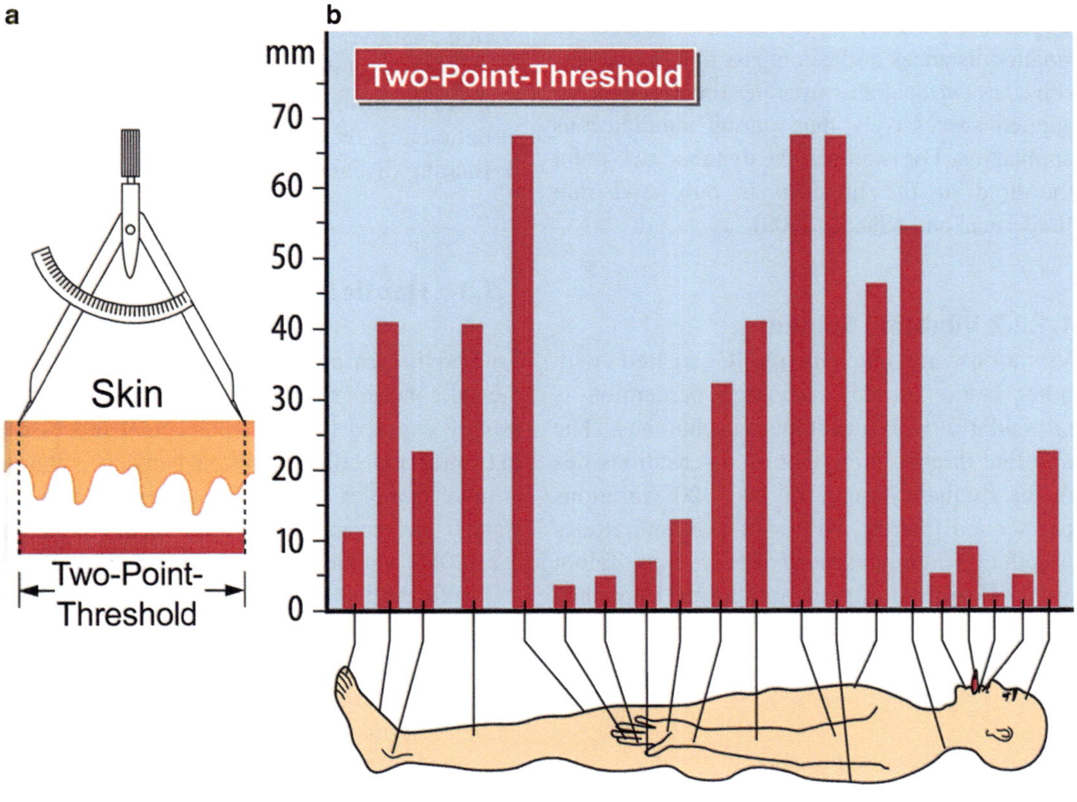

Fig. 1.3 (**a**) Test apparatus for measuring the two-point threshold. (**b**) Two-point threshold at different body sites. (Fig. translated from Birbaumer and Schmidt 2006).

1.1.2 Moving Tactile Stimuli

► **Important** There are no motionless stimuli; the speed with which a stimulus contacts the skin and deforms it is a movement itself. In addition, a living person is never entirely still; it breathes, and the body pulsates with the heartbeat. Consequently, all tactile stimuli are characterized by a dimension of more or less movement (cf. Sect. 1.1.3).

1.1.2.1 Dynamic Spatial Resolution

Surface sensitivity is usually higher if the body surface is touched with moving stimuli instead of static stimuli. Therefore, successive spatial thresholds (stimuli that follow each other in time) can be distinguished from simultaneous thresholds. For example, the dynamic two-point discrimination threshold is measured using two compass tips with a short temporal deviation. Depending on the body region, up to four times smaller distances of the compass tips can be perceived as two spatially separate stimuli if they are applied successively than during simultaneous application. For example, the dynamic two-point threshold at the fingertip is only 1–2 mm (Lederman and Klatzky 2009).

1.1.2.2 Vibration Stimuli

Vibrations are movements. Compared with other tactile stimuli, vibration perception is particularly well developed in humans. The absolute threshold for vibration sensations lies in the frequency range of 100–300 vibrations per second (Hertz), with vibration amplitudes (depth of skin indentation) of only 1 μm (Talbot et al. 1968). At higher and lower frequency ranges, higher vibration amplitudes are required to cause a vibration sensation (cf. Fig. 2.3 in Sect. 2.1.4).

► **Important** Naturally hairless skin (e.g., palms and soles) tends to be more sensitive to vibration than hairy skin (Talbot et al. 1968; Merzenich and Harrington 1969). Bone projections, nails, and teeth show the highest sensitivity to vibrational stimuli by transmitting vibrations to the surrounding skin areas (e.g., nail beds and gums).

Example

Vibration sensation (pallesthesia) can be measured by placing a vibrating tuning fork on bone projections. This **tuning fork test** (Rydell–Seifer test) is used in neurological examinations to assess deep sensibility and the ability to perceive vibrations (Rydel and Seiffer 1903; Martina et al. 1998). The examination is performed from distal (e.g., on the lower extremity at the metatarsophalangeal joint of the big toe) to proximal. The patients keep their eyes closed and indicate when they no longer feel the subsiding vibration. Decreased vibration sensation (pallhypesthesia) typically occurs due to peripheral neuropathies (e.g., due to diabetes mellitus types 1 and 2, vitamin B12 deficiency, or kidney diseases) and demyelinating diseases. ◄

1.1.3 Haptic Perception

True *tactile* sensations only occur under experimental conditions. In everyday life, humans are usually exposed to haptic perceptual processes. In contrast to tactile perception, haptic perception is more complex and enables discrimination of smaller surface and spatial differences (Libouton et al. 2010; Mueller et al. 2014; Grunwald 2001).

Haptic perceptions arise when the perceiving person actively moves. Therefore, movement information must always be processed simultaneously with touch information. However, not all motion information is relevant for haptic perception. Irrelevant motion information or other distracting stimuli (e.g., visual) can interfere with haptic perception and must be suppressed or filtered (see example).

Suppression of irrelevant information requires working memory resources (see Sect. 1.1.3.2). Because working memory resources are limited, distracting stimuli and a lack of concentration can disrupt the haptic perception process.

▶ **Important** During haptic perception, movement and position information are always present simultaneously with touch information.

Complexity of Haptic Perception

(a) The person sits in a chair with closed eyes and is instructed to recognize an object (e.g., a ball) with both hands. During the two-handed exploration of a ball, information from the skin of the fingers, muscles, connective tissue, and joints of the fingers, hands, arms, and shoulder girdle is processed for the recognition of the size, weight, and firmness of the ball. If the ball is very large or heavy, additional information from the thorax, back, and lower extremities may be relevant for detecting weight and size.

(b) Irrelevant motion information: The person in the experiment is exercising on a bicycle ergometer when the object (e.g., a ball) is handed to them. The information from muscles, tendons and joints that is required for recognition of the ball and the whole-body movements caused by cycling must be processed simultaneously. Therefore, the cycling movements must be recognized by the brain as irrelevant for object recognition, and they must be ignored. In addition, movement and sensory information that are caused by processes like breathing, blinking, and heartbeat must also be distinguished from object recognition. ◀

1.1.3.1 Absolute Haptic Threshold

A height difference of 1 µm is sufficient for a healthy adult human to perceive an elevation with their fingertip on an otherwise smooth surface (Johansson and LaMotte 1983; Louw et al. 2000, 2002); 1 µm corresponds to a height of 0.001 mm! [1 mm = 0.039 in.]. For comparison, human hair is between 30 and 100 µm thick, most pollen is between 10 and 100 µm in size, and particles of fine dust are 10 µm or smaller (particulate matter; Fig. 1.4). Furthermore, the limit of visual resolution is a particle size of about 40 µm under ideal illumination (e.g., swirled dust/pollen in sunlight). **Highly concentrated attention on exploration** and active movement of the exploring finger over the surface are crucial for reaching the absolute haptic threshold. Static (tactile) contact is insufficient for this perceptual outcome.

The movement required for haptic exploration is the reason that the distribution density of mechanoreceptors in the skin is less relevant for haptic sensitivity than for tactile sensitivity (two-point threshold). Two-point tactile discrimination requires that each of the two compass tips stimulate the receptive field of a discrete mechanoreceptor. If both compass tips stimulate the receptive field of the same receptor, this is perceived as only one point. In contrast, if two tips are moved across the skin, successively different mechanoreceptors are stimulated. Therefore, compass tips with much smaller distances can be perceived as two tips. Consequently, tactile test results cannot be used to infer haptic sensitivity. For example, age-related reduction in receptor density is associated with a reduced two-point threshold; however, active roughness discrimina-

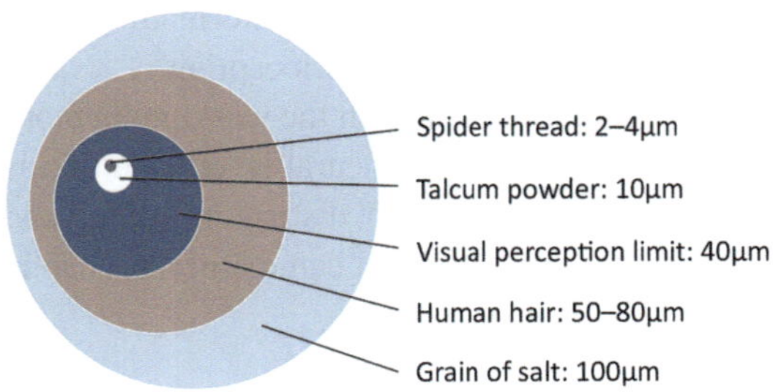

Fig. 1.4 Illustration of the relative size of a micrometer. Optimal lighting conditions (e.g., bright sunlight/backlight) are required for objects with a minimal size of about 40 µm to be perceived by the naked eye. Spider silk is visible only if light is reflected by the adhesive droplets of the silk or if the diameter of the threads is increased by dust or dew. (Illustration: Verena Kuehn)

tion (e.g., of sandpaper) remains stable as the person ages (cf. Sect. 3.1.4).

▶ **Important** To reach the absolute haptic threshold, a high degree of concentration on the exploration and active movement of the exploring finger over a surface are crucial. Static (tactile) contact is insufficient for this perceptual outcome.

1.1.3.2 Successive and Simultaneous Information Processing

Successive A distinctive feature of haptic exploration is that the shape of an object or surface must be explored piece by piece. To recognize an object or relief, many individual pieces of information, perceived **one after the other (successively)**, must be retained in memory and integrated at the neural level. Therefore, haptic perception requires that sufficient working memory resources are available. If **working memory** reaches capacity, distracting stimuli or a lack of concentration can interfere with recognition. This is likely why most individuals involuntarily close their eyes or stop talking during complex haptic exploration tasks. Furthermore, experiments have shown that the visibility of one's hand movements during exploration can interfere with the haptic recognition of complex stimuli (Mueller et al. 2013). In contrast, a fixed gaze in the direction of the exploring limb can improve attentional focus, which can facilitate haptic recognition (Tipper et al. 1998).

▶ **Important** Haptic perception requires that many separate pieces of information from exteroception, proprioception, and interoception are held in the working memory and integrated at the neural level. Due to this high cognitive demand, distracting stimuli and a lack of concentration can disrupt the haptic perception process.

Simultaneous In contrast with the successive perception of shape, some physical properties can be processed **simultaneously**. This mainly applies to an object's temperature and material (e.g., roughness, hardness, and softness).

▶ **Important** The perceptual dimensions of the haptic system (exteroception, interoception, and proprioception) influence and complement each other, and it is nearly impossible to generate sensations on just one dimension. For example, only strictly spatially limited tactile or temperature stimuli on the skin lead to exclusively exteroceptive perception. In contrast, any haptic exploration requires the integration of sensory impulses from multiple body parts; therefore, haptic exploration comprises all three perceptual dimensions.

1.1.3.3 Sensory Integration

In addition to successive information processing, the haptic recognition process is characterized by another feature. During haptic exploration, constantly changing information from the skin, musculature, connective tissue, tendons, and joints arrives at the brain from all parts of the body. The brain must sort the flood of successive and simultaneous information and assemble it meaningfully. This ability is called sensory integration (see Definition). If sensory integration is disturbed, haptic perception (among other things) is negatively affected (for more details, see Sects. 3.3.2 and 3.4.1). Therefore, tasks and tests that require haptic recognition are also used as diagnostic tools for disorders of sensory integration and body schema (for more details on body schema, see Sect. 1.4; for test and training systems, see Sect. 4.2).

▶ **Definition** **(Multi-)Sensory integration** refers to the brain's ability to order sensory stimuli (from different sensory channels, if necessary) and to link them meaningfully into an overall perception. The development of this ability begins in the womb and depends on incoming sensory stimuli. The haptic system, which is the first sense to develop in the embryo (from the seventh week of gestation), is the primary sensory input during gestation. Postnatally, sensory integration matures through the child's interaction with the environment (including haptic exploration) and their body (e.g., touch and movement stimuli). Sensory integration disorders are associated with a wide variety of learning and developmental impairments and are likely to promote the development of psychiatric and behavioral disorders (Levit-Binnun and Golland 2011; Ghassemzadeh et al. 2012). Through appropriate body and movement therapies in childhood (e.g., sensory integration therapy developed by Jean Ayres), deficits in sensory integration ability and psychomotor development can be alleviated (Ayres 1992; Bundy et al. 2007).

Conclusion

- **Tactile perceptions** occur when a motionless person is stimulated. This form of stimulation is limited due to physiological movement that cannot be prevented (e.g., due to breathing). Tactile stimuli are predominantly used under experimental conditions or in test situations (diagnostics). The smallest tactile perception thresholds can be generated by punctual pressure stimuli and require skin deformation depths of 10 μm.
- **Haptic perceptions** occur when a moving person is stimulated or a person actively touches something. For example, the absolute haptic perception threshold at the fingertip is 1 μm (equivalent to 0.001 mm or 0.00004 in.). Therefore, finer differences can be perceived during active exploration than during passive tactile or visual perception processes.
- Haptic perceptual processes require working memory capacity and cognitive resources for sensory integration. Haptic perception is complex due to the following aspects:
  - Information processing is both successive and simultaneous.
  - Movement information from all parts of the body must be processed (multisensory integration).
  - Irrelevant stimuli (motion stimuli and stimuli from other sensory channels) must be recognized as such and filtered out.

1.1.4 Hair Sensitivity

In any part of the body, the touch of a single hair can lead to a local touch sensation. This occurs because each hair follicle (hair root) is surrounded by a **network of mechanoreceptors**, in addition to the scattered receptors in the skin. Therefore, at each hair root, any deformation of the associated body hair, no matter how small, is detected (Sect. 2.1).

When determining surface sensitivity, it is usually neglected that the hairs protrude beyond the body surface, like feelers or antennae. Consequently, a touch sensation can be triggered even if there is no direct skin contact. Hair acts as an amplifier by transmitting a contact force (e.g., the weight of an insect) to a small area of skin around the hair follicle. This amplification effect can be observed especially well on shaved skin, where the perception thresholds for light touch stimuli are higher (i.e., shaved skin is less sensitive) (Frey 1896).

The exact forces required for perceptible hair deformation at different body sites have not yet been systematically investigated. However, for example, a weight of 0.4 mg (0.000014 oz) is perceptible on the hair of the middle phalanx of the index finger (Frey 1896). Anecdotally, even a 0.075 mg (0.0000026 oz) wing of a housefly falling on human forehead hairs can be perceived (Grunwald 2017; Becker-Carus and Wendt 2017). Because hair follicle receptors are especially sensitive to motion and changes in force, moving stimuli that deform several hairs in succession are likely perceptible at even lower weights.

With their large number and high sensitivity, body hair most likely fulfills a protective function for the skin, especially for body orifices (Grunwald 2017).

> **Important** The highly sensitive body hair can trigger touch sensations even before direct skin contact.

1.1.5 Interpersonal Touch

In direct interpersonal physical contact, all involved persons are senders and receivers of information about themselves and the other person. The more extensive the touch, the more information can be perceived and transmitted within moments. This applies to physical characteristics (body size, girth, and moisture) and emotional aspects. For example, during a hug, it is noticed immediately whether a person is hugging back warmly or feeling uncomfortable, stiffening, or pulling back, which will usually affect the characteristics and duration of the hug. At the same time, this will trigger thoughts and feelings in both huggers.

In the previous sections, only the sensory aspects of the haptic system (e.g., temperature, spatial resolution, and perceptual thresholds) were considered. However, tactile and haptic stimuli can also trigger emotional responses. Most emotions triggered by touch arise from the evaluation of touch stimuli and learned associations. (For more in-depth information on the psychological aspects of interpersonal touch, see Chap. 5).

> **Important** During touch, physical information (e.g., temperature, moisture, and roughness of the skin) and emotional information are conveyed and received by all involved parties.

1.1.5.1 Caressing Touches

Recent studies suggest that a specific form of skin stimulation (i.e., slow, gentle stroking) can be directly perceived as a positive emotional stimulus. The peculiarity of this stimulus compared with other sensory and mechanical stimuli is that it does not have to be evaluated in the brain as positive or negative. Instead, a special type of receptor exists in the hairy skin (C-tactile fibers; Sect. 2.1.8), which reacts specifically to stroking touch and transmits this information directly to the brain regions (insula/limbic system; Sect. 2.2.3) responsible for emotional processing (Morrison et al. 2011).

Studies in which a soft brush is stroked over hairy skin report a close correlation between the stroking speed and the positive sensation triggered by the stroking. Stroking speeds of 1–10 cm/s are perceived as most pleasant (see Fig. 1.5). Slower and faster stroking movements also lead to positive but less intense sensations (Ackerley et al. 2014b).

C-tactile fibers respond primarily to touches, that typically occur during affectionate human interaction. In addition, the C-tactile fibers respond especially strongly when slow stroking is performed at skin temperature (Ackerley et al. 2014a). Furthermore, this receptor is likely specialized to detect direct skin-to-skin contact. Therefore, it likely promotes interpersonal contact, as the positive sensations act as their own positive reinforcer.

When C-tactile fibers are activated experimentally, anxiety-relieving, calming, and pain-reducing effects have been observed. These fibers may mediate the release of oxytocin (Sect. 2.4.1) during physical contact (Walker et al. 2017).

However, like any other form of touch, the evaluation of caressing touch can be influenced by cognitive processes or emotional experiences. As a result, it can be evaluated as less pleasant or even negative. The determining factors for the emergence of pleasant sensations are a trusting relationship with the touching person, an appropriate environmental situation, and the psychological characteristics of the person being touched.

> **Important** ***NOTE:*** Some people reject gentle touch or feel uncomfortable with it. These feelings must always be taken seriously and respected.

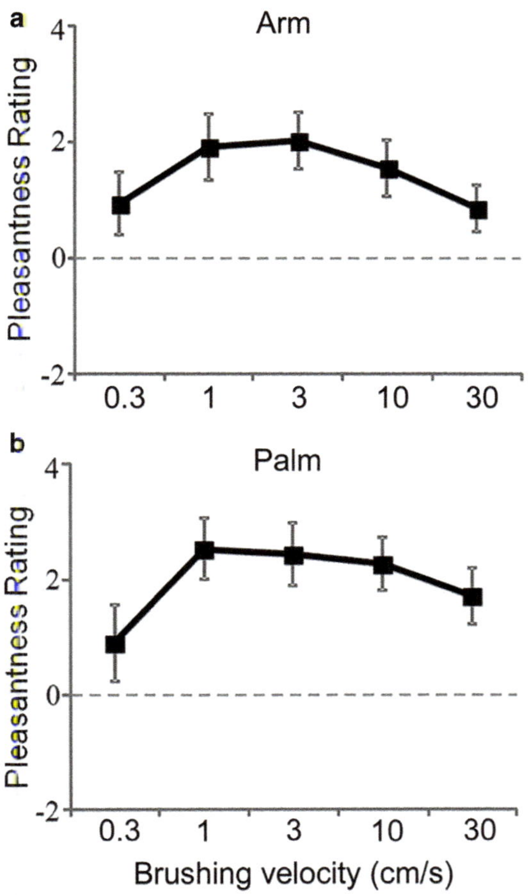

Fig. 1.5 The pleasantness of different stroking speeds on the skin. Speeds between 1 and 10 cm/s are perceived as most pleasant. In hairy skin regions (**a**), this is associated with the stimulus threshold of C-tactile fibers. In hairless skin regions (**b**), faster stroking speeds (30 cm/s) also lead to positive feelings. (From: Ackerley et al. 2014b)

In contrast with hairy skin, there are no C-tactile fibers in hairless skin, according to current knowledge. Nevertheless, positive sensations can also arise by touching hairless skin (e.g., the palm of the hand). However, there is no association between touch speed and pleasantness in hairless skin (i.e., different speeds of stroking touches on the palm are perceived consistently pleasant). In contrast with hairy skin, gentle stroking of hairless skin at fast speeds (30 cm/s) leads to positive feelings, just like at lower speeds (Ackerley et al. 2014b). It is assumed that touch on hairless skin is first transmitted to the primary sensory cortex, is passed on to association areas of the brain, and undergoes emotional evaluation in subsequent processing steps.

▶ **Important** C-tactile fibers in hairy skin contribute to pleasant sensations during skin stroking. Activation of these fibers by slow stroking touch can reduce anxiety and tension and suppress pain perception. Stroking speeds of 1–10 cm/s are perceived as particularly pleasant.

1.1.5.2 Attenuation of Self-Generated Touch

Self-touch of one's body is perceived differently and less intensively than touch from others (Chapman 1994). For example, humans cannot tickle themselves (Blakemore et al. 1998). This effect arises from a spatiotemporal prediction process. When we perform a movement, the brain assesses whether this movement could lead to self-touch, possibly with a held object (Blakemore et al. 1999). This mechanism is called the principle of reafference (Holst and Mittelstaedt 1950), and is used to predict and attenuate the sensory consequences of self-touch. Self-touch is then perceived as less intense than touch from others.

This phenomenon is most likely a protective mechanism. Studies using functional magnetic resonance imaging (fMRI) indicate that activation through self-touch and touch from others differs in certain brain areas (Boehme et al. 2019). Accordingly, the social and emotional significance of touch is analyzed more thoroughly in the case of external touch, even if it is performed with an object.

Conclusion
External touch, even with an object, is perceived more intensely than self-touch. To protect the organism, the social and emotional significance of external touch is analyzed more thoroughly than that of self-touch.

1.1.5.3 Skin Softness Illusion

To date, little is known about what motivates a person to touch another person in a way that is pleasant for the person being touched. In addition to prosocial and emotional factors and the hope of subsequently enjoying "caresses", there may be motivational aspects to touch itself. A recently discovered perceptual illusion provides evidence for this: other people's skin feels softer and more pleasant than one's own (Gentsch et al. 2015). The perceptual illusion occurs only during slow stroking movements (1–10 cm/s) and only on hairy skin areas; thus, it occurs precisely during that type of touch that is most pleasant for the touched person (cf. Sect. 2.1.8).

To create the perceptual illusion, it is crucial that the touch is performed actively and that the hand is *moved* over the hairy skin. The perceptual illusion is absent with simple static (tactile) touch.

1.1.5.4 Reduced Skin Sensitivity During Touch and Movement

During both touch and self-touch, the surface sensitivity of the respective limb is greatly reduced. This is also true for body parts that are pressed against resistance by body weight (e.g., standing or lying down). Depending on the type of stimulation, 20- to 100-fold increased perception thresholds have been measured (Boehme et al. 2019; Katz 1948). This mechanism likely prevents the pressure on the soles of the feet against the floor from being perceived as an intrusive stimulus when standing or walking. The impulse to rub a painful or itchy body area is also likely associated with this mechanism (Sect. 2.1.8).

Similar inhibitory effects on surface sensitivity are observed from voluntary limb movements (Angel and Malenka 1982; Lee and White 1974). Consequently, touch perception is reduced during active movements.

1.1.5.5 Interpersonal Touch with an Object

People can distinguish with extreme accuracy whether they are touched by human skin or an inanimate object. However, it remains unclear whether benevolent touch by an inanimate object is perceived as more or less pleasant than direct skin contact. Most studies on the perception of caressing touch are conducted using soft brushes. To date, only one study has investigated the perceptual differences between touch with an inanimate object and direct skin contact (Kress et al. 2011). In the study, the participant's forearm was stroked with either the palm of the experimenter's hand or a ruler covered with velvet. The experimenter moved the ruler across the forearm in the same stroking manner as his hand. Participants indicated that direct skin contact was more pleasant than contact with an inanimate object. In addition, direct skin contact produced stronger activation of brain areas associated with well-being (left posterior insula; fMRI scan). Therefore, direct interpersonal skin contact is immediately recognized as such and is processed differently than touch with an object. However, the effects are likely caused by the memories and emotions associated with interpersonal touch. To what extent this result can be transferred to other objects/materials (e.g., pens, gloves) or other forms of touch (e.g., poking, slapping) has not yet been investigated. However, it is likely that the emotional evaluation of touch with an object strongly depends on environmental factors, such as the person performing the touch, the situation, and the touched part of the body. Therefore, the evaluation process is like that of direct touch (for more details, see Sects. 5.1 and 5.2).

Conclusion

Interpersonal touch with direct skin contact is felt more intensely and is processed differently in the CNS than touch performed with an object. However, if the touches are similar in force and speed, the triggered feelings will also be similar.

1.1.5.6 Telecommunication: Mediated Social Touch

The developments in interactive robotics, telecommunication, virtual reality, and artificial intelligence in the last 20 years are leading to the question of whether mediated touch can mimic direct physical contact. Such technology-mediated touch differs from direct interpersonal touch in three dimensions (Huisman 2017):

1. **Spatial distance:** During telecommunication, the second person may be far away; therefore, the physical information (e.g. scent, body language) is absent that is otherwise conveyed and perceived by both participants during direct personal contact. In addition, during telecommunication, less information is available on all sensory channels about the touching person and their intentions. Nevertheless, the emotional evaluation of mediated touch - just like direct touch - depends heavily on the context in which it takes place, the gender of the touching person, and whether it is a familiar person.
2. Temporal delay: In addition to spatial distance, the mediated touch can also be **time-displaced**; it is possible to record and send a touch that can later be received as a tactile message.
3. Mediated touch differs greatly in its **physical properties** (materials, movements) from direct interpersonal skin contact. For example, actuators or robotic arms can transmit heat, pressure, or vibration stimuli to individual areas of the body (e.g., the forearm). However, these touches are usually highly simplified and limited to reduced perceptual dimensions.

Conclusion

The perception of mediated touch can be influenced by cognitive processes; depending on what information about the sender (e.g., gender, personality, or intensity of touch) is included as text or video, the emotional evaluation of the mediated touch changes (Huisman 2017). Like interpersonal touch with an object, the triggered sensations are weaker than with direct skin contact. However, mediated touch and social robots that respond to touch have the potential to support social communication over long distances (e.g., long-distance relationships), serve as a low-maintenance pet substitute (e.g., seal 'Paro' in a nursing home), or reduce fear of social contact (e.g., autism). (For more details, see Sect. 5.5.3.)

1.1.6 Temperature Perception of the Body Surface

1.1.6.1 Thermoception

Temperature stimuli are always interpreted relative to the temperature of the body surface. Stimuli with a temperature of 30–35 °C (86–95 °F) can only be perceived briefly as warm or cold until the temperature sensation adapts and is perceived as neutral. Lower (5–35 °C or 41–95 °F) and higher (30–45 °C or 86–113 °F) temperatures are permanently perceived as cold or warm, respectively. This is due to the presence of two distinct receptor types that respond to either warm or cold stimuli (Sect. 2.1.8).

Paradoxical cold sensations to heat stimuli (>45 °C or >113 °F) result from falsely responding cold receptors. In contrast, paradoxical heat sensations during extreme cold stimuli (e.g., freezing with −200 °C [−328 °F] liquid nitrogen) are caused by the disinhibition of heat-conducting neurons.

1.1.6.2 Protective Reflexes

Temperature stimuli of less than 15 °C (59 °F) or more than 45 °C (113 °F) cause pain sensations. The sudden contact with such temperature stimuli triggers protective reflexes (e.g., pulling the hand away from a hot stovetop).

1.1.6.3 Thermoregulation

The body surface temperature contributes to the regulation and maintenance of a stable core body temperature of around 37 °C (98.6 °F). For this purpose, temperature information from the musculature, internal organs, and brain is offset against that of the body surface, and physiological processes are triggered that regulate body temperature (e.g., sweating or shivering) if necessary. In addition, a drop or rise in body temperature triggers the urge to seek or create environmental conditions that enable an optimal body temperature (e.g., more or less movement, adjustment of clothing, seeking shade). (For temperature perception inside the body, see Sect. 1.2.3).

Conclusion

- External temperature stimuli are always perceived relative to one's body surface temperature.
- External temperature stimuli of less than 15 °C (59 °F) or more than 45 °C (113 °F) cause pain.

1.1.7 Pain Perception of the Body Surface

Pain and temperature sensations caused by environmental stimuli are among the best-researched dimensions of the haptic system and are described in detail in textbooks on physiology and biological psychology. For this reason, these two perceptual dimensions of exteroception and interoception will not be discussed in depth here but only presented in a cursory manner.

For information on the processing of pain and temperature stimuli *inside* the body and the development of chronic pain conditions, see Sect. 1.2.4. For information on the modulation of pain perception by touch stimuli, see Sect. 5.5.3.

1.1.7.1 Acute Pain

▶ Pain and Nociception

- **Nociception** refers to the neuronal processing that is triggered by noxious stimuli. Noxious stimuli are mechanical, thermal, or chemical stimuli that can have tissue-damaging effect.
- "**Pain** is an unpleasant sensory or emotional experience associated with actual or potential tissue damage. Pain is always a personal experience that is influenced to varying degrees by biological, psychological, and social factors. Pain and nociception are different phenomena. Pain cannot be inferred solely from activity in sensory neurons. Through their life experiences, individuals learn the concept of pain. A person's report of an experience as pain should be respected. Although pain usually serves an adaptive role, it may have adverse effects on function and social and psychological well-being. Verbal description is only one of several behaviors to express pain; the inability to communicate does not negate the possibility that a human or an animal experiences pain." (International Association for the Study of Pain 2020)
- In contrast with all other sensory stimuli, pain is almost always accompanied by negative feelings and may lead to avoidance, relieving postures, and defense and escape behaviors.
- Pain causes neurophysiological changes in the peripheral and CNSs that can contribute to chronification.

Pain and other mechanosensory events are closely linked; given sufficient intensity, all mechanical and thermal stimuli can cause pain and tissue damage. However, tissue-damaging stimuli are registered by specific receptors (nociceptors; Sect. 2.1.8) and are transmitted and processed via independent neuronal connections (Sect. 2.2). That is, despite a seemingly smooth transition from a pressure sensation to pain with increasing pressure intensity, the painful pressure stimuli are not transmitted by pressure receptors. Instead, when potentially tissue-damaging stimulation occurs, additional nociceptors are activated. Interestingly, nociceptors adapt if a stimulus is not tissue-damaging; if a tissue-damaging stimulus persists, the pain also persists.

▶ **Important** Nociceptors adapt slowly to suprathreshold, non-injurious stimulation, and they never adapt to tissue-damaging stimulation. Therefore, persistent pain is always a warning signal.

First and Second Pain

Painful stimuli of the skin are usually divided into first and second pain according to their characteristics, duration, and the nerve fibers they activate.

- **"First pain"** is sharp, well localized, and transmitted by fast-conducting Aδ fibers. This pain rapidly subsides after cessation of the pain-inducing stimulus (e.g., pinprick).
- **"Second pain"** is often mediated by inflammatory processes and transmitted by slow-conducting C-fibers. It is persistent, dull, and radiating (e.g., bruising, toothache).

1.1.7.2 Bio-psycho-social Model of Pain

From a psychological perspective, the intensity of pain perception and the associated negative feelings and expressions of emotion do not depend exclusively on the actual noxious stimulus; instead, they are influenced by a variety of other aspects of the person, situation, and environment (Fig. 1.6). Pain is a subjective perception, and its intensity cannot be measured objectively.

Social context and origin Depending on their cultural background, family tradition, and upbringing, people learn from birth what is considered an appropriate pain response. Therefore, even if pain intensity is the same, the emotional and behavioral components can vary greatly

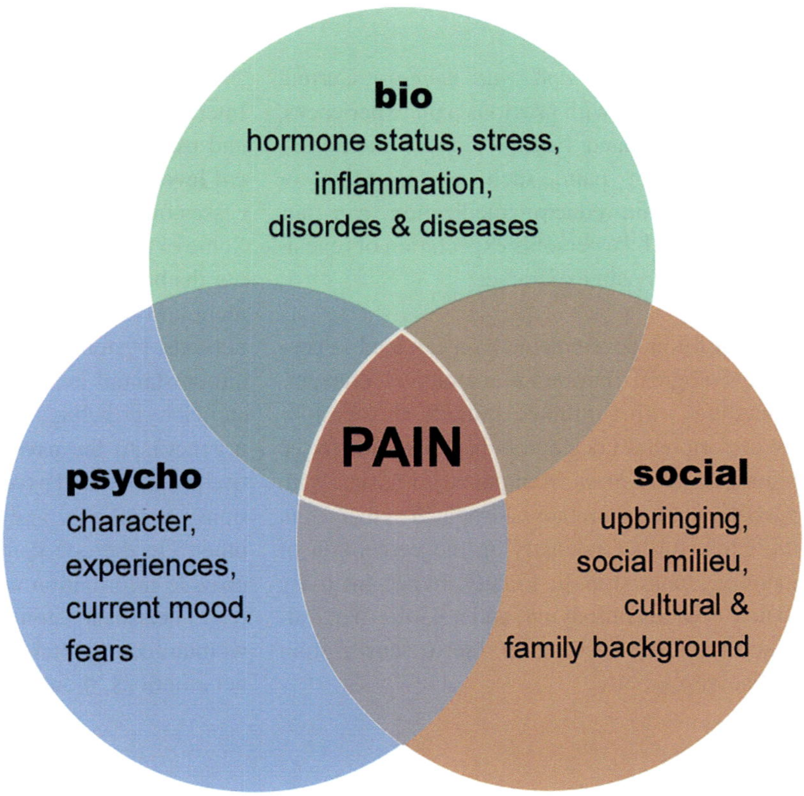

Fig. 1.6 Bio-psycho-social model of pain. How intensely a pain stimulus is felt is an interplay of biological, psychological, and social factors, including family and cultural experiences in dealing with pain. (Illustration by Anna Zender)

between individuals. In addition, pain reactions are influenced by the current social situation. As a rule, pain is expressed more openly to persons of trust in a private environment than in a public space, in competitive situations (sport, work), and possibly in treatment situations (e.g., during initial contact with a medical professional).

Psychological context The evaluation of pain depends on its cause, its accompanying circumstances, and the person's psychological state. If the cause of pain is unknown, its duration is unforeseeable, and the expected consequences for health, well-being, and social structure (e.g., workplace) are considered threatening, pain stimuli are felt more strongly. Anxious or depressed people generally have a lower pain tolerance.

Cognitive techniques, such as reinterpretation, meditation, hypnosis, and social support, can modulate or reduce the perception of pain. In addition to cognitive techniques, physical techniques (e.g., massage, touch) can also influence the perception of pain (Sect. 5.5.3).

Learning processes and pain memory Current pain is compared with previous pain experiences, and it is evaluated based on these memories. Expressions of pain, such as lamenting or demanding pain-reducing medication, can thus be influenced by a person's expectation of repeating a previous pain experience.

In addition, severe acute pain can lead to neurophysiological and brain-anatomical changes, sometimes within minutes. Initially, the sensitivity of peripheral nociceptors increases due to the release of substances from damaged tissue. With persistent pain, there are neuroplastic changes in the CNS, further intensifying the perception of incoming pain stimuli. Finally, hypersensitivity to non-noxious (allodynia) and noxious (hyperalgesia) stimuli may develop due to sensitization and neuroplasticity.

Conclusion

- Pain is a subjective phenomenon; therefore, its intensity cannot be measured objectively.
- Social situations influence pain reactions. Pain is usually expressed more openly to confidants in private settings than in public or competitive situations (e.g., sports and work).
- Pain stimuli are felt more strongly if the cause of pain is unknown, its duration is not foreseeable, and the expected consequences for health, well-being, and social structure (e.g., workplace) are considered threatening.
- Expressions of pain, such as complaining or demanding analgesic medication, may be influenced by a person's anticipation of a repetition of previous pain experiences.

1.2 Sensory Events Inside the Body (Interoception)

Interoceptive processes have both physiological and psychological relevance. At the **physiological level**, sensory information generated by processes inside the body is transmitted to the brain. Some of this information contributes to maintaining the body's homeostasis through the measurement and regulation processes of the autonomic nervous system. Other information comprises circumstantial evidence for organ activity (e.g., stomach growling, sore muscles, and urinary urgency). At the **psychological level**, interoceptive processes and psychological processes (emotions, cognitions, and behavior) influence each other. On the one hand, interoceptive processes provide information about the state of the body (e.g., heartbeat, stomach ache, and a pregnant woman feeling fetal movement), which can trigger emotions, thoughts, and actions. On the other hand, emotions, cognitions, and behavior can cause changes in organ activity (e.g., increased heart rate, and diarrhea), which in turn lead to altered interoception. (For the role of interoception in the context of psychosomatics, see Sect. 3.4.3).

1.2.1 Relevance of Interoception

Interoception (of the haptic system) refers to the processing of mechanical, thermal, and pain stimuli generated by processes inside the body in addition to their psychological evaluation. This includes:

(a) Motion stimuli due to organ activity (**visceroception**; e.g., digestion or blood flow),
(b) Movement and stretching information of the connective tissue, joints, and musculature (proprioception),
(c) Thermoception to maintain the core body temperature,
(d) Deep pain due to injuries or pathological processes, and,
(e) Chemical processes.

▶ **Important** Interoception is required for the regulation of organ functions (visceroception; Sect. 1.2.2), the adjustment of muscular tension for postural and movement control (proprioception; Sect. 1.3), as well as the maintenance of the internal environment of the body (homeostasis).

Emotions, cognitions, and behavior influence interoception and are influenced by it (cf. psychosomatics; Sect. 3.4.3).

1.2.1.1 Homeostasis

Physical stimuli influence the homeostatic processes (a) of the whole organism (e.g., body temperature and blood pressure), (b) at the organ level (e.g., bone metabolism and kidney function), and (c) at the cellular level. That means, tensile and compressive forces acting on body parts or the entire body can influence processes down to the cellular level. For example, chewing solid food stimulates cell division in the jaw bone (Ray et al. 2015) and gums (Weiss et al. 1969; Burwasser and Hill 1939), which is likely to improve the stability of teeth and reduce periodontal disease. Another example is the effect of massages on immune function and hormonal processes (Sect. 2.4).

▶ **Important**

▶ **Tensile and compressive forces acting on body parts or the entire body can influence biological processes down to the cellular level.**

1.2.1.2 Mechanosensing of Somatic Cells

All perceptions described in Sects. 1.1 and 1.2 are registered and processed by specialized mechanoreceptors. However, recent findings suggest that *every* cell of the human body has mechanosensory abilities through which it can register its environmental conditions (Discher et al. 2005). The mechanical forces acting on a cell influence its division, migration, and differentiation, the release of signal proteins, and consequently, its function or dysfunction. The mechanical forces arise from the shape, softness, and elasticity of the adjacent cells and the connective tissue between the cells (extracellular matrix). For example, stem cells develop into either bone or fat tissue depending on the mechanical cues of their microenvironment (McBeath et al. 2004). Similarly, embryonic development is guided by mechanical forces at the cellular level.

Somatic cells process mechanical forces of their microenvironment through the opening and closing of ion channels or conformational changes of proteins; the mechanosensation of somatic cells is *not* processed in the spinal cord or the brain.

▶ **Important** The mechanical forces that act on a cell influence its division, migration, and differentiation, as well as the release of signal proteins, and consequently, the cell's function or dysfunction.

Conclusion

The functions of the haptic system encompass far more than the sensitivity of the skin and fingertips. A multitude of mechanosensitive receptors are distributed throughout all body tissues, registering every physical cue of the body, both on the body surface and inside the body. Furthermore, physical forces influence the biological processes of the human body independent of whether they impinge on the body from the outside, are triggered by body movements, or arise from organ activity. The processing of mechanical stimuli by somatic cells and mechanoreceptors plays a crucial role in the accurate functioning of all organ systems.

In the following chapters, effects at the cellular level are only reported if they were triggered by (interpersonal) touch or physical activity. However, in Sect. 1.2.2, we present a small selection of the manifold processes triggered by mechanical stimuli at the cellular and organ levels.

1.2.2 Organ Activity and Visceroception

Organ activity is not automatic; it is based on constant measurement and control processes. Every process and state is controlled and regulated in millisecond cycles, if necessary. The processing of somatosensory stimuli caused by organ activity is largely unconscious and occurs via the **autonomic nervous system (sympathetic and parasympathetic)**. However, it is important to emphasize the extent of sensory information that is generated by organ activity and processed neuronally. The vagus nerve is the largest nerve of the parasympathetic nervous system and innervates most internal organs. Through activation of the parasympathetic and sympathetic nervous systems, the functions of various organs are regulated. However, only about 20% of the nerve fibers of the vagus nerve are efferent; that is, only a small portion of the vagus nerve conducts parasympathetic impulses from the brain to the organs. The **larger portion (80–90%) are afferent nerve fibers** that conduct mechanical, painful, and thermal stimuli from the organs to the brain, thereby transmitting the status of organ functions. Accordingly, organ functions are not just commissioned by the CNS; instead, stretching, pressure, and shearing forces from the organs influence the inhibitory and excitatory impulses from the CNS.

▶ **Important** Up to 90% of autonomic nerve fibers are sensory (afferent) fibers that conduct mechanical, painful, and thermal stimuli from the organs to the brain, thereby contributing to the regulation of organ activity.

Only large-scale movements (e.g., heartbeat, breathing, or swallowing) and epiphenomena of organ functions (e.g., urinary and fecal urgency, coughing, and dizziness) can be perceived consciously.

Conscious processing of sensory stimuli from inside the body is possible because the connective tissue between the organs, in addition to the smooth musculature of the organs, is permeated by mechanoreceptors and free nerve endings (Sects. 2.1 and 2.3).

1.2.2.1 Examples of Visceral Processes That Are Not Consciously Perceivable

Blood pressure and blood volume Arterial baroreceptors (Chapleau 2012; Brown 1980) measure the stretching of blood vessels and trigger the contraction of vascular smooth muscles in response (Bayliss 1902), thereby contributing to the maintenance of stable blood pressure. However, if blood pressure is persistently altered (e.g., hypertension), the receptors adapt to the new baseline value.

Venous baroreceptors primarily function to regulate blood volume, for example, during sporting activities.

Regulation of intestinal movement and heartbeat The smooth muscles of many organs exhibit spontaneous activity, which leads to regular contraction (twitching or tone) of the muscle, even without the involvement of the autonomic nervous system. For example, cardiac muscle cells exhibit the typical heartbeat pattern even when they are grown in a Petri dish.

▶ **Important** A video of the spontaneous activity of heart muscle cells in a petri dish can be viewed at youtube.com/watch?v=BefHdZTvN3M (video keywords: heart cells in a petri dish).

This is possible because smooth muscle is composed of muscle cells interspersed with additional cells, including cells of the immune system (e.g., mast cells and leukocytes), connective tissue cells (fibroblasts), and **interstitial cells of Cajal** (Fig. 1.7). Cajal cells have been studied mainly in the digestive tract, but they are found in similar forms in virtually all organs (e.g., pancreas, gallbladder, fallopian tubes, placenta, prostate, mesentery, heart) (Kostin and Popescu 2009). Cajal cells generate the pacemaker potentials responsible for spontaneous electrical and motor smooth muscle activity. Their main function is the regulation of organic movements by functioning as mediators between muscle cells and the autonomic nervous system (Sanders et al. 2014). Cajal cells and smooth muscle cells possess mechanosensitive properties (Alcaino et al. 2017). Stretching stimuli (e.g., triggered by chyme in the digestive tract) alter the pacemaker frequency of Cajal cells to ensure optimal nutrient uptake.

Cardiovascular response during exercise Heart rate, blood pressure, and cardiac output are adjusted in response to physical demand through a variety of autonomic regulation processes. One of these reflexes (**exercise pressor reflex**) is directly **triggered by the contraction of skeletal muscles** (Murphy et al. 2011; Watanabe and Hotta 2016). Muscle contractions cause mechanical stimuli that activate the finely branched free nerve endings located in the fasciae of striated muscles (Sect. 2.3). This information is transmitted and processed via the spinal cord and CNS, resulting in increased respiration and blood flow.

1.2.2.2 Examples of Perceptible Visceral Processes

Some organ functions can be directly perceived consciously due to mechanoreceptors in the organ tissue. These functions include signals from the digestive tract (transport of chyme, feeling of fullness, flatulence, and urge to defecate) and bladder (urge to urinate). Other organ movements can only be perceived if they activate mechanoreceptors in surrounding tissues (e.g., distension of the thorax due to respiratory movements, vibration due to a heartbeat). Sensations that feel systemic (e.g., shortness of breath, hunger, or nausea) are perceived only in part by mechanosensory information; such sensations are caused primarily by physiological changes and chemical signals in the CNS.

The intensity with which intraorganismic processes can be perceived differs between people. Examinations to determine interoceptive sensitivity and accuracy usually measure how accu-

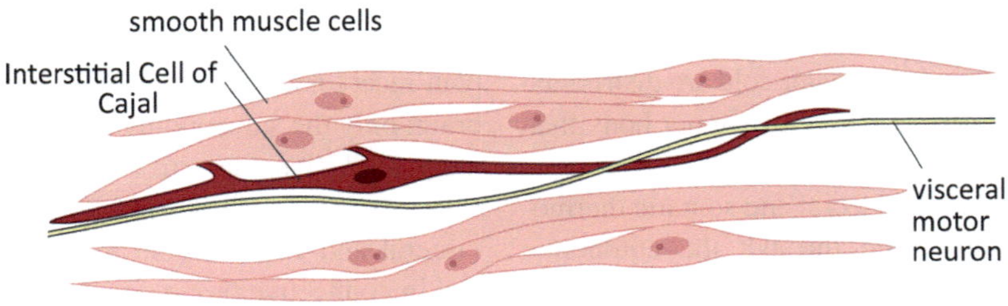

Fig. 1.7 Interstitial cell of Cajal. Cajal cells are found in smooth muscle and generate pacemaker potentials without the involvement of the autonomic nervous system. This gives rise to the spontaneous electrical and motor activity of smooth muscle. Cajal cells are mechanosensitive and change their pacing frequency when stretched. (Illustration by Verena Kuehn)

rately a person can perceive their heartbeat. Deficient interoception is associated with several psychosomatic disorders (e.g., somatoform disorder, fibromyalgia, major depression) (Sect. 3.4.3). Training (e.g., using biofeedback) can improve interoceptive sensitivity.

Conclusion

- Organ activity causes stretching, pressure, and shear forces, which are registered by mechanoreceptors and transmitted to the CNS. The forces are then processed by the CNS to control and regulate organ activity.
- Only large-scale movements (e.g., heartbeat, breathing, or swallowing) and epiphenomena of organ functions (e.g., urinary and fecal urgency, urge to cough, and dizziness) can be perceived consciously.

1.2.3 Temperature Perception Inside the Body

This section covers temperature perception inside the body; for the processing of the temperature of environmental stimuli, see Sect. 1.1.6.

Temperature-sensitive free nerve endings inside the body serve to control and maintain a constant core body temperature. It is now known that not only the hypothalamus—which functions as a regulatory center for body temperature—can perceive temperature (Simon et al. 1986). Many other areas of the body contain thermoreceptors as well, including the internal organs, spinal cord, brain stem, and skeletal muscles (Imrie and Hall 1990). Receptors that register cold are distributed about 3.5 times more frequently in our body than warm receptors.

The activation of visceral and somatic thermoreceptors is processed through the autonomic nervous system and usually triggers whole-body responses, such as sweating and freezing.

Localized temperature changes inside the body can only be consciously perceived in the mouth, pharynx, and esophagus.

1.2.4 Pain Perception Inside the Body

This section covers pain perception inside the body; for the processing of pain triggered by environmental stimuli, see Sect. 1.1.7; for modulation of pain through touch stimuli, see Sect. 5.5.3.

A distinction is usually made between deep somatic and visceral pain. **Deep somatic pain** refers to pain sensations in the musculoskeletal system (muscles, joints, connective tissue, and bones). It can occur due to arthritis, fractures, or after surgery. Deep somatic pain is usually dull and difficult to localize, and it leads to relieving postures and avoidance of movement.

In contrast, **visceral pain** is caused by the activation of free nerve endings in and around internal organs. It is usually diffuse and difficult to locate. Visceral pain can be mislocalized in the skin (head zones). A unique form of visceral pain is colic pain, which is caused by contraction of the smooth muscles of hollow organs.

1.2.4.1 Organs/Structures With and Without Nociception

Only a few structures of the human body are not sensitive to pain. These include the organ tissues (parenchyma) of the liver, spleen, lungs, stomach, and intestines (Müller 1924) and also the articular cartilage, visceral pleura (Rieger et al. 2004), the vitreous body, and the lens of the eye (Baar et al. 1987). Interestingly, there are also no pain receptors in the gray or white matter of the brain; only the surrounding meninges are heavily innervated. Pain-sensitive membranes or capsules also surround all other organs. In general, visceral and somatic pain receptors are embedded in connective tissue structures in and around the organs, striated muscle tissue, blood vessels, and bones (cf. Sect. 2.3). Additionally, the smooth musculature of hollow organs is also interspersed with pain receptors.

1.2.4.2 Chronic Pain

Pain that persists or recurs for more than 3 months is referred to as chronic pain. This pain usually does not fulfill a meaningful signaling function for acute tissue damage or persists after the physical cause has subsided. In Europe, about 19% of the total population is affected by chronic pain (Breivik et al. 2006; Reid et al. 2011). However, the prevalence of chronic pain with persistent tissue damage in Europe is only about 5% (Breivik et al. 2006). Chronic pain with persistent tissue damage includes chronic inflammatory pain, tumor pain, and neuropathic pain caused by damage or disease of the peripheral or CNS.

Arthritis, degenerative disc changes, injuries/accidents, and unknown causes are reported by the majority of the population affected by chronic pain, in most cases without clinically relevant findings. The four most common regions for chronic pain are the back, knee, head, and other joints, including the shoulder, neck, hip, and hand (Breivik et al. 2006). Current explanations for the development and persistence of chronic pain without clinical findings consist of a combination of **response stereotypies, relieving postures, and learning and memory processes**.

Response stereotypy Response stereotypies play a major role in the development and maintenance of chronic pain (without substantial organic damage). The term refers to the tendency of a specific organ to exhibit a physiological response to stressful situations; in chronic pain patients, this usually affects parts of the musculature. While all people probably show some form of response stereotypies, these are especially pronounced in patients with chronic pain and those at risk of chronic pain. The characteristic aspects are:

- **Muscular tension is prolonged**, triggering local inflammatory processes and sensitization of nociceptors. As a result, inflammation and pain lead to further tension and densification of connective tissue (see also Sect. 2.3.4), which in turn activates further nociceptors and increases pain.
- The affected persons have **difficulty perceiving the tension** in the musculature, which is why no corrective behaviors are developed.
- Chronic pain patients not only react with more muscular tension to stressful situations; they are also more **prone to classical conditioning**. Therefore, independent stimuli coinciding with the stressful event become associated with the stress. These conditioned stimuli then trigger painful muscle tension, even if they occur independently of stressful situations.

Secondary gain and relieving postures Operant learning processes (negative and positive reinforcement) and relieving postures contribute to the maintenance of chronic pain. Operant learning processes can be triggered by social attention during expressions of pain. Attention (e.g., comfort, assistance, compassion, and consideration) leads to **positive reinforcement of** the pain expressions and the pain perception. **Negative reinforcement** occurs when unpleasant situations (e.g., work) or activities (e.g., sports) can be avoided because of the pain (secondary gain). This usually occurs in combination with the adoption of **relieving postures**, whereby it is learned that avoidance leads to a reduction in pain in the short term. However, in the long term, relieving postures and a lack of exercise can lead to decreased mobility, which in turn triggers pain.

1.2.4.3 Interdisciplinary Multimodal Therapy

To break the vicious circle of pain experience, tension, inflammatory processes, and fear of further pain, multimodal therapy approaches are required. Both pharmacological and complementary strategies for pain relief are necessary, in addition to physiotherapeutic and movement therapies that enable the patient to replace relieving postures and compensatory and avoidance behaviors with new behaviors and movement patterns. Relaxation techniques, massage, biofeedback, and hypnosis can be used as complementary strategies. If necessary, concomitant psychotherapy should be considered.

Conclusion
Chronic pain is usually caused by permanent tension in the affected tissues, which is triggered by persistent or recurrent physical or psychological overload (stress, response stereotypies). Chronic pain is maintained by learning and memory processes that lead to neurophysiological changes in the brain (classical and operant conditioning and relieving postures).

1.3 Position and Motion Perception (Proprioception)

Proprioceptive processes comprise several functions that cannot be considered separately as they are mutually dependent and complementary. The main functions of proprioception include:

- Determination of the position of the body or individual body parts in space and in relation to each other;
- Perception of the movement of the body or individual body parts; and,
- Detection of tensile, compressive, and weight forces.

These functions are crucial for a person to be able to stand and walk upright and to perceive, without visual support, the spatial position of their own body and its moving parts. This is true when the body is in a resting position and during active and passive movement. For example, a healthy person can unerringly touch any part of their body, even with closed eyes.

Therefore, depending on their severity, disorders of proprioception can have **profound effects on motor function, coordination, and speech**. Depending on which part of the nervous system (receptors, peripheral nerves, or CNS) causes the disorder, different abilities are affected to different degrees. For example, peripheral nerve damage to the lower extremities (e.g., diabetic polyneuropathy) can cause gait unsteadiness and a lack of force control, which can also impact braking and accelerating while driving. In the case of a focal brain injury (e.g., after a stroke), the control of muscle groups and the subsequent execution of movements (e.g., walking, speaking) may be impaired. Furthermore, sensory integration disorders (Sect. 1.1) and body schema disorders (Sect. 1.4) may also be accompanied by altered proprioceptive ability.

► **Definition** Proprioception refers to the ability of an organism to map the position and movement of the limbs appropriately at all times in relation to its body and in relation to the external environment. Proprioception is essential for all active and passive movements and haptic processes. The ability to perceive and control the movement of body parts is sometimes referred to as "kinesthesia" in older literature.

Proprioception is the **basis for all explorative and all motor activities**; therefore, proprioceptive processes are part of both exteroception and interoception. Proprioceptive processes contribute to **exteroception**, for example, when objects are touched. Even when only the fingertips are brushing over a surface, a variety of proprioceptive information is simultaneously generated by arm movement and head and body posture, and this information must be neuronally processed. Indeed, recent findings suggest that when finger skin sensitivity fails, proprioceptive information is sufficient to recognize relief figures (Symmons et al. 2008). In contrast, if objects are held in hand and explored, information about the weight and size of the object, in addition to the surface information, is always included in the recognition process. Weight and size are conveyed primarily via the muscle and tendon receptors of the fingers, arms, and shoulder girdle. Depending on the size and weight of the object, mechanoreceptors of the back, glutes, and legs may also be activated (e.g., when lifting or pushing against an object). For example, if palpation is performed as part of a diagnostic or treatment procedure, the entire body may be used to apply force to the patient's body. This may even be the case when only the hands are in contact with the patient's body. In addition, complex manual therapy treatments require that the practiced techniques are performed with reliable postures of the arms, shoulders, and back.

Proprioceptive processes contribute to **interoception**, as every movement triggers sensations in muscles, tendons, and joints. The condition of the musculoskeletal system can be inferred based on these sensations (e.g., strain or pain). Furthermore, different body postures can trigger compression effects on internal organs (e.g., the gastrointestinal tract) when a person is in a squatting position.

Some authors label a subgroup of mechanoreceptors as **"proprioceptors,"** which usually refers to muscle spindles and Golgi tendon organs (cf. Sect. 2.1). However, this designation is misleading and gives the impression that there are specialized mechanoreceptors that are exclusively responsible for proprioceptive processes while no other receptors are involved. However, this is not the case. Muscle spindles and Golgi tendon organs are specifically responsible for the adaptation of force and stretch control. This contributes to proprioceptive processes and protects the musculoskeletal system from overload and overstretching. Other **mechanoreceptors of the joints, skin, and connective tissue** contribute to proprioception by providing additional information about the stretching or flexion of body limbs. For example, joint movement activates the stretch receptors of the skin (Edin 2001). The involvement of skin receptors in proprioception is one explanation for why knee and ankle braces can help improve balance and strength.

1.3.1 Weight and Forces

The ability to squeeze, push, and pull with regulated forces and to determine weight forces acting on the body or its parts also relies on proprioceptive processes. Muscular receptors, tendon stretch receptors, joint receptors, and receptors in the skin and connective tissue are responsible for these complex actions.

1.3.2 Posture and Fine Motor Skills

Posture, automated movements, and fine motor skills are controlled by the cerebrum and deeper structures, such as the basal ganglia, brainstem, and cerebellum. Constant measurement and control processes are required for these movements to occur in a coordinated and goal-directed manner. Mechanoreceptors and the vestibular system provide the necessary information to enable coordinated movement sequences (e.g., walking, climbing stairs, playing tennis, chewing, and speaking). Without proprioceptive feedback, movements occur in an unstructured manner. Proprioceptive feedback is essential, even to enable upright standing or sitting and head posture.

▶ **Important** Proprioceptive information is relevant for posture, force regulation, coordinated movement patterns, and fine motor skills.

1.3.3 Role of the Vestibular System

A sub-process of proprioception, which determines the spatial position of the head relative to the body and the position of the entire body relative to space, is established in association with the vestibular system in the inner ear. Therefore, with every change in body position, proprioception and the vestibular system work together to determine the position in space. This process occurs with every movement (e.g., turning the head, bending over, or walking). In addition, skin receptors contribute to the determination of which way is up by signaling which parts of the body are in contact with the floor or another surface.

Conclusion

Proprioception describes the perception of movements and positional changes of the entire body and positional changes of individual body parts; it forms the indispensable basis for postural and movement control of all movement processes of the body, including speech production.

1.4 Body Schema

Any living being that moves in three-dimensional space must constantly be informed about the three-dimensional structure of its body. The basis for this is the **neural body representation**, also referred to as the body schema. Through the body schema, the organism is informed *at all times* about the spatial constitution of its body (e.g., size, circumference, and shape of the whole body and its limbs) (Bretas et al. 2020; Vallortigara 2020; Brecht 2017; Magnani and Sedda 2017). This process is necessary for movement planning and eye-hand coordination, among other things. For example, successfully catching a ball or avoiding an obstacle is only possible if one's body shape and range of motion are adequately estimated. Moreover, the body schema is the neurobiological basis for locating body parts and performing targeted movements, even in complete darkness or in cases of blindness. Therefore, adequate proprioception of the body and its limbs is only possible if the neural body representation is accurate.

The body schema **almost exclusively uses information from the haptic system.** Visual information can briefly, but not permanently, alter the body schema in the form of illusions or during tool use (Braun et al. 2014; Haans et al. 2012; Baccarini et al. 2014; Serino et al. 2016; Aymerich-Franch and Ganesh 2016; Hornburger et al. 2019; Romano et al. 2019; Sun and Tang 2019; Olgiati et al. 2017; Martel et al. 2016; Laessoe et al. 2017). The molecular, biological, neuronal, and cortical aspects of the body schema have not yet been fully understood scientifically.

▶ **Important** Information about the **three-dimensional shape of one's body** is a product of neural activity that is not accessible to consciousness and is referred to as body schema (Berlucchi and Aglioti 1997; Holmes and Spence 2004).

The body schema is not accessible to consciousness or language. Therefore, the neurobiological process that enables the emergence and adaptation of the body schema cannot be observed or commented on. An everyday ability can be used to illustrate this—the inner workings of memory, which are equally fundamental for humans but also elude direct observation. Every human organism can store and retrieve information as memory content. However, *how* the neurobiological processes of information storage and retrieval take place cannot be consciously observed by the organism itself. Therefore, we can only observe in ourselves and other people that we can remember and retrieve information. However, the underlying processes of memory—information selection, storage, linkage, search, and retrieval—are not accessible to self-observation or language.

In contrast with the body schema, **body image** (Sect. 1.5) is defined as a conscious perception process of the subjectively perceived condition and emotional evaluation of one's body. Body image disorders can occur independently or in connection with body schema disorders.

1.4.1 Phantom Limbs and Body Schema

Phantom sensations are indirect evidence of the presence of a body schema. A person may perceive an amputated body part both in its spatial shape and in its various motor and sensory functions, despite the body part no longer existing objectively. Sensations of movement, in addition to the somatosensory sensations of the amputated body part, may occur. However, this phenomenon only occurs in patients who have abruptly lost a body part. In cases of gradual change (e.g., in the course of leprosy), neither phantom sensations nor phantom pain occur (Malaviya 2003; Simmel 1956). The slow process of nerve degeneration enables concomitant restructuring of somatosensory representations in the cortex and adaptation of the body schema to the actual existing shape. Flor and colleagues were able to demonstrate that the extent of cortical reorganization correlates with the extent of phantom pain (Flor et al. 1995); less phantom pain is reported when more cortical adaptation has taken place.

▶ **Important** Phantom sensations usually only occur after the sudden loss of a body part.

Persons with **congenital limb deficiency** (CLD) (i.e., in whom limbs were not fully or not at all formed during embryonic development) also generally do not report phantom sensations (Saadah and Melzack 1994; Farry 2009). In the context of the sensory feedback hypothesis of body schema development (see Sect. 1.4.2), these observations suggest that no cortical representation of the corresponding limbs was formed in affected individuals because sensorimotor stimulation did not occur in utero. However, interestingly, in some affected individuals with CLD, complete phantom limbs emerged after injury, surgery, or myoelectric stimulation of the deficient limb. Malzack and colleagues (Melzack et al. 1997) hypothesized that phantom limb sensations occur because of a genetically determined neural matrix in the body. Critics of this perspective argue that phantom sensations in cases of congenital limb defects may develop postnatally through learning processes or the use of prosthetic limbs (Price 2006; Della Sala 2007).

1.4.2 Ontogenesis of the Body Schema

Current research seeks to elucidate which psychological and neurobiological mechanisms of postnatal multisensory integration contribute to the formation of the body schema and thus bodily self-awareness (Ramachandran and Brang 2009; Altschuler and Ramachandran 2007; Spence et al. 2004; Brownell and Slaughter 2012). Central to these theories is the assumption that the body schema develops postnatally through multisensory integration processes (Stein et al. 2014; Stein and Rowland 2020; Meijer et al. 2019). This argument is based exclusively on animal studies (cats and mice) that investigated the integration of visual stimuli with other sensory systems. To understand the limitations of this theory, one must remember that both cats and mice are born with their eyes shut.

Other researchers assume that the body schema exists prenatally as an innate, genetically determined neural matrix and that postnatally, sensory inputs from various sensory systems are constantly aligned with this matrix (Maravita et al. 2003).

In contrast, the authors of this book hypothesize that **prenatal sensorimotor feedback during fetal development** is crucial to the development of the body schema (Yamada et al. 2016). With reference to various study data, we hypothesize that the neural representation of one's own body is **a lifelong adaptive process** (Fox and Wong 2005; Hepper et al. 1997, 1998; Hepper 1997).

Spontaneous movements of the limbs and head occur long before purposeful movements of the fetus are observable. The embryo experiences its first sensory stimuli through these spontaneous muscle impulses and the movements of the mother. Through the movements of the mother, the embryo, and later the fetus, is passively moved in the amniotic fluid, thereby coming into contact with its environment (uterus and umbilical cord). As early as the seventh week of pregnancy, the **spontaneous body movements** of the embryo lead to sensory feedback about its body boundaries, range of motion, and environment. Between the 10th and 12th weeks of pregnancy, the fetus begins actively touching its body and its environment and sucking on the thumb (Sect. 3.1.1 Development in utero). Therefore, we hypothesize that sensorimotor perception plays a crucial role in the development of body schema and body awareness. In particular, spontaneously occurring sensorimotor events are prerequisites for the ability to plan and execute goal-directed movements. The execution of **goal-directed**

movements requires the coordinated interaction of muscle fibers and millions of touch-sensitive receptors while maintaining and controlling all other bodily and sensory functions. We assume that the *purposeful* movements of a fetus toward its own body and the environment require the presence of an adequate body schema. Therefore, it is unlikely that the development of a body schema would begin after birth.

The complexity of fetal movements and behaviors supports the assumption that a complete body representation exists in utero (Piontelli 2010; Bystrova 2009; Hepper 1996; Hepper et al. 1997). These movements include sucking movements of the thumb, which are performed without visual control. Of note, as the fetus develops, the mouth opens at the initiation of the arm movement rather than after the mouth has been touched by the fingers. This process can be interpreted as the intentional coordination of arm and mouth movements. Similarly, fetuses regularly touch their faces, and the duration and frequency of this behavior correspond to the emotional status of the mother (Reissland et al. 2009, 2014, 2015; Reissland and Burt 2010; Reissland and Francis 2010).

For the prenatal development of the human body schema, it can be assumed that both genetically encoded information about the body structure *and* constant multisensory integration processes are relevant. The multisensory integration of the various sensory information from exteroception, proprioception, and interoception is processed in the fetal brain, not only into a neural representation of its own body but also into a **neural representation of the external world.** Movement, self-touch, and physical contact within the confines of the uterus represent constant stimuli for the fetus (Yamada et al. 2016). The multisensory relevance of the haptic system for the development of neural body representation is supported by its extremely early development (cf. Sect. 3.1.1 and Fig. 3.1).

> **Important** The ontogeny of the body schema begins in utero and is based on multisensory integration processes from movement and touch stimuli. Genetically encoded information about body structure is combined with various sensory information from exteroception, proprioception, and interoception to form a neural body representation.

The details of how the neurobiological development of neural body representation based on genetic dispositions and sensory inputs from the haptic system occurs are not yet known. However, it is clear that visual and auditory information are not necessary for this process, nor would they be available during this developmental period. As evidence for this statement, individuals born blind or deaf with neurotypical cognitive abilities are usually unimpaired in their motor and proprioceptive performance without supporting visual information. If the development of a body schema was dependent on visual or auditory information, severe motor impairments would occur in individuals born blind or deaf; however, this is not the case (Nelson et al. 2018; Aggius-Vella et al. 2017; Nava et al. 2014; Petkova et al. 2012). The motor development of blind people without other cognitive impairments is slower but not otherwise limited compared to that of non-visually impaired people (Bakke et al. 2019; Wagner et al. 2013; Jeka et al. 1996; Mahon et al. 2010; Ricciardi et al. 2014; Sonksen et al. 1984; Tröster and Brambring 1993).

1.4.3 Body Schema and Growth Processes

The adaptation of neural body representation is required during growth (Butti et al. 2020; Franchak 2019; Guilbert et al. 2018; Marshall and Meltzoff 2015; Brownell and Slaughter 2012; Raimo et al. 2021). The rapid body growth of humans before and after birth is accompanied by the further maturation of sensory systems and all neural structures (Berlucchi and Aglioti 1997; Waters et al. 1997). Due to constant body growth, the spatial structure of a growing human changes successively. Proportions and the size and weight ratios of the body and limbs—including the head—change dramatically, especially during the first few years after birth. The range of motion of the body changes, as does the position of the body in relation to gravity (crawling, walking). This process of physical change, which is inherent in human biology, requires continuous adaptation of the body schema to the changing physical conditions. Through this process, outdated neural networks of the existing body schema must be adapted to the new physical conditions. It can be assumed that these neonatal adaptations are driven by multisensory integration processes in the haptic system. This is supported by findings on **psychomotor development**, which is directly associated with the sensory and motor stimulation of the growing organism (Howard et al. 2020; Azim and Seki 2019; Follmann et al. 2018; Khazipov and Milh 2018; Brooks and Thaler 2017; Mele et al. 2017; Franklin et al. 2016; Moreno-López et al. 2016; Gizzi et al. 2015; Seidler and Meehan 2015; Weiss et al. 2014; Tomasino et al. 2013; Canu et al. 2012; Dalton and Bergenn 2012; Manto and Huisman 2018; Waldie and Mosley 2000; Raimo et al. 2021). However, despite these observations, little is known about the process of adaptation of the body schema to growth processes. Studies suggest that predominantly **socially mediated physical contact and active interaction with the environment** contribute to the adaptation of the body schema to the growing body during child development (Bonandrini 2014; Brownell and Slaughter 2012; Buhler 2013; Marshall and Meltzoff 2015; Shi et al. 2013; Sheffield et al. 2009). Likewise, sufficient motor activity is indispensable for the formation of an adequate neural body representation (Assaiante 2012; Assaiante et al. 2014; Jones et al. 2011).

▶ **Important** The body schema is subject to a lifelong process of adaptation to successive changes in the body (e.g., growth and weight changes). Social physical contact, active movement, and physical interaction with the environment are crucial for changes in the body's schema.

1.4.4 Disorders of the Body Schema

Like all vital biological processes, a person's neural body representation can be disturbed. In these cases, affected individuals experience the physical dimensions of their entire body or its limbs as spatially distorted or feel that body parts do not belong to their body (e.g., neglect, body dysmorphic disorder, body identity integrity disorder, and schizophrenia).

For example, people with right-hemispheric damage (e.g., after a stroke) regularly perceive the left side of their body as no longer belonging to their body. This form of neurological disorder is called **neglect.** One of the numerous consequences of a right-sided stroke is motor neglect of the left arm and the left leg, which leads to significant restrictions of movement and action for the affected person (Rubio and van Deusen 1995; White et al. 2010; Preston and Newport 2011). Although the sensitivity to touch on the left side of the body remains intact, the sensory impulses cannot be integrated into the body schema of the patient (Coslett 1998). It is not uncommon for these patients to request that caregivers remove their arm or leg, which appear alien to them, from the bed with the explanation that they belong to their neighbor or someone else. The patients are often affected by anosognosia, that is, they do not recognize their condition or deficit. In approximately 70% of those affected, neglect symptoms regress without specific treatment. The mechanisms underlying this process are not yet fully understood.

▶ **Important** Body schema disorders are associated with various brain disorders and are difficult to treat.

In the absence of a stroke, it is still possible for people to feel like individual body parts or sensory channels (hearing or vision) do not belong to their bodies. Such body schema disorders usually begin in early childhood and are referred to in the literature as **body integrity identity disorder (BIID)** (Blom et al. 2012; Skoruppa et al. 2013; Stirn et al. 2010). The otherwise physically healthy and cognitively unimpaired patient perceives defined body areas (e.g., legs, arms, and forearms) as foreign objects that do not belong to their body. The limbs perceived as foreign are experienced as disturbing and psychologically stressful. Therefore, patients are usually convinced that surgical removal of the limbs—or even surgically induced paralysis—is indispensable to alleviating their suffering. Due to the small number of cases of BIID and insufficient knowledge of the causes of this disorder, these patients are often not treated within the medical system. Therefore, it is not uncommon for the affected patients to try to achieve the desired physical changes by self-injury or self-amputation.

Equally difficult in its prognosis is another pathological form of body representation called **body dysmorphic disorder** (Albertini and Phillips 1999; Buhlmann et al. 2004; Phillips 2004). In this condition, patients are convinced that their face or another part of their body is disfigured. However, the perception of physical disfigurement is not associated with actual disfigurement. Therefore, the slightest unevenness of the facial skin is experienced as severe disfigurement by the patient, which usually leads to social withdrawal. The course of the disease is accompanied by severe depression, which leads to suicide attempts in many cases. The feeling of supposedly severe physical disfigurement is immune to factual arguments from social or professional environments. Likewise, patients cannot recognize their sensations or behavior as pathological. An average of 8–12 years passes before patients receive psychotherapeutic treatment for the first time; during this period, patients try to alleviate their suffering through cosmetic operations. Cognitive-behavioral psychotherapy is successful in treating the disorder in some cases.

As with the disorders outlined thus far, body schema disturbance in patients with **anorexia nervosa** and its development are not yet sufficiently understood. Anorexic patients perceive their body or parts of it as fat or unshapely, although there is no objective reason for this assessment. Out of excessive fear of weight gain and the associated physical disfigurement, the affected patients reduce their food intake to a few grams per day. The consequence of this food restriction is rapid weight loss with severe secondary physical diseases, which lead to death in 10–15% of cases. Like patients with neglect, patients with anorexia nervosa are unable to recognize the pathological value of their physical and mental conditions. Even when the patient's physical deterioration requires intensive medical care, patients are unable to comprehend why these life-saving measures and inpatient treatment are necessary. Psychotherapeutic or psychopharmacological interventions can lead to positive changes in anxiety and obsessive-compulsive symptomatology in affected individuals. However, their inadequate experience of their bodies remains unchanged, even after years of psychotherapeutic treatment (Ben-Tovim et al. 2001; Ben-Tovim and Walker 1995; Grunwald 2008). Therefore, the body schema disorder in the context of anorexia nervosa represents a **central element in the chronification and maintenance of the disease.** To date, substantial changes in the body schema have only been described after body-oriented psychotherapeutic interventions. Here, the therapeutic setting focuses on raising awareness of the body's experience and improving the patient's perception of the spatial dimensions of the body. One body-oriented, neurobiological approach was developed by the author. In this approach, **movement-induced body stimulations**—triggered by a custom-made neoprene suit—activate right parietal cortex areas in affected patients (Grunwald and Weiss 2005; Grunwald 2008). As a result of this cortical activation, the patients experience the spatial structure of their bodies more adequately. To date, only a small number of patients have been treated with this approach. Therefore, no conclusions can be drawn about the long-term effects of such interventions.

Focal dystonias are neurological disorders that affect motor function and cause involuntary contractions in specific muscle groups. One predominant form is focal hand dystonia, which involves alterations in the neural body representation of the fingers and hands (Furuya and Hanakawa 2016; Karnath 2012). The disorder often occurs in professional musicians who repeatedly perform rapid and forceful finger movements over a long period of practice. Due to motor overload, the neural representation areas of individual fingers overlap in these patients, which leads to cramps and incorrect execution of movement sequences. The functional overlay arises due to excessive hand and finger use when the neuronal associations of the individual fingers are frequently stimulated simultaneously. When rapidly and repetitively playing the piano or guitar, the neuronal association of one finger remains active when the next finger is already in motion. Focal hand dystonia can cause severe limitations, such that professional musicians can no longer practice their profession. Successful therapeutic interventions use training processes in which the unaffected fingers are restricted in their mobility through splints. The additional afferent information generated in this way is used by the brain to reorganize the neural representation areas, causing a decline in symptoms (Candia et al. 1999, 2002; Pantev et al. 2001; Elbert et al. 1998).

Schizophrenia is a mental illness associated with severe brain disorders that are divided into at least two symptom domains: (a) Schizophrenic disorders with positive symptoms range from severe disturbances of perception to hallucinations. Characteristics include thought disorders, delusions, and depersonalization/derealization experiences. (b) Schizophrenic disorders with negative symptoms are characterized by reductions in normal experience. Among the many symptoms are apathy, lethargy, social withdrawal, and motor symptoms. In recent experimental studies, patients with positive symptoms have been found to have a markedly disturbed body schema (Graham et al. 2014; de Vignemont 2017). Among other phenomena, the patients experience the **"rubber hand illusion"** much more vividly than healthy people and have difficulty recognizing the illusory character of the perception. The rubber hand illusion is a sensory illusion in which the impression is created that an artificial hand belongs to one's own body. For the experiment, one hand is covered with a cloth, and an artificial hand is placed visibly next to it. Then, both the covered, real hand and the visible, fake hand are stroked with a brush at the same rhythm and speed. As a result, the more or less vivid illusion of having three hands is created.

1.4.5 Cortical Localization of the Body Schema

The neural network underlying the human body schema is not yet fully understood. Nevertheless, certain brain regions have been identified whose damage regularly leads to body schema disorders. Clinical-neuropsychological findings support the assumption that generally, damage to the right hemisphere (in dominant right-handers with left-hemispheric language processing) is necessary to cause body schema disorders (Kolb and Whishaw 2008). Specifically, **damage to the right parietal cortex** or **right insular cortex** corresponds to various symptoms of body schema disturbance and to the inability to recognize one's pathological state (anosognosia). The right parietal cortex is functionally considered a central multisensory integration processor (see also Sect. 2.2.3). These neuron populations order and integrate external and internal sensory stimuli, among other tasks. The tasks of the right insular cortex include the neural processing of interoceptive information such as hunger, pain, thirst, pleasure, and fear. Furthermore, various authors posit that the right insular cortex integrates polymodal information and thereby contributes to conscious body perception (Karnath and Baier 2010; Baier and Karnath 2008; Craig 2009, 2011).

▶ **Important** Body schema disorders are associated with damage to the right parietal cortex and insula.

1.5 Body Image

The conscious experience and evaluation of the body's attributes is called body image (Gallagher 1986). Body image is influenced by both body schema and emotional and cognitive processes. Body image is an adaptive process that can be **neutral, positive, or negative in terms of body evaluation.** For example, we can reflect on and discuss whether we currently perceive our body or parts of it as attractive or unattractive, too thin or too fat, or beautiful or ugly. These evaluations are not determined by objective facts but by subjective feelings, which are influenced by the body schema and by social circumstances, experiences, and emotional and cognitive processes. For example, healthy people are more likely to judge their bodies more critically in a gym or swimming pool than in the vicinity of a choir. In addition to the social environment, age and cultural context are central factors that influence body image.

The term body image is used extremely heterogeneously in the literature to describe a variety of body-related phenomena, both as an umbrella term and to denote individual aspects of perception. In recent years, early attempts have been made to systematize the conceptualizations (Rohricht et al. 2005; Joraschky 1995). Accordingly, the term body image subsumes the **psychological aspects of body experience** derived from **perceptual, cognitive, affective, and behavioral components** (Smolak 2004; Legenbauer and Vocks 2005; Martin and Svaldi 2015). Perceptual information about the properties of the body and its characteristics is gathered from *all* sensory channels. These perceptual aspects are processed cognitively, compared with desired ideal images, and subsequently evaluated. The evaluation of physical appearance has consequences for self-esteem and lifestyle. Body-related cognitions can cause either positive or negative moods and emotions and can fundamentally influence the behavior of individuals.

To operationalize body image for research purposes, emotional expressions (body satisfaction) and the associated behaviors are predominantly assessed.

> ▶ **Important** Body image denotes the psychological aspects of body experience, which are composed of perceptual, cognitive, affective, and behavioral components.

1.5.1 Positive Body Image

Ideally, a positive body image prevails in a person, regardless of their actual size, shape, social conventions, or possible deficiencies. This person feels comfortable in their body and is satisfied with their appearance, which in turn has a positive effect on their behavior and **self-esteem** (Howald 2016). Positive behavioral effects include balanced eating and exercise habits, which positively influence body image and self-worth in a self-perpetuating cycle (Wertheim et al. 2009). Healthy, positive self-esteem is associated with better self-confidence in social interactions, self-respect, and increased productivity. People with positive self-esteem generally have a better sense of well-being and are less likely to suffer from depression than people with negative self-esteem (Howald 2016). Consequently, a positive body image is important for a person's healthy physical development, identity formation, and maintenance of physical and mental health (Dittmar 2009; Wertheim et al. 2009).

1.5.2 Negative Body Image and Body Image Disturbance

To our knowledge, no individual is born with a negative body image. Instead, body image can be influenced by both external factors and physical changes. External change factors include (repeated) derogatory (body) comments by significant others (e.g., parents or peers) and impactful life events (e.g., sexual harassment, experiences of violence) (Smolak 2004; Thompson and Stice 2001; Striegel-Moore and Cachelin 1999). Changes in body image triggered by changes in body shape or functionality are usually caused by illnesses or accidents (Rumsey et al. 2004). In the literature, a distinction is made between **body dissatisfaction**, which is also common among healthy people, and clinically relevant **body image disturbance**. These conditions are manifestations of the same dimension. While body dissatisfaction can vary between contexts and only intermittently (or weakly) affect behavior, body image disturbances are positively correlated with depression, social phobia, and eating disorders (Cash et al. 2004). A body image disturbance is characterized by one or more severely impaired body image dimensions (see definition; Legenbauer and Vocks 2005; Tuschen-Caffier 2015; Martin and Svaldi 2015).

▶ **Definition Body image disturbances** are characterized by:

- Body schema disorder: deficient perception of body dimensions or body features (e.g., color, texture, and size of a body part);
- Intense negative evaluation and exaggeration of the perceived flaw, with negative consequences for self-worth;
- Persistent suffering, shame, and anxiety caused by the perceived flaw (often exacerbated in social situations); and,
- Restrictions on social and professional life due to avoidance of certain situations, eating disorders, cosmetic surgery, social withdrawal, or suicide attempts.

Moderate-to-severe, **temporary**, negative body image is reported by women depending on the monthly hormone cycle. This phenomenon encompasses increased body dissatisfaction and misperceptions of the size or proportions of one's body or body areas. It can be accompanied by an increased fear of negative social evaluation and of emitting an odor due to menstruation (Jappe and Gardner 2009; Carr-Nangle et al. 1994; Ruggieri and Valeri 1981; Kaczmarek and Trambacz-Oleszak 2016; Teixeira et al. 2013).

1.5.3 Body Schema Influences Body Image, Not Vice Versa

The subjective evaluation and attitude toward one's body and its external appearance are unconsciously influenced by the information provided by the body schema. The body schema and its influence on body image are not directly observable or accessible to consciousness. Furthermore, the processes of the body schema are not perceivable or measurable by external observers. Only the dimensions of the body image can be described or measured. It is reasonable to assume a relationship between body schema and body image on a neurobiological level, as evidenced by clinical observations and the often extreme severity of body image disturbances, which can be changed only marginally or not at all through cognitive psychotherapy. Severe body image disturbances can be observed in patients with anorexia nervosa (Grunwald et al. 2004; Grunwald 2005), body dysmorphic disorders (Albertini and Phillips 1999; Bjornsson et al. 2010), BIID (Blom et al. 2012; Giummarra et al. 2011), phantom limbs (Bromage and Melzack 1974), and neglect (Coslett 1998). These disorders were previously described as body schema disorders (Sect. 1.4.4). Patients with phantom limbs experience their bodies as complete and experience limbs that are objectively not present. In contrast, neglect patients ignore one side of their body despite its objective and physical presence. Patients with anorexia nervosa experience much bigger body dimensions than they objectively are. Patients with body dysmorphic disorder experience their body, or parts of it, as disfigured without any objective findings to support their experience. Patients with BIID experience parts of their body as not belonging to them, although they use them functionally and successfully in everyday life. An inherent aspect of body image disturbance is that the patients suffer from a body they perceive as distorted and wish to change their experience through treatment. The level of suffering can become so strong over time that it can be accompanied by depression or suicidal tendencies if the experience remains unchanged. It is crucial to understand that such body image disturbances cannot be changed through therapeutically intended confrontation with objective facts (e.g., mirror confrontation) in any of these patient groups. Despite repeated assertions (e.g., by clinical staff or by relatives), it is not possible for the affected person to consciously correct their distorted perception of their bodies. Most often, these patients are also unable to recognize the pathological state of their body image (anosognosia). Body image disturbances associated with these disorders can only be successfully treated to a limited extent (Butters and Cash 1987; Phillips 1996;

Rosen 1996; Ben-Tovim et al. 2001; Fernandez-Aranda et al. 1999). Often, patients achieve cognitive access to their body image disturbance after years of treatment; however, the impaired body experience does not change substantially. Because extreme forms of body image disturbance are not substantially treatable by language-based or confrontational therapies, it can be assumed that there is a direct neurobiological relationship between body schema and body image. In the case of the aforementioned disorders, the body schema dominates the processing levels of the body image, which becomes evident through measurable distortions of the body image. Therefore, a disorder of the body schema usually results in a disturbance in body image. However, a temporary disturbance in body image (i.e., body dissatisfaction) is not necessarily an indication that the body schema is also changed or disturbed.

This statement is important considering that temporary, negative evaluations of one's own body are a common phenomenon. Temporarily perceiving oneself as unattractive or even ugly (i.e., having a negative body image) is a common and clinically irrelevant state (Hargreaves and Tiggemann 2004; Agliata and Tantleff-Dunn 2004). A temporarily negative body image and dissatisfaction with one's appearance can be influenced by external factors (e.g., social encounters, visiting the beach, trying on new clothes; cf. Sect. 1.5.2) and are often the starting point for participating in sporting activities or phases of more conscious eating. Ordinarily, body dissatisfaction subsides after some time, either because perceptible changes can be observed or because the focus of attention changes over time. However, if the dissatisfaction with one's body is permanent and persists for months or years, the body image disturbance may be clinically relevant and could be caused by an impaired body schema.

From the authors' point of view, the treatment resistance of body image disturbances is an indication that they are caused by a neurobiological dysfunction in neural body representation. In the reverse case, we believe that emotional and cognitive body image is not able to influence a fundamental biological process, like body schema. In this respect, we argue that temporary body image disturbances do not have a significant influence on the body schema.

▶ **Important** Disorders of the body schema regularly entail disturbances of the body image. However, a temporary disturbance of body image cannot cause changes in neural body representation.

Summary

The **haptic system** comprises all mechanosensory processes in humans. Mechanosensory processes can result from single or combined exteroceptive, proprioceptive, and interoceptive processes, including pain and temperature perception (Table 1.2). The perceiving person can either actively explore or passively receive a stimulus. Perceptual processes of the haptic system and psychological processes (e.g., evaluations, expectations, and emotions) influence each other.

Table 1.2 Submodalities of the haptic system

Submodality	Receptors	Afferent nerve fibers	Exteroception	Interoception
Mechanoreception	Free nerve endings and encapsulated mechanoreceptors	Ia, Ib, II/Aβ, IV/C	x	x
Proprioception	Encapsulated mechanoreceptors	Ia, Ib, II	x	x
Thermoception	Free nerve endings	III/Aδ, IV/C	x	x
Nociception	Free nerve endings	III/Aδ, IV/C	x	x
Visceroception	Free nerve endings and encapsulated mechanoreceptors	II, III, IV		x

For a description of afferent nerve fibers, see Sect. 2.2. (Table adapted from Treede and Baumgärtner 2019)

The **somatosensory system** is the neural network of the haptic system; its structures process all extero-, intero-, and proprioceptions as well as temperature perception. However, only the physiological aspects of perception are subsumed under somatosensation, without regard for the accompanying psychological processes. The term somatosensation is not only used in medical/physiological/neurophysiological literature but also in some textbooks of biological psychology.

Haptics, as a **technical term,** designates the interdisciplinary field of science that includes the study of the haptic system of humans and its applications.

Haptic as a **physical property** refers to the material, object, and surface attributes that can be detected through haptic exploration.

Haptic perception as a **skill** refers to the performance and thresholds of the human haptic system.

Mechanosensation is caused by the activation of mechanosensory receptors and refers to the perception of all changes in the body caused by physical forces like pressure, strain, vibration, and friction. This includes forces that act on the body from the outside and those that occur inside the body.

Exteroception refers to external perception. In the case of the haptic system, this includes mechanical stimuli (pressure, vibration, friction, and stretch), temperature, and pain stimuli. Exteroception comprises the active exploration of objects, one's body, and the environment (**haptic perception**) and passively impinging mechanical/temperature stimuli on the body (**tactile perception**). For exteroceptive processes, both the surface sensitivity of the skin and mechanoreceptors inside the body are relevant (e.g., during explorative actions; cf. **proprioception**).

Interoception refers to internal perception. Regarding the haptic system, interoception includes all mechanical stimuli as well as temperature and pain stimuli inside the body, including stimuli that arise from organ functions (**visceroception**) and stretching and movement stimuli of the muscles, tendons, and joints (proprioception).

Proprioception refers to the ability to perceive the position and movement of the body and its parts. This includes the control of movement, force, and posture. Proprioception is crucial for the perception of tensile, compressive, and weight forces acting on either the entire body or its parts. Proprioception is the basis for all voluntary motor processes, including speech and food intake. All exploratory actions (haptic perception) require proprioception for controlled movements. Therefore, proprioception is closely related to exteroception.

► **Important** A clear distinction between the perceptual dimensions (exteroception, interoception, and proprioception) of the haptic system is only possible to a limited extent because they influence and complement each other. Only strictly localized tactile or temperature stimuli produce exclusively exteroceptive perception. In contrast, active haptic exploration processes integrate information from all parts of the body, thereby encompassing aspects of all three perceptual dimensions. Proprioceptive processes form the basis for haptic exploration of the external world (exteroception) and are concurrently part of interoception due to signals from muscles and joints.

The **body schema** is the neural representation of the human body (also called neural body representation) in its three-dimensional form. It is a product of neuronal activity (sensory integration processes) that is not accessible to consciousness and that adapts to physical growth or tool use. The body schema is genetically predetermined and uses mechanosensory information to adapt; it can also be temporarily altered by visual information.

▶ **Body image** is defined as the emotional perception, evaluation, and attitude toward the properties and external appearance of one's body.

References

Ackerley R, Wasling HB, Liljencrantz J, Olausson H, Johnson RD, Wessberg J. Human C-tactile afferents are tuned to the temperature of a skin-stroking caress. J Neurosci. 2014a;34(8):2879–83. https://doi.org/10.1523/JNEUROSCI.2847-13.2014.

Ackerley R, Carlsson I, Wester H, Olausson H, Wasling HB. Touch perceptions across skin sites: differences between sensitivity, direction discrimination and pleasantness. Front Behavioral Neurosci. 2014b;8:54. https://doi.org/10.3389/fnbeh.2014.00054.

Aggius-Vella E, Campus C, Finocchietti S, Gori M. Audio spatial representation around the body. Front Psychol. 2017;8:1932. https://doi.org/10.3389/fpsyg.2017.01932.

Agliata D, Tantleff-Dunn S. The impact of media exposure on males' body image. J Soc Clin Psychol. 2004;23(1):7–22.

Albertini R, Phillips KA. Thirty-three cases of body dysmorphic disorder in children and adolescents. J Am Acad Child Adolesc Psychiatry. 1999;38:453–9.

Alcaino C, Farrugia G, Beyder A. Mechanosensitive piezo channels in the gastrointestinal tract. Curr Top Membr. 2017;79:219–44. https://doi.org/10.1016/bs.ctm.2016.11.003.

Altschuler EL, Ramachandran VS. A simple method to stand outside oneself. Perception. 2007;36(4):632–4. https://doi.org/10.1068/p5730.

Angel RW, Malenka RC. Velocity-dependent suppression of cutaneous sensitivity during movement. Exp Neurol. 1982;77(2):266–74. https://doi.org/10.1016/0014-4886(82)90244-8.

Assaiante C. Action and representation of action during childhood and adolescence: a functional approach. Neurophysiol Clin. 2012;42(1–2):43–51. https://doi.org/10.1016/j.neucli.2011.09.002.

Assaiante C, Barlaam F, Cignetti F, Vaugoyeau M. Body schema building during childhood and adolescence: a neurosensory approach. Neurophysiol Clin. 2014;44(1):3–12. https://doi.org/10.1016/j.neucli.2013.10.125.

Aymerich-Franch L, Ganesh G. The role of functionality in the body model for self-attribution. Neurosci Res. 2016;104:31–7. https://doi.org/10.1016/j.neures.2015.11.001.

Ayres AJ. Bausteine der kindlichen Entwicklung. Die Bedeutung der Integration der Sinne für die Entwicklung des Kindes. Zweite Auflage ed. Berlin: Springer; 1992.

Azim E, Seki K. Gain control in the sensorimotor system. Curr Opin Physiol. 2019;8:177–87. https://doi.org/10.1016/j.cophys.2019.03.005.

Baar HA, Mohr U, Schara J, Winkelmüller W, editors. Schmerzbehandlung in Praxis und Klinik. Berlin: Springer; 1987.

Baccarini M, Martel M, Cardinali L, Sillan O, Farnè A, Roy AC. Tool use imagery triggers tool incorporation in the body schema. Front Psychol. 2014;5:492. https://doi.org/10.3389/fpsyg.2014.00492.

Baier B, Karnath H-O. Tight link between our sense of limb ownership and self-awareness of actions. Stroke. 2008;39(2):486–8. https://doi.org/10.1161/STROKEAHA.107.495606.

Bakke HA, Cavalcante WA, Santos de Oliveira I, Sarinho SW, Cattuzzo MT. Assessment of motor skills in children with visual impairment: a systematic and integrative review. Clin Med Insights Pediatr. 2019;13:1179556519838287. https://doi.org/10.1177/1179556519838287.

Bayliss WM. On the local reactions of the arterial wall to changes of internal pressure. J Physiol. 1902;28(3):220–31. https://doi.org/10.1113/jphysiol.1902.sp000911.

Becker-Carus C, Wendt M. Allgemeine Psychologie. Eine Einführung. 2., vollständig überarbeitete und erweiterte Neuauflage. Berlin: Springer; 2017.

Ben-Tovim DI, Walker MK. Body image, disfigurement and disability. J Psychosom Res. 1995;39(3):283–91.

Ben-Tovim DI, Walker K, Gilchrist P, Freeman R, Kalucy R, Esterman A. Outcome in patients with eating disorders: a 5-year study. Lancet. 2001;357(9264):1254–7. https://doi.org/10.1016/S0140-6736(00)04406-8.

Berlucchi G, Aglioti S. The body in the brain: neural bases of corporeal awareness. Trends Neurosci. 1997;20(12):560–4.

Birbaumer N-P, Schmidt RF. Biologische Psychologie. 6., vollst. überarb. und erg. Aufl. Heidelberg: Springer Medizin; 2006.

Bjornsson AS, Didie ER, Phillips KA. Body dysmorphic disorder. Dialogues Clin Neurosci. 2010;12(2):221–32.

Blakemore SJ, Wolpert DM, Frith CD. Central cancellation of self-produced tickle sensation. Nat Neurosci. 1998;1(7):635–40. https://doi.org/10.1038/2870.

Blakemore SJ, Frith CD, Wolpert DM. Spatio-temporal prediction modulates the perception of self-produced stimuli. J Cogn Neurosci. 1999;11(5):551–9. https://doi.org/10.1162/089892999563607.

Blom RM, Hennekam RC, Denys D. Body integrity identity disorder. PLoS One. 2012;7(4):e34702. https://doi.org/10.1371/journal.pone.0034702.

Boehme R, Hauser S, Gerling GJ, Heilig M, Olausson H. Distinction of self-produced touch and social touch at cortical and spinal cord levels. Proc Natl Acad Sci. 2019;116(6):2290–9. https://doi.org/10.1073/pnas.1816278116.

Bonandrini B. The development of the body schema. Soins Psychiatr. 2014;(292):39–43.

Braun N, Thorne JD, Hildebrandt H, Debener S. Interplay of agency and ownership. The intentional binding and rubber hand illusion paradigm combined. PLoS One. 2014;9(11):e111967. https://doi.org/10.1371/journal.pone.0111967.

Brecht M. The body model theory of somatosensory cortex. Neuron. 2017;94(5):985–92. https://doi.org/10.1016/j.neuron.2017.05.018.

Breivik H, Collett B, Ventafridda V, Cohen R, Gallacher D. Survey of chronic pain in Europe: prevalence, impact on daily life, and treatment. Eur J Pain. 2006;10(4):287–333. https://doi.org/10.1016/j.ejpain.2005.06.009.

Bretas RV, Taoka M, Suzuki H, Iriki A. Secondary somatosensory cortex of primates: beyond body maps, toward conscious self-in-the-world maps. Exp Brain Res. 2020;238(2):259–72. https://doi.org/10.1007/s00221-020-05727-9.

Bromage PR, Melzack R. Phantom limbs and the body schema. Can Anaesth Soc J. 1974;21(3):267–74. https://doi.org/10.1007/BF03005731.

Brooks J, Thaler A. The sensorimotor system minimizes prediction error for object lifting when the object's weight is uncertain. J Neurophysiol. 2017;118(2):649–51. https://doi.org/10.1152/jn.00232.2017.

Brown AM. Receptors under pressure. An update on baroreceptors. Circ Res. 1980;46(1):1–10. https://doi.org/10.1161/01.res.46.1.1.

Brownell CA, Slaughter V, editors. Early development of body representations. Cambridge: Cambridge University Press; 2012.

Buhler K. The mental development of the child. A summary of modern psychological theory. Hoboken: Taylor and Francis; 2013. Online verfügbar unter. http://gbv.eblib.com/patron/FullRecord.aspx?p=1542871.

Buhlmann U, McNally RJ, Etcoff NL, Tuschen-Caffier B, Wilhelm S. Emotion recognition deficits in body dysmorphic disorder. J Psychiatr Res. 2004;38(2):201–6.

Bundy AC, Lane S, Murray EA. Sensorische Integrationstherapie. Theorie und Praxis. Sonderausgabe der 3, vollständig überarbeiteten Auflage; 2007.

Burwasser P, Hill TJ. The effect of hard and soft diets on the gingival tissues of dogs. J Dent Res. 1939;18(4):389–93. https://doi.org/10.1177/00220345390180040801.

Butters JW, Cash TF. Cognitive-behavioral treatment of women's body-image dissatisfaction. J Consult Clin Psychol. 1987;55(6):889–97.

Butti N, Montirosso R, Giusti L, Borgatti R, Urgesi C. Premature birth affects visual body representation and body schema in preterm children. Brain Cogn. 2020;145:105612. https://doi.org/10.1016/j.bandc.2020.105612.

Bystrova K. Novel mechanism of human fetal growth regulation: a potential role of lanugo, vernix caseosa and a second tactile system of unmyelinated low-threshold C-afferents. Med Hypotheses. 2009;72(2):143–6.

Candia V, Elbert T, Altenmüller E, Rau H, Schäfer T, Taub E. Constraint-induced movement therapy for focal hand dystonia in musicians. Lancet. 1999;353(9146):42. https://doi.org/10.1016/S0140-6736(05)74865-0.

Candia V, Schäfer T, Taub E, Rau H, Altenmüller E, Rockstroh B, Elbert T. Sensory motor retuning: a behavioral treatment for focal hand dystonia of pianists and guitarists. Arch Phys Med Rehabil. 2002;83(10):1342–8. https://doi.org/10.1053/apmr.2002.35094.

Canu M-H, Coq J-O, Barbe MF, Dinse HR. Plasticity of adult sensorimotor system. Neural Plast. 2012;2012:768259. https://doi.org/10.1155/2012/768259.

Carr-Nangle RE, Johnson WG, Bergeron KC, Nangle DW. Body image changes over the menstrual cycle in normal women. Int J Eat Disord. 1994;16(3):267–73. https://doi.org/10.1002/1098-108x(199411)16:3<267::aid-eat2260160307>3.0.co;2-y.

Cash TF, Phillips KA, Santos MT, Hrabosky JI. Measuring "negative body image". Validation of the body image disturbance questionnaire in a nonclinical population. Body Image. 2004;1(4):363–72. https://doi.org/10.1016/j.bodyim.2004.10.001.

Chapleau MW. Chapter 33: Baroreceptor reflexes. In: Robertson D, Biaggioni I, Burnstock G, Low PA, Paton JF, editors. Primer on the autonomic nervous system. 3rd ed. Amsterdam: Elsevier; 2012. p. 161–5.

Chapman CE. Active versus passive touch: factors influencing the transmission of somatosensory signals to primary somatosensory cortex. Can J Physiol Pharmacol. 1994;72(5):558–70. https://doi.org/10.1139/y94-080.

Coslett HB. Evidence for a disturbance of the body schema in neglect. Brain Cogn. 1998;37(3):527–44. https://doi.org/10.1006/brcg.1998.1011.

Craig AD. How do you feel—now? The anterior insula and human awareness. Nat Rev Neurosci. 2009;10(1):59–70.

Craig AD. Significance of the insula for the evolution of human awareness of feelings from the body. Ann N Y Acad Sci. 2011;1225:72–82.

Dalton TC, Bergenn VW. Early experience, the brain, and consciousness. In: An historical and interdisciplinary synthesis. Hoboken: Taylor and Francis; 2012.

de Vignemont F. Beyond differences between the body schema and the body image: insights from body hallucinations. Conscious Cogn. 2017;53:115–21. https://doi.org/10.1016/j.concog.2017.06.006.

Della Sala S. Tall tales about the mind and brain separating fact from fiction. Oxford: Oxford University Press; 2007.

Discher DE, Janmey P, Wang Y-L. Tissue cells feel and respond to the stiffness of their substrate. Science. 2005;310(5751):1139–43. https://doi.org/10.1126/science.1116995.

Dittmar H. How do "body perfect" ideals in the media have a negative impact on body image and behaviors? Factors and processes related to self and identity. J Soc Clin Psychol. 2009;28(1):1–8.

Edin B. Cutaneous afferents provide information about knee joint movements in humans. J Physiol. 2001;531(Pt 1):289–97. https://doi.org/10.1111/j.1469-7793.2001.0289j.x.

Elbert T, Candia V, Altenmüller E, Rau H, Sterr A, Rockstroh B, et al. Alteration of digital representations in somatosensory cortex in focal hand dystonia. Neuroreport. 1998;9(16):3571–5. https://doi.org/10.1097/00001756-199811160-00006.

Farry K. Phantom limb development in congenitally upper limb-deficient individuals. J Prosthet Orthot. 2009;21:145. https://doi.org/10.1097/JPO.0b013e3181b15dff.

Fernandez-Aranda F, Dahme B, Meermann R. Body image in eating disorders and analysis of its relevance: a preliminary study. J Psychosom Res. 1999;47(5):419–28.

Flor H, Elbert T, Knecht S, Wienbruch C, Pantev C, Birbaumer N, et al. Phantom-limb pain as a perceptual correlate of cortical reorganization following arm amputation. Nature. 1995;375(6531):482–4. https://doi.org/10.1038/375482a0.

Follmann R, Goldsmith CJ, Stein W. Multimodal sensory information is represented by a combinatorial code in a sensorimotor system. PLoS Biol. 2018;16(10):e2004527. https://doi.org/10.1371/journal.pbio.2004527.

Fox K, Wong ROL. A comparison of experience-dependent plasticity in the visual and somatosensory systems. Neuron. 2005;48(3):465–77. https://doi.org/10.1016/j.neuron.2005.10.013.

Franchak JM. Development of affordance perception and recalibration in children and adults. J Exp Child Psychol. 2019;183:100–14. https://doi.org/10.1016/j.jecp.2019.01.016.

Franklin DW, Batchelor AV, Wolpert DM. The sensorimotor system can sculpt behaviorally relevant representations for motor learning. eNeuro. 2016;3(4):ENEURO.0070-16.2016. https://doi.org/10.1523/ENEURO.0070-16.2016.

Furuya S, Hanakawa T. The curse of motor expertise: use-dependent focal dystonia as a manifestation of maladaptive changes in body representation. Neurosci Res. 2016;104:112–9. https://doi.org/10.1016/j.neures.2015.12.001.

Gallagher S. Body-image and body schema—a conceptual clarification. J Mind Behav. 1986;7(4):541–4.

Gentsch A, Panagiotopoulou E, Fotopoulou A. Active interpersonal touch gives rise to the social softness illusion. Curr Biol. 2015;25(18):2392–7. https://doi.org/10.1016/j.cub.2015.07.049.

Ghassemzadeh H, Mojtabai R, Karamghadiri N, Noroozian M, Sharifi V, Ebrahimkhani N. Neuropsychological and neurological deficits in obsessive-compulsive disorder: the role of comorbid depression. IJCM. 2012;3(3):200–10. https://doi.org/10.4236/ijcm.2012.33040.

Giummarra MJ, Bradshaw JL, Nicholls MER, Hilti LM, Brugger P. Body integrity identity disorder: deranged body processing, right fronto-parietal dysfunction, and phenomenological experience of body incongruity. Neuropsychol Rev. 2011;21(4):320–33. https://doi.org/10.1007/s11065-011-9184-8.

Gizzi L, Tamburella F, Iosa M, Dominici N. Neuro-motor control and feed-forward models of locomotion in humans. Lausanne: Frontiers Media SA; 2015.

Graham KT, Martin-Iverson MT, Holmes NP, Jablensky A, Waters F. Deficits in agency in schizophrenia, and additional deficits in body image, body schema, and internal timing, in passivity symptoms. Front Psychiatry. 2014;5:126. https://doi.org/10.3389/fpsyt.2014.00126.

Grunwald M, Beyer L. (Hrsg.). Der bewegte Sinn: Grundlagen und Anwendungen zur haptischenWahrnehmung. Basel: Birkhäuser. 2001. ISBN: 978-3-7643-6516-5.

Grunwald M. Inducing sensory stimulation in treatment of anorexia nervosa. QJM. 2005;98(5):379–80. https://doi.org/10.1093/qjmed/hci061.

Grunwald M. Haptic perception in anorexia nervosa. In: Grunwald M, editor. Human haptic perception: basics and applications. Basel: Birkhäuser; 2008. p. 335–51.

Grunwald M. Homo hapticus. Warum wir ohne Tastsinn nicht leben können. München: DroemerKnaur; 2017.

Grunwald M. Haut als sensorisches System. Der Schmerzpatient. 2019;2(2):76–83. https://doi.org/10.1055/a-0823-0732.

Grunwald M, Weiss T. Inducing sensory stimulation in treatment of anorexia nervosa. QJM. 2005;98(5):379–80.

Grunwald M, Weiss T, Assmann B, Ettrich C. Stable asymmetric interhemispheric theta power in patients with anorexia nervosa during haptic perception even after weight gain: a longitudinal study. J Clin Exp Neuropsychol. 2004;26(5):608–20. https://doi.org/10.1080/13803390409609785.

Guilbert J, Jouen F, Molina M. Motor imagery development and proprioceptive integration: which sensory reweighting during childhood? J Exp Child Psychol. 2018;166:621–34. https://doi.org/10.1016/j.jecp.2017.09.023.

Haans A, Kaiser F, Bouwhuis DG, Ijsselsteijn WA. Individual differences in the rubber-hand illusion. Predicting self-reports of people's personal experiences. Acta Psychol. 2012;141(2):169–77. https://doi.org/10.1016/j.actpsy.2012.07.016.

Hargreaves DA, Tiggemann M. Idealized media images and adolescent body image. "Comparing" boys and girls. Body Image. 2004;1(4):351–61.

Hepper PG. Fetal behavior: who so sceptical? Ultrasound Obstet Gynecol. 1996;8(3):145–8. https://doi.org/10.1046/j.1469-0705.1996.08030145.x.

Hepper PG. Fetal habituation: another Pandora's box? Dev Med Child Neurol. 1997;39(4):274–8.
Hepper PG, Shannon EA, Dornan JC. Sex differences in fetal mouth movements. Lancet. 1997;350(9094):1820. https://doi.org/10.1016/S0140-6736(05)63635-5.
Hepper PG, McCartney GR, Shannon EA. Lateralised behaviour in first trimester human foetuses. Neuropsychologia. 1998;36(6):531–4.
Holmes NP, Spence C. The body schema and the multisensory representation(s) of peripersonal space. Cogn Process. 2004;5(2):94–105. https://doi.org/10.1007/s10339-004-0013-3.
Hornburger H, Nguemeni C, Odorfer T, Zeller D. Modulation of the rubber hand illusion by transcranial direct current stimulation over the contralateral somatosensory cortex. Neuropsychologia. 2019;131:353–9. https://doi.org/10.1016/j.neuropsychologia.2019.05.008.
Howald FW. Positives Körperbild. Grundbegriffe, Einflussfaktoren und Auswirkungen. Themenblatt, S. 1–8. Online verfügbar unter. 2016. https://gesundheitsfoerderung.ch/grundlagen/publikationen/psychische-gesundheit.html. zuletzt geprüft am 26.10.2018.
Howard IS, Franklin S, Franklin DW. Asymmetry in kinematic generalization between visual and passive lead-in movements are consistent with a forward model in the sensorimotor system. PLoS One. 2020;15(1):e0228083. https://doi.org/10.1371/journal.pone.0228083.
Huisman G. Social touch technology: a survey of haptic technology for social touch. IEEE Trans Haptics. 2017;10(3):391–408. https://doi.org/10.1109/TOH.2017.2650221.
Imrie MM, Hall GM. Body temperature and anaesthesia. Br J Anaesth. 1990;64(3):346–54. https://doi.org/10.1093/bja/64.3.346.
Jappe LM, Gardner RM. Body-image perception and dissatisfaction throughout phases of the female menstrual cycle. Percept Mot Skills. 2009;108(1):74–80. https://doi.org/10.2466/PMS.108.1.74-80.
Jeka JJ, Easton RD, Bentzen BL, Lackner JR. Haptic cues for orientation and postural control in sighted and blind individuals. Percept Psychophys. 1996;58(3):409–23.
Johansson RS, LaMotte RH. Tactile detection thresholds for a single asperity on an otherwise smooth surface. Somatosens Res. 1983;1(1):21–31. https://doi.org/10.3109/07367228309144538.
Johansson RS, Vallbo AB, Westling G. Thresholds of mechanosensitive afferents in the human hand as measured with von Frey hairs. Brain Res. 1980;184(2):343–51. https://doi.org/10.1016/0006-8993(80)90803-3.
Jones RA, Riethmuller A, Hesketh K, Trezise J, Batterham M, Okely AD. Promoting fundamental movement skill development and physical activity in early childhood settings: a cluster randomized controlled trial. Pediatr Exerc Sci. 2011;23(4):600–15.
Joraschky P. Das Körperschema und das Körper-Selbst. In: Brähler E, editor. Körpererleben. Ein subjektiver Ausdruck von Körper und Seele ; Beiträge zur psychosomatischen Medizin. 2nd ed. Gießen: Psychosozial-Verl. (Edition Psychosozial); 1995. p. 34–49.
Kaczmarek M, Trambacz-Oleszak S. The association between menstrual cycle characteristics and perceived body image: a cross-sectional survey of Polish female adolescents. J Biosoc Sci. 2016;48(3):374–90. https://doi.org/10.1017/S0021932015000292.
Karnath H-O, editor. Kognitive Neurowissenschaften. Mit 28 Tabellen. 3., aktualisierte u. erw. Aufl. Berlin: Springer; 2012.
Karnath H-O, Baier B. Right insula for our sense of limb ownership and self-awareness of actions. Brain Struct Funct. 2010;214(5–6):411–7. https://doi.org/10.1007/s00429-010-0250-4.
Katz D. Gestaltpsychologie. 2. erw. ed. Basel: Schwabe & Co.; 1948.
Khazipov R, Milh M. Early patterns of activity in the developing cortex: focus on the sensorimotor system. Semin Cell Dev Biol. 2018;76:120–9. https://doi.org/10.1016/j.semcdb.2017.09.014.
Kolb B, Whishaw IQ. Fundamentals of human neuropsychology. New York: Worth Publishers; 2008.
Kostin S, Popescu LM. A distinct type of cell in myocardium: interstitial Cajal-like cells (ICLCs). J Cell Mol Med. 2009;13(2):295–308. https://doi.org/10.1111/j.1582-4934.2008.00668.x.
Kress IU, Minati L, Ferraro S, Critchley HD. Direct skin-to-skin versus indirect touch modulates neural responses to stroking versus tapping. Neuroreport. 2011;22(13):646–51. https://doi.org/10.1097/WNR.0b013e328349d166.
Laessoe U, Barth L, Skeie S, McGirr K. Manipulation of the body schema—unilateral manual stimulation of lower extremity influences weight distribution in standing position. J Bodyw Mov Ther. 2017;21(3):612–7. https://doi.org/10.1016/j.jbmt.2016.09.013.
Lederman SJ, Klatzky RL. Haptic perception: a tutorial. Atten Percept Psychophys. 2009;71(7):1439–59. https://doi.org/10.3758/app.71.7.1439.
Lee RG, White DG. Modification of the human somatosensory evoked response during voluntary movement. Electroencephalogr Clin Neurophysiol. 1974;36(1):53–62. https://doi.org/10.1016/0013-4694(74)90136-9.
Legenbauer T, Vocks S. Wer schön sein will, muss leiden? Wege aus dem Schönheitswahn ; ein Ratgeber. Göttingen: Hogrefe; 2005.
Levit-Binnun N, Golland Y. Finding behavioral and network indicators of brain vulnerability. Front Hum Neurosci. 2011;6:10. https://doi.org/10.3389/fnhum.2012.00010.
Libouton X, Barbier O, Plaghki L, Thonnard JL. Tactile roughness discrimination threshold is unrelated to tactile spatial acuity. Behavioural Brain Research, 2010;208(2):473–8. https://doi.org/10.1016/j.bbr.2009.12.017.
Louw S, Kappers AM, Koenderink JJ. Haptic detection thresholds of Gaussian profiles over the whole range of spatial scales. Exp Brain Res. 2000;132(3):369–74. https://doi.org/10.1007/s002210000350.

Louw S, Kappers AML, Koenderink JJ. Haptic discrimination of stimuli varying in amplitude and width. Exp Brain Res. 2002;146(1):32–7. https://doi.org/10.1007/s00221-002-1148-z.

Magnani FG, Sedda A. Paying the price for body evolution: the role of evolution in disorders of body representation. Med Hypotheses. 2017;98:81–6. https://doi.org/10.1016/j.mehy.2016.11.013.

Mahon BZ, Schwarzbach J, Caramazza A. The representation of tools in left parietal cortex is independent of visual experience. Psychol Sci. 2010;21(6):764–71. https://doi.org/10.1177/0956797610370754.

Malaviya GN. Sensory perception in leprosy-neurophysiological correlates. Int J Lepr Other Mycobact Dis. 2003;71(2):119–24. https://doi.org/10.1489/1544-581x(2003)71<119:spilc>2.0.co;2.

Manto M, Huisman TAGM. The cerebellum from the fetus to the elderly: history, advances, and future challenges. Handb Clin Neurol. 2018;155:407–13. https://doi.org/10.1016/B978-0-444-64189-2.00027-5.

Maravita A, Spence C, Driver J. Multisensory integration and the body schema: close to hand and within reach. Curr Biol. 2003;13(13):R531–9. https://doi.org/10.1016/s0960-9822(03)00449-4.

Marshall PJ, Meltzoff AN. Body maps in the infant brain. Trends Cogn Sci. 2015;19(9):499–505. https://doi.org/10.1016/j.tics.2015.06.012.

Martel M, Cardinali L, Roy AC, Farnè A. Tool-use: an open window into body representation and its plasticity. Cogn Neuropsychol. 2016;33(1–2):82–101. https://doi.org/10.1080/02643294.2016.1167678.

Martin A, Svaldi J. Körperbild und Körperbildstörungen. Psychotherapeut. (2015);(60):475–6.

Martina IS, van Koningsveld R, Schmitz PI, van der Meché FG, van Doorn PA. Measuring vibration threshold with a graduated tuning fork in normal aging and in patients with polyneuropathy. European Inflammatory Neuropathy Cause and Treatment (INCAT) group. J Neurol Neurosurg Psychiatry. 1998;65(5):743–7. https://doi.org/10.1136/jnnp.65.5.743.

McBeath R, Pirone DM, Nelson CM, Bhadriraju K, Chen CS. Cell shape, cytoskeletal tension, and RhoA regulate stem cell lineage commitment. Dev Cell. 2004;6(4):483–95. https://doi.org/10.1016/s1534-5807(04)00075-9.

Meijer GT, Mertens PEC, Pennartz CMA, Olcese U, Lansink CS. The circuit architecture of cortical multisensory processing: distinct functions jointly operating within a common anatomical network. Prog Neurobiol. 2019;174:1–15. https://doi.org/10.1016/j.pneurobio.2019.01.004.

Mele S, Ghirardi V, Craighero L. Facial expressions as a model to test the role of the sensorimotor system in the visual perception of the actions. Exp Brain Res. 2017;235(12):3771–83. https://doi.org/10.1007/s00221-017-5097-y.

Melzack R, Israel R, Lacroix R, Schultz G. Phantom limbs in people with congenital limb deficiency or amputation in early childhood. Brain. 1997;120(Pt 9):1603–20.

Merzenich MM, Harrington TH. The sense of flutter-vibration evoked by stimulation of the hairy skin of primates: comparison of human sensory capacity with the responses of mechanoreceptive afferents innervating the hairy skin of monkeys. Exp Brain Res. 1969;9(3):236–60. https://doi.org/10.1007/BF00234457.

Moreno-López Y, Olivares-Moreno R, Cordero-Erausquin M, Rojas-Piloni G. Sensorimotor integration by corticospinal system. Front Neuroanat. 2016;10:24. https://doi.org/10.3389/fnana.2016.00024.

Morrison I, Björnsdotter M, Olausson H. Vicarious responses to social touch in posterior insular cortex are tuned to pleasant caressing speeds. J Neurosci. 2011;31(26):9554–62. https://doi.org/10.1523/JNEUROSCI.0397-11.2011.

Mueller S, Winkelmann C, Krause F, Grunwald M. Occupation-related long-term sensory training enhances roughness discrimination but not tactile acuity. Exp Brain Res. 2014;232(6):1905–14. https://doi.org/10.1007/s00221-014-3882-4.

Müller LR. Die Empfindungen in unseren inneren Organen. In: Müller LR, editor. Die Lebensnerven. Berlin: Springer; 1924. p. 495–524.

Mueller SM, Grunwald M. Haptische Wahrnehmungsleistungen: Effekte bei erfahrenen und unerfahrenen Physiotherapeuten. Manuelle Medizin, 2013;51(6):473–8. https://doi.org/10.1007/s00337-013-1068-y

Murphy MN, Mizuno M, Mitchell JH, Smith SA. Cardiovascular regulation by skeletal muscle reflexes in health and disease. Am J Physiol Heart Circ Physiol. 2011;301(4):H1191–204. https://doi.org/10.1152/ajpheart.00208.2011.

Nava E, Steiger T, Röder B. Both developmental and adult vision shape body representations. Sci Rep. 2014;4:6622. https://doi.org/10.1038/srep06622.

Nelson JS, Kuling IA, Gori M, Postma A, Brenner E, Smeets JBJ. Spatial representation of the workspace in blind, low vision, and sighted human participants. i-Perception. 2018;9(3):2041669518781877. https://doi.org/10.1177/2041669518781877.

Olgiati E, Maravita A, Spandri V, Casati R, Ferraro F, Tedesco L, et al. Body schema and corporeal self-recognition in the alien hand syndrome. Neuropsychology. 2017;31(5):575–84. https://doi.org/10.1037/neu0000359.

Pantev C, Engelien A, Candia V, Elbert T. Representational cortex in musicians. Plastic alterations in response to musical practice. Ann N Y Acad Sci. 2001;930:300–14.

Petkova VI, Zetterberg H, Ehrsson HH. Rubber hands feel touch, but not in blind individuals. PLoS One. 2012;7(4):e35912. https://doi.org/10.1371/journal.pone.0035912.

Phillips KA. Body dysmorphic disorder: diagnosis and treatment of image ugliness. Clin Psychiatry. 1996;57(8):61–4.

Phillips KA. Psychosis in body dysmorphic disorder. J Psychiatr Res. 2004;38(1):63–72.

Piontelli A. Development of normal fetal movements. The first 25 weeks of gestation. Milan: Springer-Verlag; 2010.

Preston C, Newport R. Evidence for dissociable representations for body image and body schema from a patient with visual neglect. Neurocase. 2011;17(6):473–9. https://doi.org/10.1080/13554794.2010.532504.

Price EH. A critical review of congenital phantom limb cases and a developmental theory for the basis of body image. Conscious Cogn. 2006;15(2):310–22. https://doi.org/10.1016/j.concog.2005.07.003.

Raimo S, Iona T, Di Vita A, Boccia M, Buratin S, Ruggeri F, et al. The development of body representations in school-aged children. Appl Neuropsychol Child. 2021;10(4):327–39. https://doi.org/10.1080/21622965.2019.1703704.

Ramachandran VS, Brang D. Sensations evoked in patients with amputation from watching an individual whose corresponding intact limb is being touched. Arch Neurol. 2009;66(10):1281–4. https://doi.org/10.1001/archneurol.2009.206.

Ray TJ, McGraw WS, Sun Z, Jeon M, Johnson T, Cheffins K, et al. Mandibular bone mineral density variation in three west African Cercopithecoid monkey species: associations with diet and feeding behavior. Arch Oral Biol. 2015;60(12):1714–20. https://doi.org/10.1016/j.archoralbio.2015.09.011.

Reid KJ, Harker J, Bala MM, Truyers C, Kellen E, Bekkering GE, Kleijnen J. Epidemiology of chronic non-cancer pain in Europe: narrative review of prevalence, pain treatments and pain impact. Curr Med Res Opin. 2011;27(2):449–62. https://doi.org/10.1185/03007995.2010.545813.

Reissland N, Burt M. Bi-directional effects of depressed mood in the postnatal period on mother-infant non-verbal engagement with picture books. Infant Behav Dev. 2010;33(4):613–8.

Reissland N, Francis B. The quality of fetal arm movements as indicators of fetal stress. Early Hum Dev. 2010;86(12):813–6.

Reissland N, Hopkins B, Helms P, Williams B. Maternal stress and depression and the lateralisation of infant cradling. J Child Psychol Psychiatry Allied Discip. 2009;50(3):263–9.

Reissland N, Francis B, Aydin E, Mason J, Schaal B. The development of anticipation in the fetus: a longitudinal account of human fetal mouth movements in reaction to and anticipation of touch. Dev Psychobiol. 2014;56(5):955–63. https://doi.org/10.1002/dev.21172.

Reissland N, Francis B, Kumarendran K, Mason J. Ultrasound observations of subtle movements: a pilot study comparing foetuses of smoking and nonsmoking mothers. Acta Paediatr. 2015;104(6):596–603.

Ricciardi E, Handjaras G, Pietrini P. The blind brain: how (lack of) vision shapes the morphological and functional architecture of the human brain. Exp Biol Med (Maywood). 2014;239(11):1414–20. https://doi.org/10.1177/1535370214538740.

Rieger C, Hardt H, Sennhauser FH, Wahn U, Zach M, editors. Pädiatrische Pneumologie. 2. Auflage ed. Berlin: Springer; 2004.

Rohricht F, Seidler KP, Joraschky P, Borkenhagen A, Lausberg H, Lemche E, et al. Consensus paper on the terminological differentiation of various aspect of body experience. Psychother Psychosom Med Psychol. 2005;55(3–4):183–90. https://doi.org/10.1055/s-2004-834551.

Romano D, Uberti E, Caggiano P, Cocchini G, Maravita A. Different tool training induces specific effects on body metric representation. Exp Brain Res. 2019;237(2):493–501. https://doi.org/10.1007/s00221-018-5405-1.

Rosen JC. Body image assessment and treatment in controlled studies of eating disorders. Int J Eat Disord. 1996;20(4):331–43.

Rubio KB, van Deusen J. Relation of perceptual and body image dysfunction to activities of daily living of persons after stroke. Am J OccupTher. 1995;49(6):551–9.

Ruggieri V, Valeri C. Variations in perception of right and left halves of the body during the menstrual cycle. Percept Mot Skills. 1981;52(3):931–6. https://doi.org/10.2466/pms.1981.52.3.931.

Rumsey N, Clarke A, White P, Wyn-Williams M, Garlick W. Altered body image. Appearance-related concerns of people with visible disfigurement. J Adv Nurs. 2004;48(5):443–53. https://doi.org/10.1111/j.1365-2648.2004.03227.x.

Rydel A, Seiffer W. Untersuchungen über das Vibrationsgefühl oder die sog. „Knochensensibilität" (Pallästhesie). Archiv f. Psychiatrie. 1903;37(2):488–536. https://doi.org/10.1007/bf02228367.

Saadah ES, Melzack R. Phantom limb experiences in congenital limb-deficient adults. Cortex. 1994;30(3):479–85. https://doi.org/10.1016/s0010-9452(13)80343-7.

Sanders KM, Ward SM, Koh SD. Interstitial cells: regulators of smooth muscle function. Physiol Rev. 2014;94(3):859–907. https://doi.org/10.1152/physrev.00037.2013.

Seidler RD, Meehan SK. A multidisciplinary approach to motor learning and sensorimotor adaptation. Lausanne: Frontiers Media SA; 2015.

Serino S, Pedroli E, Keizer A, Triberti S, Dakanalis A, Pallavicini F, et al. Virtual reality body swapping: a tool for modifying the Allocentric memory of the body. Cyberpsychol Behav Social Netw. 2016;19(2):127–33. https://doi.org/10.1089/cyber.2015.0229.

Sheffield A, Waller G, Emanuelli F, Murray J, Meyer C. Do schema processes mediate links between parenting and eating pathology? Eur Eating Disorders Rev. 2009;17(4):290–300. https://doi.org/10.1002/erv.922.

Shi Y, Apker G, Buneo CA. Multimodal representation of limb endpoint position in the posterior parietal cortex. J Neurophysiol. 2013;109(8):2097–107. https://doi.org/10.1152/jn.00223.2012.

Simmel ML. Phantoms in patients with leprosy and in elderly digital amputees. Am J Psychol. 1956;69(4):529–45.

Simon E, Pierau FK, Taylor DC. Central and peripheral thermal control of effectors in homeothermic temperature regulation. Physiol Rev. 1986;66(2):235–300. https://doi.org/10.1152/physrev.1986.66.2.235.

Skoruppa S, Stirn AV, Pantel J. Body Integrity Identity Disorder - der Wunsch körperbehindert zu sein. Eine fMRT Studie. Frankfurt am Main, Johann Wolfgang Goethe-Univ., Diss. Frankfurt am Main: Univ.-Bibliothek Frankfurt am Main. Online verfügbar unter. 2013. http://nbn-resolving.de/urn:nbn:de:hebis:30:3-314378.

Smolak L. Body image in children and adolescents. Where do we go from here? Body Image. 2004;1(1):15–28. https://doi.org/10.1016/S1740-1445(03)00008-1.

Sonksen PM, Levitt S, Kitsinger M. Identification of constraints acting on motor development in young visually disabled children and principles of remediation. Child Care Health Dev. 1984;10(5):273–86.

Spence C, Pavani F, Maravita A, Holmes N. Multisensory contributions to the 3-D representation of visuotactile peripersonal space in humans: evidence from the crossmodal congruency task. J Physiol Paris. 2004;98(1–3):171–89. https://doi.org/10.1016/j.jphysparis.2004.03.008.

Stein BE, Rowland BA. Chapter 3 - Neural development of multisensory integration. In: Sathian K, Ramachandran VS, editors. Multisensory perception. New York: Academic Press; 2020. p. 57–87. Online verfügbar unter. http://www.sciencedirect.com/science/article/pii/B9780128124925000036.

Stein BE, Stanford TR, Rowland BA. Development of multisensory integration from the perspective of the individual neuron. Nat Rev Neurosci. 2014;15(8):520–35. https://doi.org/10.1038/nrn3742.

Stirn A, Thiel A, Oddo S, Nieder TO Body integrity identity disorder (BIID). Störungsbild, Diagnostik, Therapieansätze. 1. Aufl. Weinheim: Beltz; 2010.

Striegel-Moore RH, Cachelin FM. Body image concerns and disordered eating in adolescent girls: risk and protective factors. In: Johnson NG, Roberts MC, Worell J, editors. Beyond appearance. A new look at adolescent girls. 1st ed. Washington, DC: American Psychological Association; 1999. p. 85–108.

Sun Y, Tang R. Tool-use training induces changes of the body schema in the limb without using tool. Front Hum Neurosci. 2019;13:454. https://doi.org/10.3389/fnhum.2019.00454.

Symmons MA, Richardson BL, Wuillemin DB. Components of haptic information: skin rivals kinaesthesis. Perception. 2008;37(10):1596–604. https://doi.org/10.1068/p5855.

Talbot WH, Darian-Smith I, Kornhuber HH, Mountcastle VB. The sense of flutter-vibration: comparison of the human capacity with response patterns of mechanoreceptive afferents from the monkey hand. J Neurophysiol. 1968;31(2):301–34. https://doi.org/10.1152/jn.1968.31.2.301.

Teixeira ALS, Dias MRC, Damasceno VO, Lamounier JA, Gardner RM. Association between different phases of menstrual cycle and body image measures of perceived size, ideal size, and body dissatisfaction. Percept Mot Skills. 2013;117(3):892–902. https://doi.org/10.2466/24.27.PMS.117x31z1.

Thompson JK, Stice E. Thin-ideal internalization. Mounting evidence for a new risk factor for body-image disturbance and eating pathology. Curr Dir Psychol Sci. 2001;10(5):181–3.

Tipper SP, Lloyd D, Shorland B, Dancer C, Howard LA, McGlone F. Vision influences tactile perception without proprioceptive orienting. Neuroreport. 1998;9(8):1741–4.

Tomasino B, Maieron M, Guatto E, Fabbro F, Rumiati RI. How are the motor system activity and functional connectivity between the cognitive and sensorimotor systems modulated by athletic expertise? Brain Res. 2013;1540:21–41. https://doi.org/10.1016/j.brainres.2013.09.048.

Treede RD, Baumgärtner U. Das somatosensorische System. In: Brandes R, Lang F, Schmidt RF, editors. Physiologie des Menschen. Mit Pathophysiologie. 32. Auflage: Springer-Lehrbuch; 2019. p. 644–65.

Tröster H, Brambring M. Early motor development in blind infants. J Appl Dev Psychol. 1993;14:83–106. https://doi.org/10.1016/0193-3973(93)90025-Q.

Tuschen-Caffier B. Körperbildstörungen. In: Herpertz S, de Zwaan M, Zipfel S, editors. Handbuch Essstörungen und Adipositas. 2., überarb. Aufl. Berlin: Springer-Verlag; 2015. p. 141–7.

Vallortigara G. The rose and the fly. A conjecture on the origin of consciousness. Biochem Biophys Res Commun. 2020;564:170. https://doi.org/10.1016/j.bbrc.2020.11.005.

von Frey M. Untersuchungen uber die Sinnesfunktionen der menschlichen Haut. Druckempfindung und Schmerz. Abhandl. d. Kgl. Sächs. Ges. d. Wiss. Math.-phys. Cl. Leipzig: Hirzel; 1896.

von Holst E, Mittelstaedt H. Das Reafferenzprinzip. Naturwissenschaften. 1950;37(20):464–76. https://doi.org/10.1007/bf00622503.

Wagner MO, Haibach PS, Lieberman LJ. Gross motor skill performance in children with and without visual impairments—research to practice. Res Dev Disabil. 2013;34(10):3246–52. https://doi.org/10.1016/j.ridd.2013.06.030.

Waldie KE, Mosley JL. Developmental trends in right hemispheric participation in reading. Neuropsychologia. 2000;38(4):462–74. https://doi.org/10.1016/s0028-3932(99)00091-3.

Walker SC, Trotter PD, Swaney WT, Marshall A, Mcglone FP. C-tactile afferents: cutaneous mediators of oxytocin release during affiliative tactile interactions? Neuropeptides. 2017;64:27–38. https://doi.org/10.1016/j.npep.2017.01.001.

Watanabe N, Hotta H. Heart rate changes in response to mechanical pressure stimulation of skeletal muscles are mediated by cardiac sympathetic nerve activity. Front Neurosci. 2016;10:614. https://doi.org/10.3389/fnins.2016.00614.

Waters NS, Klintsova AY, Foster TC. Insensitivity of the hippocampus to environmental stimulation during postnatal development. J Neurosci. 1997;17(20):7967–73.

Weiss R, Stahl SS, Tonna EA. The effects of diets of different physical consistencies on the periodontal proliferative activity in young adult rats. J Periodontal Res. 1969;4(4):296–9. https://doi.org/10.1111/j.1600-0765.1969.tb01983.x.

Weiss C, Tsakiris M, Haggard P, Schütz-Bosbach S. Agency in the sensorimotor system and its relation to explicit action awareness. Neuropsychologia. 2014;52:82–92. https://doi.org/10.1016/j.neuropsychologia.2013.09.034.

Wertheim EH, Paxton SJ, Blaney S. Body image in girls. In: Smolak L, Kevin Thompson J, editors. Body image, eating disorders, and obesity in youth. Assessment, prevention, and treatment. 2nd ed. Washington, DC: American Psychological Association; 2009. p. 47–76.

White RC, Davies AMA, Kischka U, Davies M. Touch and feel? Using the rubber hand paradigm to investigate self-touch enhancement in right-hemisphere stroke patients. Neuropsychologia. 2010;48(1):26–37.

Yamada Y, Kanazawa H, Iwasaki S, Tsukahara Y, Iwata O, Yamada S, Kuniyoshi Y. An embodied brain model of the human foetus. Sci Rep. 2016;6:27893. https://doi.org/10.1038/srep27893.

Anatomical and Physiological Basics

2

Stephanie Margarete Mueller and Martin Grunwald

Contents

S. M. Mueller (✉) · M. Grunwald
Haptic Research Lab, Paul-Flechsig-Institute for Brain Research, Leipzig University, Leipzig, Germany
e-mail: s.mueller@medizin.uni-leipzig.de; mgrun@medizin.uni-leipzig.de

S. M. Mueller et al., *Human Touch in Healthcare*, https://doi.org/10.1007/978-3-662-67860-2_2

2.1 Types and Functions of Mechanoreceptors

Almost all tissues in the human body contain cells that are sensitive to mechanical stimuli (mechanoreceptors). Depending on their localization, these mechanoreceptors register stimuli that impinge on the body from the outside, are caused by the body's movements, or arise due to organ activity. There are **several hundred such receptors in every cubic centimeter of body tissue**, and they vary greatly in their design and function. Thus far, no systematic count has been attempted of all the mechanosensory units in the entire human body. However, cautious extrapolations can be made based on selective analyses (Grunwald 2017, 2019):

- Rough estimations suggest that there are between six million and 250 million receptive units **in the skin** alone in the adult human body. Indeed, the body surface is covered with about five million hairs, and the root of each hair is surrounded by at least one free nerve ending. Some authors assume that there may be up to 50 receptors of different types in the immediate vicinity of each hair root (Sect. 1.1.4). The skin areas with the highest density of encapsulated mechanoreceptors are the palms and the soles of the feet, which have approximately 17,000 encapsulated mechanoreceptors each (Halata and Baumann 2008). In addition, the hairless skin of the palms and soles also contains numerous free nerve endings (approximately 100/mm^2). The highest density of free nerve endings can be found in the cornea of the eye, with 3500–7000 units/mm^2.
- Furthermore, there are mechanosensory units **inside the body**. For example, an adult human possesses about 5 kg of loose connective tissue in which, according to conservative estimates, approximately 100 million free nerve endings are distributed. In addition, there are an unknown number of other encapsulated mechanoreceptors inside the body and about 65,000 muscle and tendon receptors.

In summary, approximately 300–700 million mechanosensory units are distributed throughout the body.

Depending on the classification, about 10 different types of mechanoreceptors can be distinguished (Grunwald 2017, 2019). Different mechanoreceptors are usually specialized for different stimulus qualities.

This chapter aims to describe all the types of mechanoreceptors, their localizations, and their functions in order to draw attention to their ubiquity in the human body. Up to the present, textbooks and other sources have presented only the mechanoreceptors of the skin, the mechanoreceptors of a specific body region (e.g., the hand), or mechanoreceptors with a specific function (e.g., joint position). Unfortunately, this segmentation obscures the true extent of mechanosensory processes and the scope of haptic system functions.

2.1.1 Spatial Resolution, Receptive Fields, and Adaptation

2.1.1.1 Rest Potential/Standby Mode

All primary mechanoreceptors have in common that they are the terminals of **afferent nerve fibers**. Afferent nerve fibers carry sensory information from the body and its surface to the spinal cord or brain. (In contrast, **efferent pathways** send signals from the brain to the periphery.) Some mechanoreceptors form complex encapsulated structures, while others are finely pointed nerve endings located between body tissues. Regardless of their different structures, all mechanoreceptors generate a resting potential. The resting potential (approximately −70 mV; also called **membrane potential**) functions as a standby mode that allows for the fast processing of incoming stimuli. The receptor cells must actively maintain their resting potential through ion channels and ion pumps. Therefore, mechanoreceptors are not only activated by an incoming stimulus but are in a state of readiness at all times. Even though the individual is not consciously aware of this, the states of millions of mechanoreceptors are evaluated every second. Even if an individual does not move or is not touched, the brain processes a massive flood of impulse streams from the body's receptors. Most probably, it is this constant background noise that gives humans the feeling of a cohesive body and that forms the biological basis of self-consciousness (Grunwald 2017). (For more in-depth information on body representation, see Sect. 1.4.)

2.1.1.2 Action Potential

When a mechanical stimulus encounters a corresponding receptor, an action potential is generated. Action potentials are very short-lasting changes in membrane potential that serve to transmit stimuli via the axons to other nerve cells. An action potential is generated by the opening of sodium channels in the cell membrane. Through these channels, positively charged sodium ions flow into the interior of the cell, converting the negative resting potential into a positive charge (approximately +30 mV; depolarization). After a short time, the sodium channels close again, and the potassium channels are opened. Positively charged potassium ions flow out of the cell through these channels, which restore the resting potential (repolarization).

2.1.1.3 Adaptation

When a stimulus mechanically deforms a mechanoreceptor, an action potential is generated. The decreasing sensitivity of a receptor in the presence of a persistent stimulus is called adaptation. A distinction can be made between mechanoreceptors whose excitation lasts for a long time (slowly adapting, SA) and those that only transmit an action potential when a change in stimulus occurs (rapidly adapting, RA). A mechanoreceptor that responds to vibration stimuli is, thus, RA, since a vibration can also be described as a repeated stimulus change. Conversely, SA receptors are those that register, for example, long-lasting pressure stimuli.

2.1.1.4 Receptive Fields and Spatial Resolution

The density of mechanoreceptors in the body varies depending on the function and body area. Some receptor types are clustered at body orifices or exploration areas (e.g., hand, feet, tongue), while others are specific to certain tissues (e.g., in the muscles). However, the sensitivity of the tissue depends not only on receptor density but also on the receptive field of the mechanoreceptors. **The receptive field** describes the size of the area registered by a single receptor (cf. Fig. 2.1). Depending on the stimulus quality, smaller or larger areas are mechanically deformed on contact. For example, a sharp, punctual pressure stimulus deforms a much smaller area than a vibratory stimulus, which also causes the surrounding tissue to vibrate. The combination of the receptive field size and distribution density of the receptors determines the **spatial resolution capacity** of the respective body region. For example, in body regions that have more receptors with small receptive fields, it is possible to perceive punctual stimuli more precisely. Usually, spatial resolution is measured by employing tactile stimuli on the body surface (see Sect. 1.1.1). Therefore, receptive field sizes have only been determined for mechanoreceptors of the skin. Correspondingly, no data on the size of the receptive fields exists for muscle spindles and Golgi tendon organs.

▶ **Important**

- SA-I receptors (Merkel cells) are slow-adapting and have small receptive fields. Therefore, they enable the recognition of spatial details (e.g., Braille reading).
- SA-II receptors (Ruffini corpuscles) adapt slowly and have large receptive fields. They respond primarily to sustained stretch stimuli (e.g., feeling the weight of a backpack on the shoulders and back).
- RA-I receptors (Meissner corpuscles) are rapid-adapting and have small receptive fields. They are sensitive to motion and stimulus changes (e.g., detecting the roughness of a surface).
- RA-II (or PC) receptors (Pacinian corpuscles) adapt very rapidly and have large receptive fields. They predominantly respond to vibration and acceleration stimuli (e.g., the microvibrations of writing with a pen on paper).

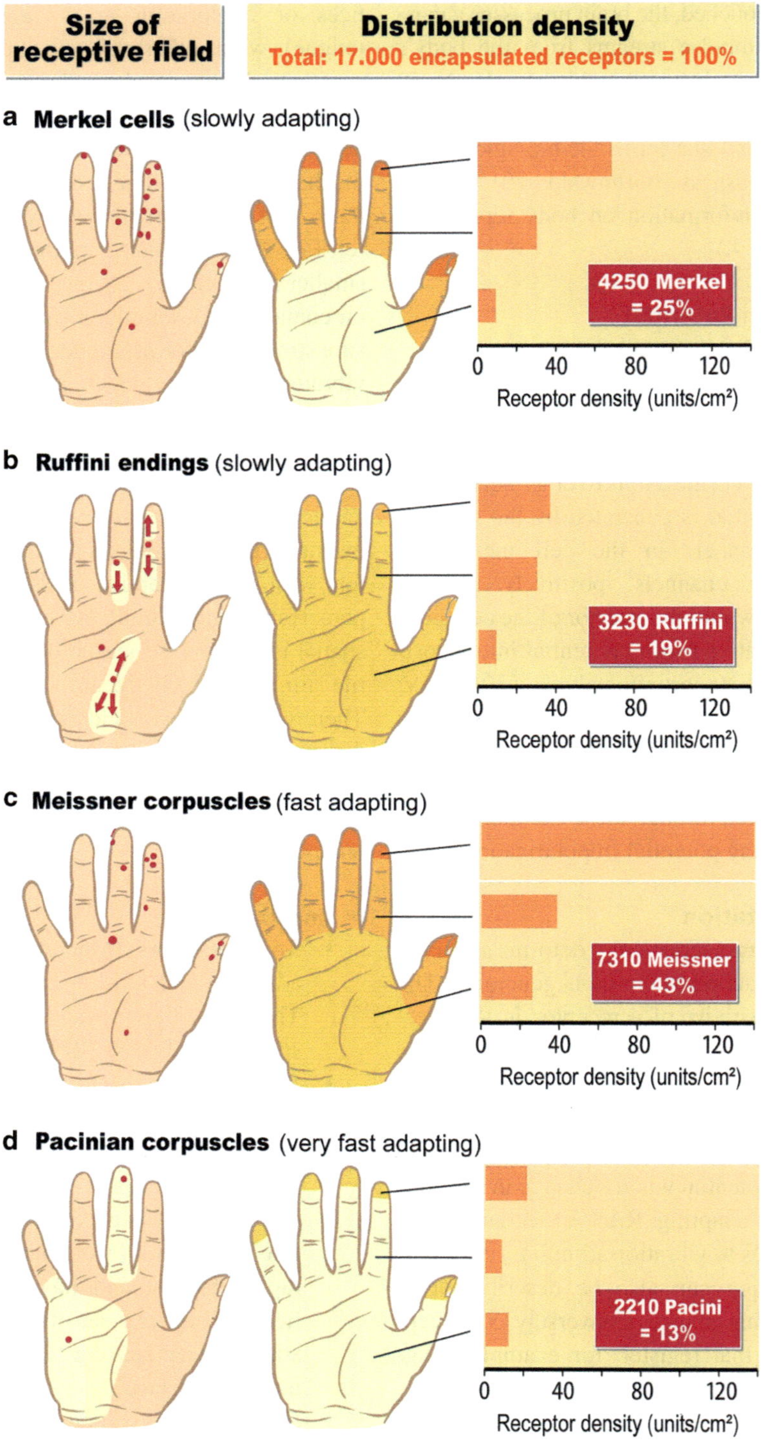

Fig. 2.1 (**a–d**) The receptive fields and innervation density of the skin of the human palm. The left side of the figure shows the receptive fields of the encapsulated skin receptors: Merkel and Meissner's cells have very small fields; Ruffini and Pacini corpuscles have large ones. The right side of the figure shows the innervation density: the light areas mark low receptor density; the darker areas mark higher receptor density. (Fig. from Birbaumer and Schmidt 2006, p. 326)

► **Important** In regions with higher spatial resolution, the receptors with small receptive fields are present in larger numbers (Meissner cells, Merkel cells, and free nerve endings).

The distribution density of mechanoreceptors with large receptive fields (Ruffini and Pacini corpuscles) is relatively constant across the body surface.

Pacinian corpuscles (large receptive fields) and free nerve endings (very small receptive fields) are distributed throughout all body tissues.

2.1.2 Meissner Corpuscles

Meissner corpuscles, named after their discoverer, Georg Meissner (1829–1905, German anatomist and physiologist), are encapsulated mechanoreceptors. They have an oval shape, a length of approximately 120 µm, and a width of approximately 50 µm. **Schwann cells** are stacked within the capsular envelope (see Fig. 2.2). These are innervated by multiple myelinated axons of 3–5 µm thickness.

2.1.2.1 Localization and Receptor Density

Unlike most other receptor types, Meissner corpuscles are localized exclusively in the skin and, thus, contribute to surface sensitivity. Meissner corpuscles are located in the papillary layer (see Fig. 1.1. in Sect. 1.1) of hairless skin as well as in the vicinity of hair follicles in hairy skin (hair follicle receptors). These receptors are prevalent on the tips of the fingers and toes, on the palms of the hands and soles of the feet, and on the mouth, nipples, and anus.

Up to 15 of these receptors can be found in 1 mm^2 of hairless skin. However, the number of Meissner corpuscles decreases with age. The highest receptor density is present in childhood, and this density decreases by 50% from childhood to middle adulthood. The causes of this process are currently unknown. It is assumed that the decrease in spatial resolution at an older age is partly due to the decrease in the number of Meissner's corpuscles. (For detailed changes over the lifespan, see Sect. 3.1).

2.1.2.2 Characteristics

Meissner corpuscles are also called tactile corpuscles. They are rapidly adaptive (RA-I), and they respond to pressure stimuli, moving skin deformations, and stimulus changes (e.g., beginning and end of a sustained pressure; tapping). The receptive threshold of Meissner corpuscles are single pressure stimuli with a skin indentation of only 10 µm. They also respond to low-frequency vibrations with an optimum of 20–30 Hz. This receptor type does not respond to higher-frequency vibrations or constant-pressure stimuli.

The receptive fields (see Fig. 2.1) of Meissner corpuscles are relatively small (5–8 mm; Vega-Bermudez and Johnson 1999), but the distribution density of the receptors is very high. Therefore, they allow the discrimination of stimuli that are close to each other (**e.g., static two-point threshold** Sect. 1.1.1). Accordingly, they play a central role in object recognition and surface exploration. In addition, due to their fast adaptability to moving skin deformations, they register the slippage (friction) of held objects and, thus, contribute fundamentally to force control when holding and manipulating objects.

Synopsis

Meissner Corpuscles

- Adapt quickly to light pressure stimuli (RA-I).
- Respond to low-frequency vibration, moving stimuli, and stimulus changes.
- Do not respond to high-frequency vibrations or sustained pressure stimuli.
- Have a density of up to 15 Meissner receptors in 1 mm^2 of hairless skin, although the number decreases sharply with age.
- Occurrence: exclusively in the skin and around the hair follicles.

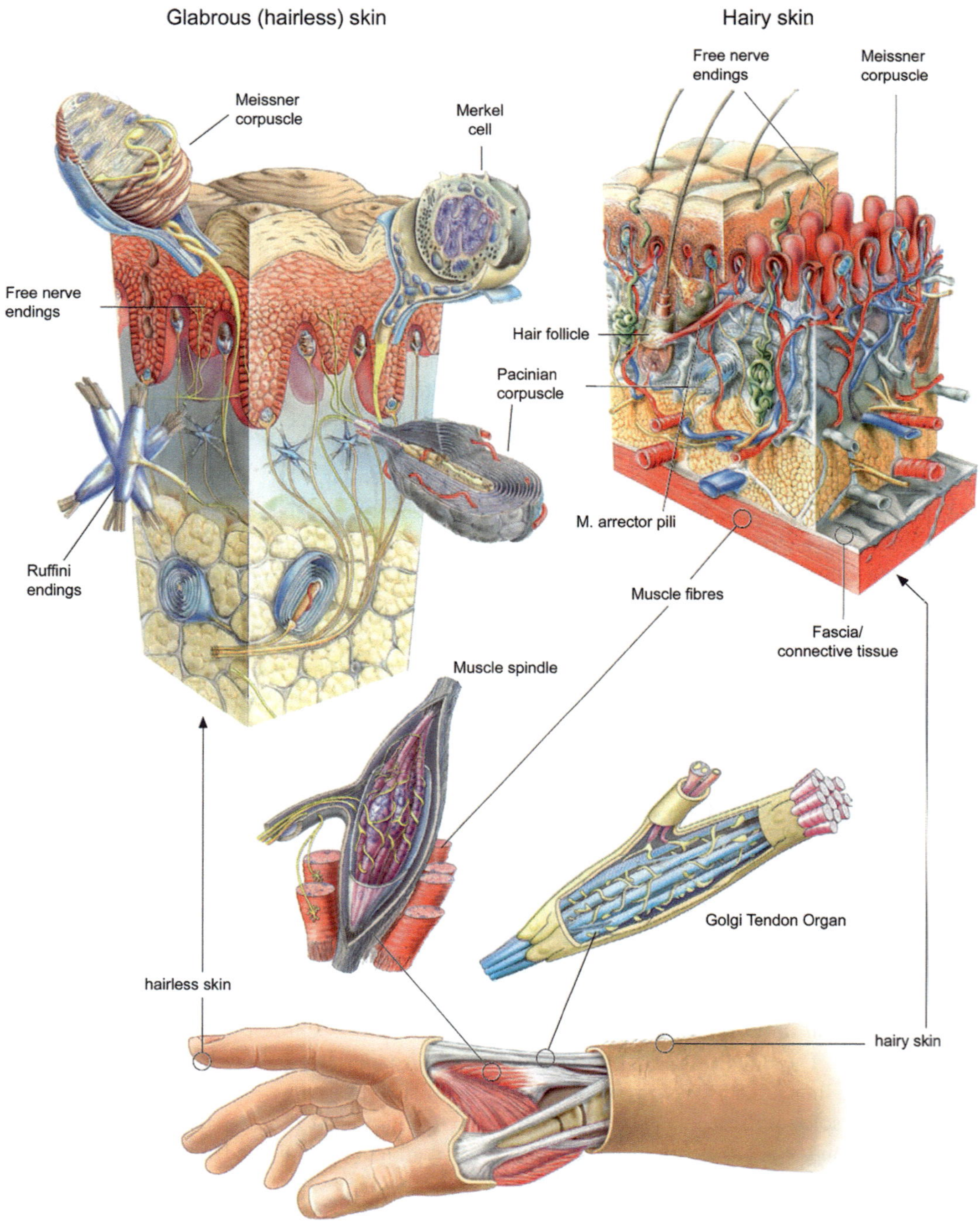

Fig. 2.2 Receptors of the haptic system. Illustration Julius Ecke. (Fig. from Grunwald and Mueller 2017, p. 259)

2.1.3 Merkel Cells

Merkel cells were discovered by the German anatomist Friedrich Merkel (1845–1919) in 1875. These cells are in the shape of small oval discs, are approximately 10 µm in size, and usually occur in groups of up to 19 cells. Each group of Merkel cells is supplied by a joint myelinated nerve fiber of 3–5 µm in diameter (Baumann et al. 2011).

2.1.3.1 Localization and Receptor Density

Apart from Meissner corpuscles, Merkel cells are the only mechanoreceptors that occur exclusively in the skin. They are located in the stratum basale of the epidermis (see Fig. 2.2), around the hair follicles, and in mucous membranes (e.g., in the mouth and esophagus). Merkel cells are less abundant compared to Meissner corpuscles. Approximately 20 of these receptors have been found per 1 cm^2 of human digital skin. Furthermore, in the skin of other body parts, they are even rarer (Fradette et al. 2003).

2.1.3.2 Characteristics

Merkel cells respond to pressure stimuli applied vertically to the skin and adapt slowly (SA-I). They primarily signal the duration and strength of sustained pressure stimuli. Their receptive fields are 5–20 mm in size, depending on the depth of the pressure; specifically, with deeper skin indentations (50–500 μm) by the pressure stimulus, the receptive field becomes wider (Vega-Bermudez and Johnson 1999). If even greater pressure depths (>0.5 mm) are reached, the stretch receptors of the deeper skin layers (Ruffini corpuscles) and, possibly, the muscle spindles of the musculature are also activated.

▶ **Important** Merkel cells are crucial for surface discrimination. For example, studies on the representation of Braille dots (Braille reading) by different receptor types showed that the small elevations were best registered by Merkel cells (Phillips et al. 1990).

2.1.3.3 Special Attributes

Merkel cells contain so-called neurosecretory granules and may be part of the **diffuse neuroendocrine system** (DNES). The DNES comprises cells that are individually scattered in the surface epithelium of various organs, and these cells can produce as well as store hormones. However, their physiological functions are controversial. Merkel cells may possibly play a role in the formation of hair follicles and sweat glands (Abraham and Mathew 2019).

2.1.3.4 Variants

Particularly large clusters of about 50 Merkel cells are called *Pinkus Iggo domes*.

Synopsis

Merkel Cells

- Are very slow at adapting to pressure stimuli (SA-I).
- Contribute to high-resolution surface discrimination (e.g., Braille).
- Occurrence: exclusively in the skin (including the mucous membranes and at the hair follicles).

2.1.4 Vater Pacini Corpuscles

The encapsulated mechanoreceptors that are known today as Pacinian or Vater-Pacini corpuscles were first described in 1741 by Abraham Vater (German anatomist, 1684–1751) and rediscovered in 1840 by Filippo Pacini (Italian anatomist, 1812–1883). With a length of up to 2 mm and a width of up to 1 mm, they are the largest known mechanoreceptors besides the muscle spindles. They consist of a centrally located axon of 6–10 μm in thickness surrounded by 20–60 onion-peel-shaped lamellae (cf. Fig. 2.2).

2.1.4.1 Localization

Pacinian corpuscles are distributed throughout the body. In the skin, they are located in the deeper layers: in the reticular layer of the dermis and in the subcutis (cf. Fig. 1.1. in Sect. 1.1). Inside the body, they are mainly found in the connective tissue around the organs, in and around the musculature (fasciae), and in the joint capsules, tendons, ligaments, aponeuroses, periosteum, middle ear, peritoneum, mesentery, pancreas, and the genital region (Schiebler et al. 1995). They have also been identified in the adventitia and the immediately adjacent tissues of the vascular walls (Thoma 1889).

2.1.4.2 Characteristics

Pacinian corpuscles are very fast-adapting receptors (RA-II) that respond predominantly to vibrations in the range of 10–1000 Hz (Fig. 2.3) and to accelerations of movements. They are most sensitive to frequencies around 200 Hz but also respond to vibrations with amplitudes as low as 20 nm (nanometer! → 0.001 millimeter = 1000 nm).

The receptive fields of Vater-Pacini corpuscles are large and diffuse, which gives them low spatial resolution. In addition, vibrations are generally transmitted through body tissues (especially via the bones, teeth, fingernails, and toenails), meaning that incoming vibratory stimuli usually activate several receptors. These activated receptors can sometimes be located far away from the actual contact point of the vibration stimulus.

▶ **Important** Depending on the intensity, vibration can affect a variety of physiological functions, both positively and negatively. Prolonged vibration usually leads to tissue damage and functional impairment (Griffin 2004). The presence of vibration-sensitive receptors in all body areas indicates their signaling function as protection and warning sensors.

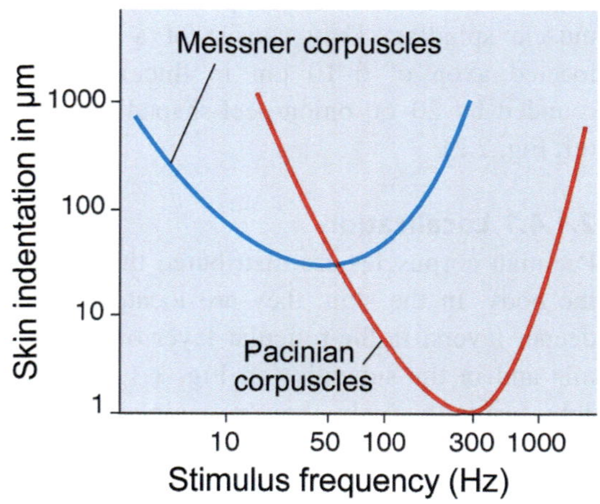

Fig. 2.3 Vibration detection of Meissner and Pacinian corpuscles. The curves show the minimum required stimulus properties (frequency and vibration amplitude) at which action potentials are generated. The vibration amplitudes are shown as a skin indentation in micrometers. Pacinian corpuscles respond most strongly to high-frequency stimuli, starting at very low amplitudes. Meissner corpuscles respond more strongly to low-frequency stimuli. (Fig. from Bear et al. 2018, p. 441, based on Talbot et al. 1968)

2.1.4.3 Variants

In addition to the large Vater-Pacini corpuscles, other forms of lamellar corpuscles exist that likely serve similar functions.

End-bulbs of Krause are also encapsulated mechanoreceptors (Michailow 1907). They are found mainly in the epithelium of mucous membranes, including the mouth, nose, urinary bladder, rectum, and the edge of the cornea and conjunctiva in the eye.

Golgi-Mazzoni corpuscles resemble Vater-Pacini receptors in their lamellar structure but have two or more axons and several inner bulbs. Thus far, they have been identified mainly in the genital region and in the joint capsules.

Synopsis
Vater-Pacini corpuscles are:

- Very fast adapting (RA-II).
- Acceleration and vibration receptors.
- Occurrence: throughout the body.

2.1.5 Ruffini Endings

Ruffini endings, which are encapsulated mechanoreceptors, were named after the Italian anatomist Angelo Ruffini (1864–1929). Ruffini endings (or Bulbous corpuscles) consist of a cylindrical connective tissue capsule that surrounds a nerve fiber of 5–10 µm thickness and long collagen fibers. In some Ruffini endings, several fiber cylinders cross in the middle, meaning each cylinder points in a different direction (cf. Fig. 2.2). The size of Ruffini endings varies between 50 and 300 µm.

2.1.5.1 Localization and Receptor Density

Ruffini endings are located in the reticular layer of hairy and hairless skin (cf. Fig. 1.1. in Sect.

1.1), in the intermuscular connective tissue, and in the joint capsules, fasciae, aponeuroses, and tendons. They have also been localized in the dura mater, iris, and ciliary body of the eye (Vogt 2012). Little is known about the number of Ruffini endings in various body tissues. One study detected approximately 60 Ruffini endings in the human shoulder joint and associated ligaments (Gohlke et al. 1998).

2.1.5.2 Characteristics

Ruffini endings adapt very slowly (SA-II) and respond mainly to long-lasting stretch stimuli of the skin, tendons, and joints. Their receptive fields are large, and consequently, their spatial resolution is low.

As they adapt slowly and are located deep in the skin, they play an essential role in detecting forces that, if prolonged, can lead to tissue damage. In tendons, ligaments, and joint capsules, they contribute to the perception of movements and changes in the position of the limbs (proprioception).

▶ **Important** In addition to muscle spindles and Golgi tendon organs, Ruffini endings are crucial for proprioception (Sect. 1.3) and the stability of the joints.

Synopsis
Ruffini endings are:

- Very slow adapting (SA-II).
- Sensitive to skin stretching and joint activity.
- Occurrence: in the deeper layers of the skin, as well as in joints, connective tissues, and tendons.

2.1.6 Muscle Spindles

Muscle spindles (cf. Fig. 2.2) consist of a spindle-shaped connective tissue capsule that encloses muscle fibers (“intrafusal fibers”). The spindles are 2–10 mm long and 0.2 mm thick (Halata and Baumann 2008). Muscle spindles lie parallel to the surrounding muscle fibers (“extrafusal fibers”) and are closely connected to them. When the length of the muscle changes, the muscle spindles are compressed or stretched. The sensory information from the muscle spindles is transmitted via afferent nerve pathways (Ia and II) and controlled by efferent pathways (γ-motoneuron) (For more details on neural innervation, see Sect. 2.2).

2.1.6.1 Localization and Receptor Density

Muscle spindles occur in all skeletal (striated) muscles but not in smooth or cardiac muscle tissues. In addition, the density of muscle spindles is significantly higher in small muscles than in large muscles (Peck et al. 1984).

2.1.6.2 Characteristics

Muscle spindles adapt very slowly; they detect the static length of a muscle, as well as the speed of the change in its length, and they also respond to both passive and active stretches (see Fig. 2.4). Muscle spindles play a central role in maintaining muscle tone and mediating the interaction of antagonistic muscle groups. In addition, muscle stretch reflexes, such as the patellar reflex, are triggered by the sudden activation of muscle spindles. Muscle spindles are, thus, crucial for movement control and maintaining posture (i.e., head position, sitting, walking).

Furthermore, the abundance of muscle spindles in small muscles suggests that they provide important information for fine-tuning movement sequences. Accordingly, they enable fine motor control of eye movements, as well as laryngeal movements, which are necessary for speech production. The muscle spindles of the finger musculature are essential for executing complex and graded grasping movements (Goodwin and Wheat 2008).

Synopsis
Muscle spindles are:

- Slow adaption to muscle stretching.

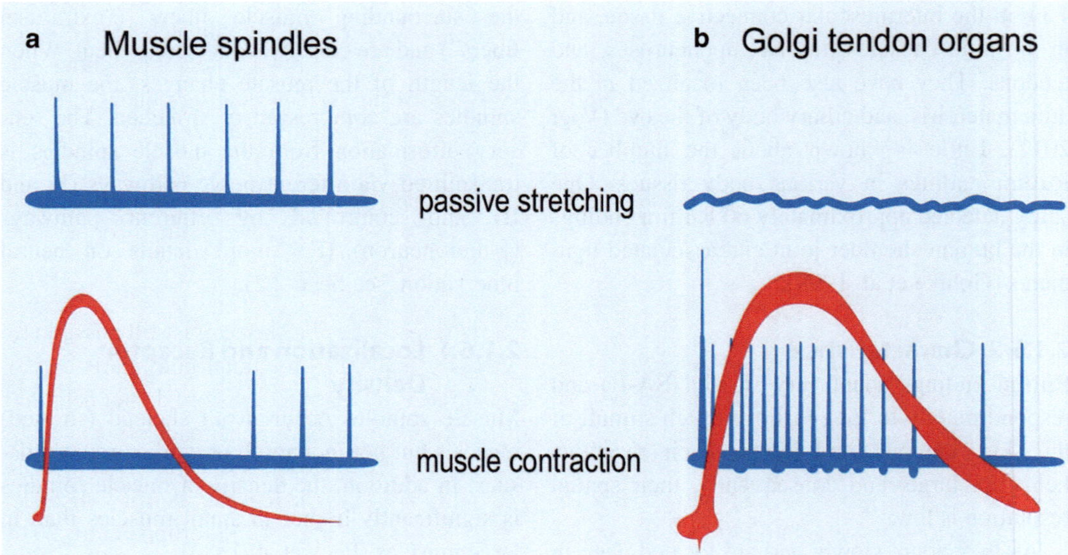

Fig. 2.4 (**a**, **b**) Action potentials of muscle spindles and Golgi tendon organs during stretch and contraction. The *curved line* represents the force progression during a single muscle contraction. Each *vertical line* is an action potential. (**a**) The type Ia afferent from the muscle spindle is activated by mild stretching. In contrast, no action potentials are generated at the muscle spindle during muscle contraction. (**b**) The type Ib afferent from the Golgi tendon organ does not respond to stretch but is activated by mild active muscle contraction. (Fig. from Treede and Baumgärtner 2019, p. 659)

- Relevant for movement control, the maintenance of posture, and the fine-tuning of movement sequences.
- More common in small muscles than in large muscles.
- Occurrence: in the striated musculature.

2.1.7 Golgi Tendon Organs

Golgi tendon organs were named after Camillo Golgi (Italian physician and histologist, 1843–1926). They consist of a bundle of collagenous fibers enclosed in a connective tissue capsule and reach a size of about 1.5 mm in length and 120 μm in width. The afferent nerve terminals of the Golgi tendon organs wrap around the collagenous fibers of tendons like a braid and branch between them. Each Golgi tendon organ is supplied by at least three myelinated nerve tracts (Ib afferents). (For more details, see Sect. 2.2. and Fig. 2.5).

2.1.7.1 Localization

Golgi tendon organs are located in the tendons of striated muscles, especially at the junctions between muscles and tendon fibers. They are also located in the joint capsules and ligaments.

2.1.7.2 Characteristics

Golgi tendon organs adapt slowly. They respond to muscular tension changes triggered by active muscle contraction (cf. Fig. 2.4). Through their neuronal circuitry in the spinal cord, the impulses from the Golgi tendon organs can inhibit the α-motoneurons of the same muscle and activate their antagonists. Therefore, this reflex pathway, which lowers the tone of the muscle, protects the tendons of an overly contracted muscle from extension and tearing.

▶ **Important** Together with information from the muscle spindles and other mechanoreceptors in connective tissue and in and around the joints, the impulses from the Golgi tendon organs form the basis of

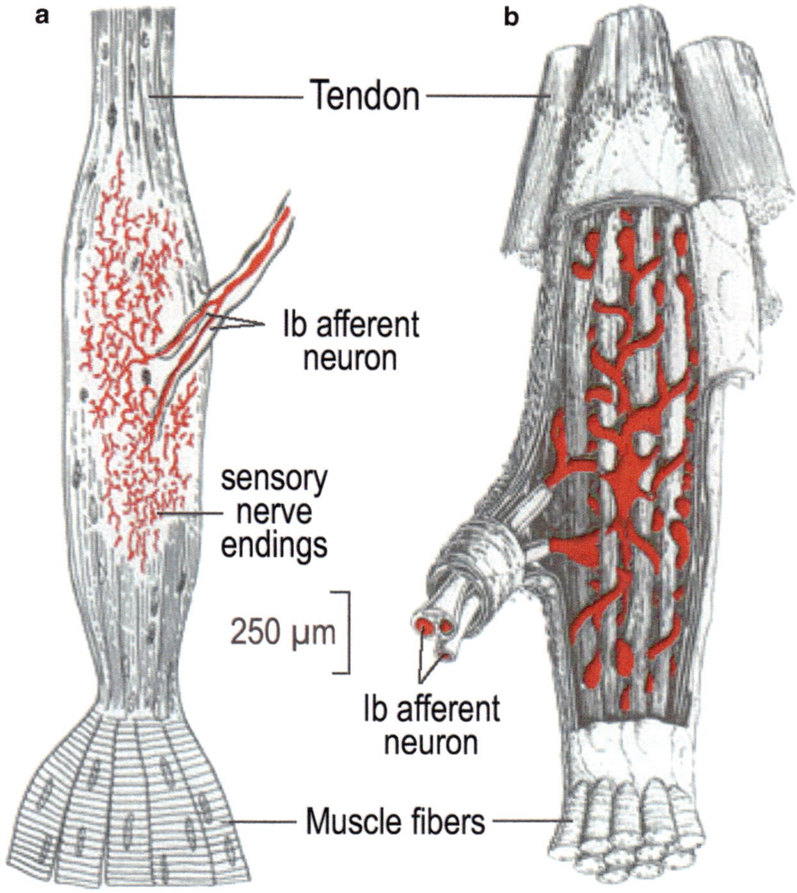

Fig. 2.5 Structure of a Golgi tendon organ. (**a**) Drawing of a Golgi tendon organ based on a light microscopic image by Santiago Ramón y Cajal (1906). The Golgi organ consists of unmyelinated nerve endings (red) that lie between collagen strands and unite to form myelinated Ib fibers. (**b**) Depiction of nerve endings (red) arising between collagen strands forming a type Ib fiber. (Fig. from Lehmann-Horn 2017, p. 128)

coordinated muscular activity and of the perception of movement and the position of the limbs in space (proprioception).

Synopsis
Golgi tendon organs are:

- Slowly adapting receptors.
- Activated by active muscle contraction.
- Occurrence: in dense connective tissues (e.g., tendons and joint capsules).

2.1.8 Free Nerve Endings

All the mechanoreceptors described so far have in common that they are supplied by fast-conducting nerve fibers with thick myelin sheaths (for more details, see Sect. 2.2) and are surrounded by a connective tissue capsule (encapsulated receptors). Conversely, the sensory terminals of slow-conducting Aδ- and C-fibers do not usually form capsules but form unencapsulated, finely branched "free" nerve endings (Fig. 2.2) (Knoche 1951; Jabonero 1967). With a diameter of 1–3 μm, free nerve endings are the smallest and simplest sensitive units of the human body (Cauna 1980).

2.1.8.1 Localization and Receptor Density

Free nerve endings are distributed throughout the body in almost all tissues. For example, 1 mm^2 of human finger skin (stratum granulosum; see Figs. 1.1 and 2.2) can contain up to 100 free nerve endings (Cauna 1980); furthermore, 1 mm^2 of the cornea of the eye can even contain 3500 to 7000 (!) (Bergua 2017). This means that free nerve endings are not only the smallest but also the most densely distributed mechanoreceptors in the human body.

In addition to being found in the skin, free nerve endings are also found around the hair follicles, in loose and dense connective tissue, in mucous membranes, in the smooth muscle tissue of the internal organs, in striated muscles, in blood vessels, and in the transparent cornea of the eye.

2.1.8.2 Characteristics

For a long time, free nerve endings were regarded primarily as pain receptors (nociceptors). It is now known that they are responsible for processing various mechanical, chemical, and thermal stimuli. Some free nerve endings respond to multiple stimulus modalities, whereas others are only sensitive to specific stimuli (e.g., cold).

Pain (see also Sects. 1.1.7 and 1.2.4) Nociceptors adapt very slowly in the case of non-damaging stimulation. However, they never adapt if stimulation is tissue-damaging! The most pain-sensitive region of the human body is the cornea of the eye. Even a pressure stimulus of only 0.2 g/mm^2 is felt as unpleasant or painful there (Krückmann 1895). Other areas of the body are not sensitive to pain at all. This applies to the brain and most organs of the abdominal cavity. However, organs without nociceptors are usually surrounded by highly pain-sensitive and protective connective tissue layers (e.g., meninges and pleura).

▶ **Important** Nociceptors do not adapt during tissue-damaging stimulation!

Temperature (see also Sects. 1.1.6 and 1.2.3) Some free nerve endings respond selectively to cold stimuli, whereas others respond selectively to heat stimuli (thermoreceptors). Cold receptors respond within a sensitivity range of approximately 5–35 °C (41–95 °F). Conversely, warm receptors detect heat stimuli in the range of 30–45 °C (86–113 °F). Both warm and cold stimuli are always processed as compared to body temperature. In the range of 30–35 °C (86–95 °F), thermoreceptors adapt relatively quickly, meaning that cold or warm sensations disappear after a short time. However, temperatures outside this zone of indifference are permanently perceived (no adaptation) as warm or cold. Temperature stimuli of less than 15 °C (59 °F) or more than 45 °C (113 °F) excite nociceptive nerve endings and are perceived as cold or heat pain.

▶ **Important** Cold receptors are about three times more abundant in humans compared to warm receptors.

Itching Some free nerve endings (probably C-fibers) of the skin and mucous membranes respond selectively to chemical substances (e.g., histamines). These substances can be released locally or systemically due to inflammation, mosquito bites, or internal diseases. The contact of such nerve endings with these substances results in itching sensations.

▶ **Important** Stimuli, such as pressure, heat, or cold, can temporarily mask itching or pain sensations.

Cardiovascular Reflex (Exercise Pressor Reflex) Free nerve endings in the fasciae of skeletal muscles (so-called interstitial muscle receptors) are stimulated by muscle movement (e.g., during exercise). This stimulation leads to a reflexive adaptation of the heart rate and cardiac output to physical load (Mitchell and Schmidt 2011; Watanabe and Hotta 2016). Therefore, during physical exercise, the heart rate increases not only due to the higher oxygen demand but also due to this sensory reflex.

Gentle Touch (Stroking) (see also Sect. 1.1.5) Some C-fiber terminals are selectively activated by slow stroking touch (1 cm/s to 10 cm/s) (Nordin 1990). These so-called tactile C-fibers, which are located only in hairy skin, are associated with the pleasant sensations that can be elicited by social touch. In addition, according to some authors, these free nerve endings contribute to the positive emotional and anxiety-relieving effects of touch (Walker et al. 2017). In contrast, they are not involved in processing the physical properties of stimuli (e.g., temperature, intensity, and direction of movement).

Visceroception (see also Sect. 1.2) The perceptible results of the stimulation of the free nerve endings of the internal organs include, for example, the detection of foreign bodies in the trachea or bronchi and the triggering of the cough reflex. In the gastrointestinal tract and urinary bladder, free nerve endings measure tissue stretching and, thus, convey a feeling of fullness, the urge to urinate, or the urge to defecate.

However, not all stimuli processed by free nerve endings can be perceived consciously. In particular, the processing of mechanical stimuli that arise in the course of organ activity is not usually consciously perceived. In the smooth muscle tissues and mucous membranes of the internal organs, free nerve endings contribute to the registration of pressure, stretch, tension, and shear stimuli that influence the function of the organs and are relevant for their homeostasis. One example of visceral nerve endings is the baroreceptors of the blood vessels. These receptors constantly measure the dilation of the blood vessels and contribute to maintaining stable blood pressure through the baroreceptor reflex.

The relevance of sensory information for the correct functioning of the internal organs is regularly underestimated. However, it should be emphasized that up to 90% of the nerve fibers of the parasympathetic vagus nerve of the abdominal and thoracic viscera are afferent (sensory) nerve fibers.

Synopsis

Free nerve endings are:

- Very slow to non-adaptive.
- Activated by pain, temperature, light stroking touch, itching (chemical), tissue stretching, and visceral stimuli.
- Not all stimuli processed by free nerve endings are consciously perceptible.
- Occurrence: in all body tissues.

2.1.9 Hair Cells of the Auditory and Vestibular Systems

The hair cells of the inner ear also belong to the category of mechanoreceptors. All the receptors that have been described so far are primary sensory cells with a connected axon. In contrast, hair cells are called secondary sensory cells. They are pure epithelial receptor cells that do not have an axon but transmit their receptor potentials via a synaptic connection to consecutive nerve cells.

The hair cells of the **auditory system** are located in the organ of Corti in the cochlea. These hair cells are excited by sound (mediated by the corresponding vibration of the basilar membrane; see Fig. 2.6).

The hair cells of the **vestibular system** are located in the semicircular ducts and otolithic organs and are excited by rotational and linear acceleration, respectively.

2.1.10 Summary

See Table 2.1.

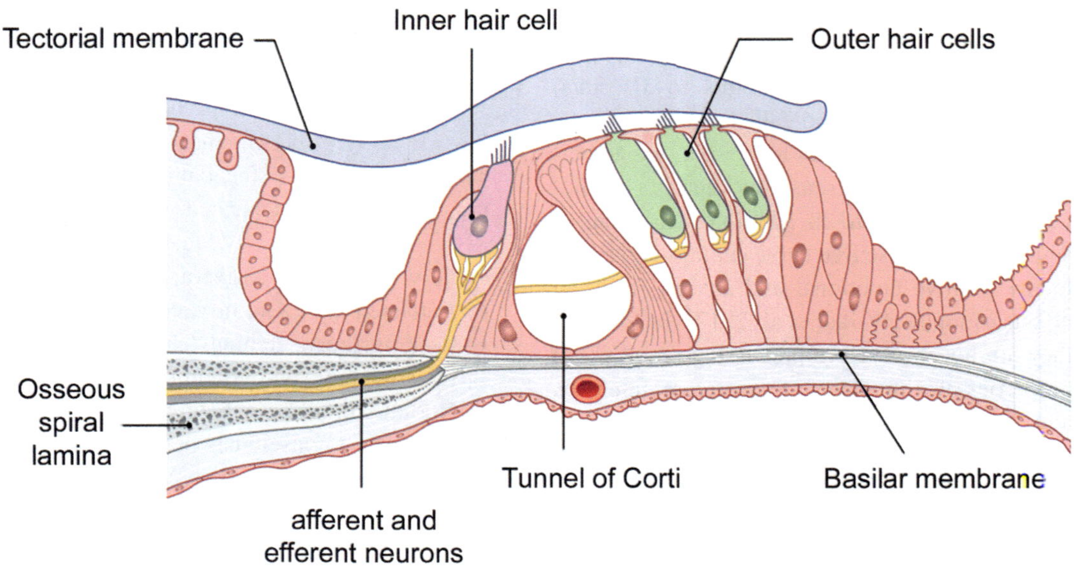

Fig. 2.6 Hair cells of the auditory system (organ of Corti). Incoming sound waves cause the tympanic membrane to oscillate. These oscillations are amplified by the ossicles (i.e., the malleus, incus, and stapes) and transmitted to the lymphatic fluid in the inner ear—the cochlea. The hair cells that enable hearing are located on the inner wall of the cochlea. The oscillating lymph fluid sets the basilar membrane of the cochlea in motion, causing the stereocilia of the hair cells to be displaced against the tectorial membrane. The bending of the stereocilia triggers electrical nerve impulses that are transmitted to the brain. Hair cells at different locations in the cochlea are activated by different oscillation frequencies, from which different sounds are derived. (Fig. simplified, after Amunts et al. 2010, p. 706)

Table 2.1 Function and localization of the mechanoreceptors in the human body

Receptors	Adaptation	Type of afferent nerve fiber	Occurrence	Perception dimensions	Receptive field/ spatial resolution (tactile)
Meissner corpuscles	Fast adapting (RA-I)	Aβ	Exclusively in the skin and around hair follicles	Touch, stimulus changes, slow vibration	Small receptive field; high resolution
Merkel cells	Slow adapting (SA-I)	Aβ	Exclusively in the skin and mucous membranes	Sustained pressure stimuli	Small receptive field; high resolution
Vater-Pacini corpuscles	Very fast adapting (RA-II)	II/Aβ	Throughout the body	Acceleration, high-frequency vibration	Large receptive field; low resolution
Ruffini endings	Very slow adapting (SA-II)	II/Aβ	Skin, joints, tendons, and muscular connective tissue	Stretch	Large receptive field; low resolution
Muscle spindles	Slowly adapting	Ia, II	Striated musculature; more frequent in small muscles than in large ones	Stretch	–
Golgi tendon organs	Slowly adapting	Ib	Tendons, ligaments, and joint capsules	Active muscle contraction	–
Free nerve endings	Very slow adapting	III/Aδ, IV/C	Throughout the body	Pain, temperature, itching, soft touch, stretching, shearing forces	Small receptive field; high resolution

2.2 Neural Processing of the Haptic System

2.2.1 Peripheral Sensory Fibers

Different types of mechanoreceptors are innervated by nerve fibers (afferent neurons) of different diameters and myelin sheath thicknesses. These afferent nerve fibers are assigned to four different classes according to their diameter (see Fig. 2.7). Axons that are thicker have faster conduction velocities. Indeed, thicker axons are usually surrounded by several layers of myelin sheath, which are interrupted by nodes of Ranvier. These nodes of Ranvier enable the faster saltatory (jumping) conduction of action potentials. Neurons with thick myelin insulation conduct action potentials at a speed of up to 130 m/s, which is equivalent to nearly 500 km/h (31 mph). Conversely, axons without a myelin sheath or with a very thin myelin sheath conduct action potentials at a speed of 0.5–30 m/s.

Axons from the skin		Aβ	Aδ	C
Axons from inside the body	Group I	II	III	IV
Diameter (in μm)	13–20	6–12	1–5	0,2–1,5
Speed (m/s)	80–120	35–75	5–30	0,5–2
Receptors/ sensory function	Primary muscle spindle afferents; Golgi tendon organs	Secondary muscle spindle afferents; encapsulated mechanoreceptors	Free nerve endings: pain, temperature, mechanosensory	Free nerve endings: pain, temperature, itching, pleasant touch

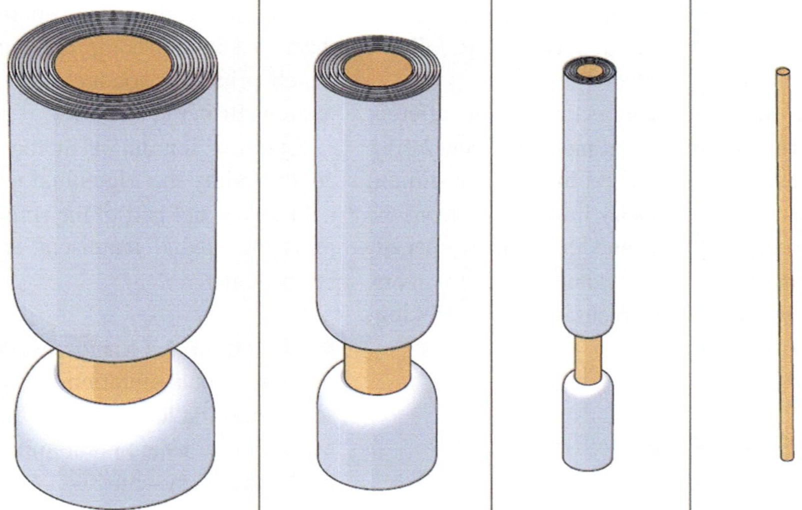

Fig. 2.7 Size differences of primary afferent nerve fibers. Axons with a larger diameter and a thicker myelin layer have a faster conduction velocity. The thickest afferent axons (type I) are exclusively connected to muscle spindles and tendon organs. There is no equivalent in the skin. The classifications were introduced by Erlanger and Gasser, as well as Lloyd and Hunt. (Fig. modified from Bear et al. 2018)

▶ **Important** Axons with larger diameters and thicker myelin sheaths show faster conduction velocity.

Depending on whether the afferent nerve fibers form mechanoreceptors in the skin or within the body, the different classes of neurons are designated either by letters (axons of the skin: Aβ-, Aδ-, and C-fibers) or by Roman numerals (axons of musculature and viscera: types I, II, III, and IV) (see Fig. 2.7).

The fastest-conducting nerve fibers are those of the muscle spindles and Golgi tendon organs, and they are called type I fibers. All other encapsulated mechanoreceptors are connected to Aβ- or type II fibers.

In contrast, the type III (Aδ-fibers) and type IV (C-fibers) nerve tracts conduct information only slowly. Type III (Aδ) fibers are surrounded by a very thin myelin layer and, consequently, conduct somewhat faster than type IV (C) fibers. C-fibers are unmyelinated.

These slow-conducting classes of afferent fibers form free nerve endings (see Sect. 2.1.8). They transmit pain, temperature, and itch stimuli, as well as mechanosensory information from the viscera (interoception) and the skin. A specialized form of C-fibers, called C-tactile fibers, respond specifically to pleasant (slow stroking) touch (Löken et al. 2009).

2.2.2 Spinal Cord

Afferent sensory nerve fibers from the skin, connective tissue, muscles, and viscera enter the spinal cord through the dorsal root. In the posterior horn of the spinal cord, mechanosensory afferents form two ascending pathways to the brain (Fig. 2.8): the lemniscal system and the spinothalamic system (Stopford 1929). Additionally, the posterior horn contains interneurons that form synaptic connections with the efferent motor neurons of the anterior horn and trigger the **spinal reflexes** (see Fig. 2.9). These include muscle and skin reflexes (**somatic reflexes**), organ functions such as bladder emptying (**visceral reflexes**), and **mixed reflexes** involving both somatic and visceral tissues (e.g., Head zones or the abdominal rigidity of the acute abdomen).

In the medulla oblongata and thalamus, information from the ascending pathways is modified and supplemented by information from other systems. For instance, interneurons connect to descending pathways from the cortex and subcortical areas as well as between the collateral ascending pathways (e.g., between fibers of the spinothalamic and lemniscal systems).

2.2.2.1 The Lemniscal System (Epicritic Sensation)

The **lemniscal system** (also known as the dorsal column-medial lemniscus pathway) consists mainly of thickly myelinated axons that predominantly conduct sensory information from the encapsulated mechanoreceptors of the trunk and extremities. Additionally, approximately 25% of the dorsal column comprises unmyelinated fibers, which primarily conduct pain perception information (Briner et al. 1988).

Epicritic sensations in the facial region are conducted by the trigeminal nerve. The trigeminal nerve is not part of the spinal cord; instead, it joins the medial lemniscus at the level of the brain stem.

▶ **Definition** Mechanosensations such as pressure, touch, vibration, and proprioception are sometimes called **epicritic sensations**. These body sensations are predominantly conducted by the lemniscal system.

The first-order neuron population sends information from the mechanoreceptors in the periphery via the dorsal root into the dorsal column of the spinal cord (Amunts et al. 2010). One spinal ganglion is formed on each side of the spinal cord segment. In the spinal ganglion, the cell bodies of the first-order neurons are bundled. The peripheral processes of all the neurons of a spinal ganglion enter the spinal cord through a common dorsal root and innervate a circumscribed skin area called a dermatome (Fig. 2.10). Indeed, each dorsal root is strictly associated with a particular dermatome and the underlaying tissue. The

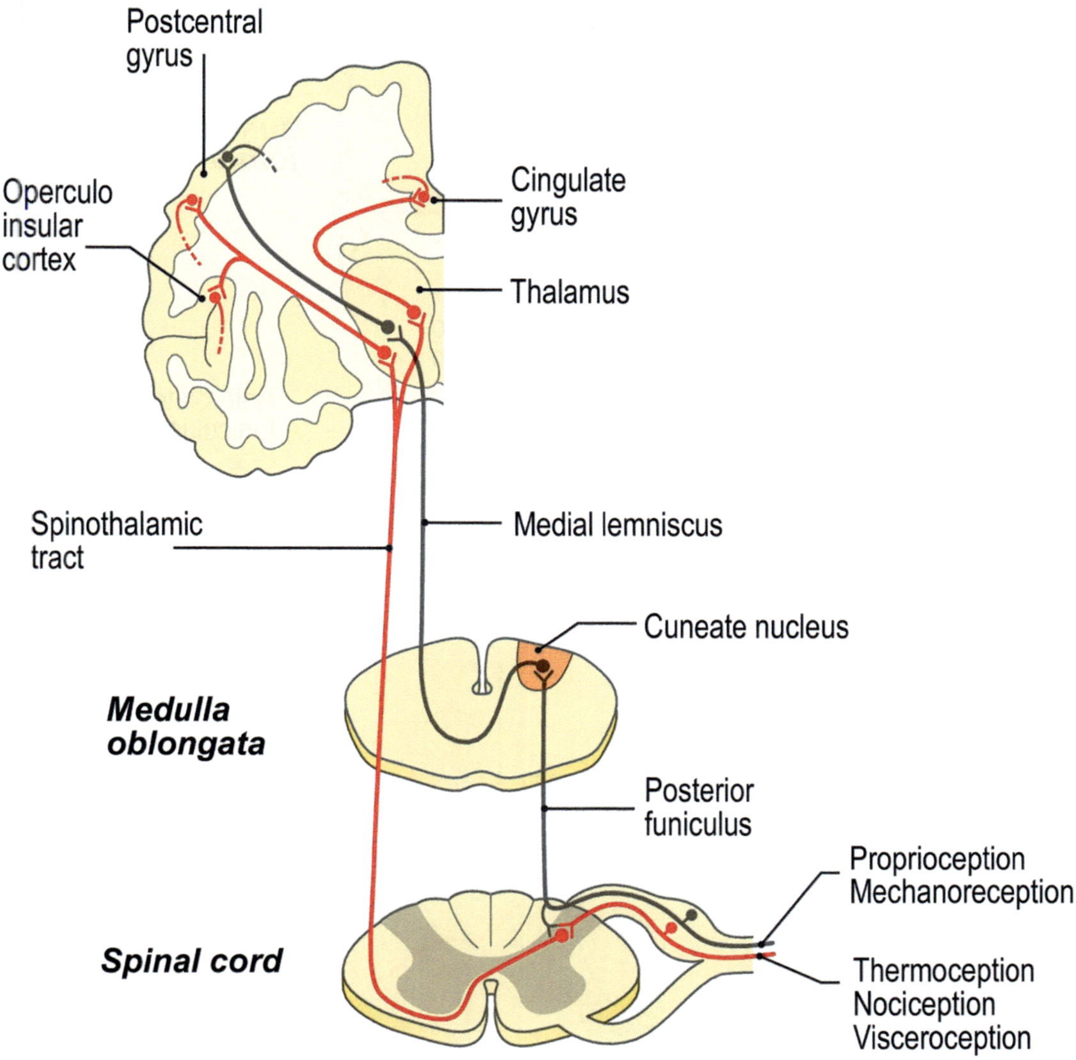

Fig. 2.8 The neural pathways of the haptic system. Black: pathways and nuclei of the lemniscal system (mechanosensation and proprioception). Red: pathways and nuclei of the spinothalamic system (thermoreception, nociception, and visceroception). (Fig. from Treede and Baumgärtner 2019, p. 644)

somatosensory information in the dorsal column is organized as a somatotopic map according to the dermatomes. In particular, from medial to lateral, the dorsal column represents the lower limbs, the lower half of the trunk, the upper half of the trunk, the upper limbs, and finally, the neck (Amunts et al. 2010).

▶ **Definition** The topographical representation of the body's periphery in the central nervous system is called **somatotopy.**

The first-order neurons synapse with the second-order neurons in the medulla oblongata (dorsal column nuclei). This connection means that the path from a mechanoreceptor in the periphery to the medulla oblongata in the lower part of the brainstem is formed by just a single nerve fiber.

In the brainstem, the axons cross to the opposite side and form synapses with the third-order neurons in the thalamus. Next, the signals reach the contralateral cerebral cortex (primary

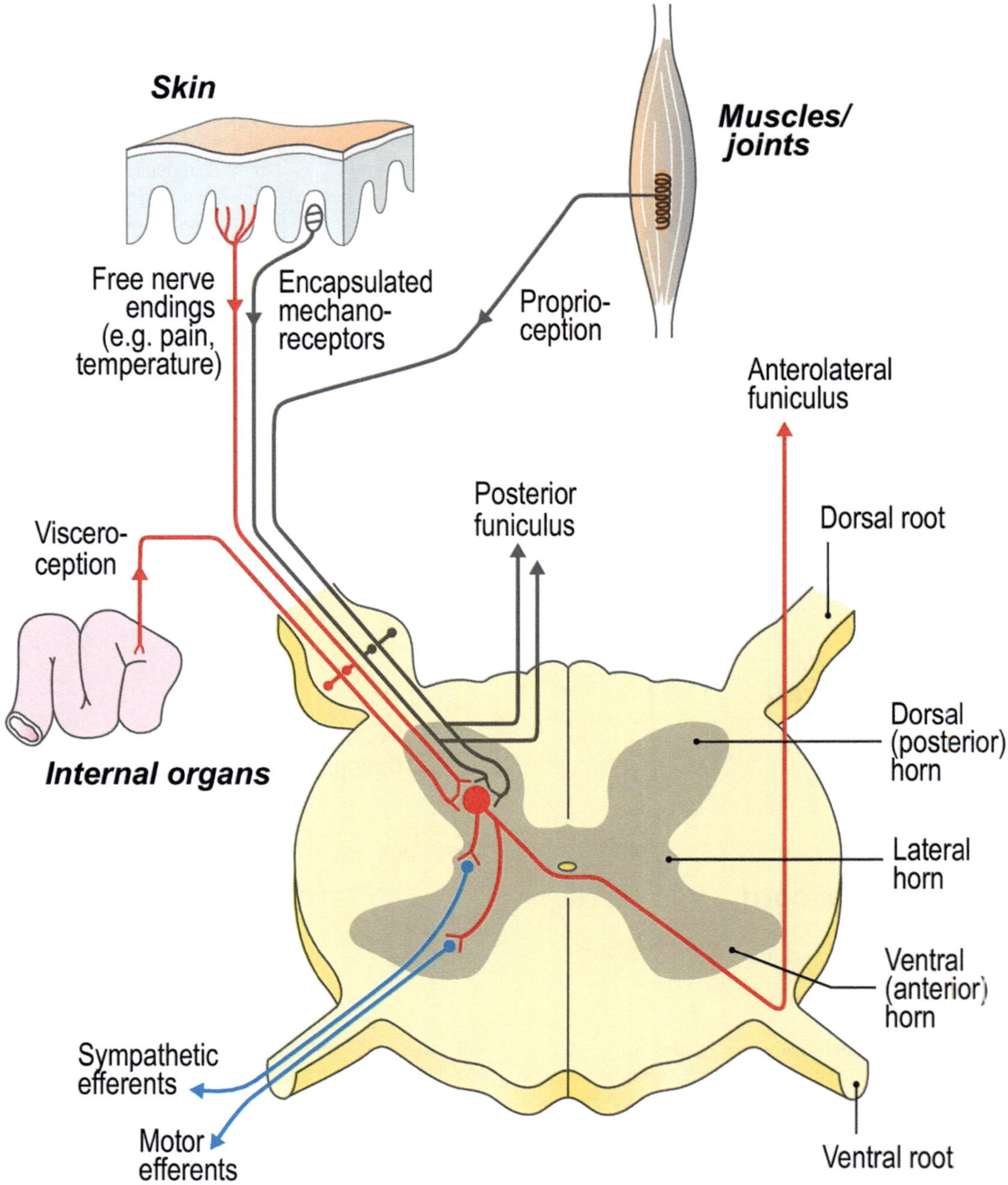

Fig. 2.9 Interconnections of neural pathways in the spinal cord. Afferent nerve fibers from the skin, locomotor system, and viscera enter the spinal cord through the dorsal root and form excitatory synapses with neurons in the posterior horn. These connections also result in the convergence of different types of afferents (black: lemniscal system, red: spinothalamic system). In addition to the activation of ascending pathways, there are also spinal motor and autonomic reflexes (blue). (Fig. from Treede and Baumgärtner 2019, p. 649)

somatosensory cortex) via the third-order neurons. From there, association fibers (fourth-order neurons) connect to other cortex areas (including the secondary somatosensory cortex, insula, frontal cortex, and association areas; see Sect. 2.2.3).

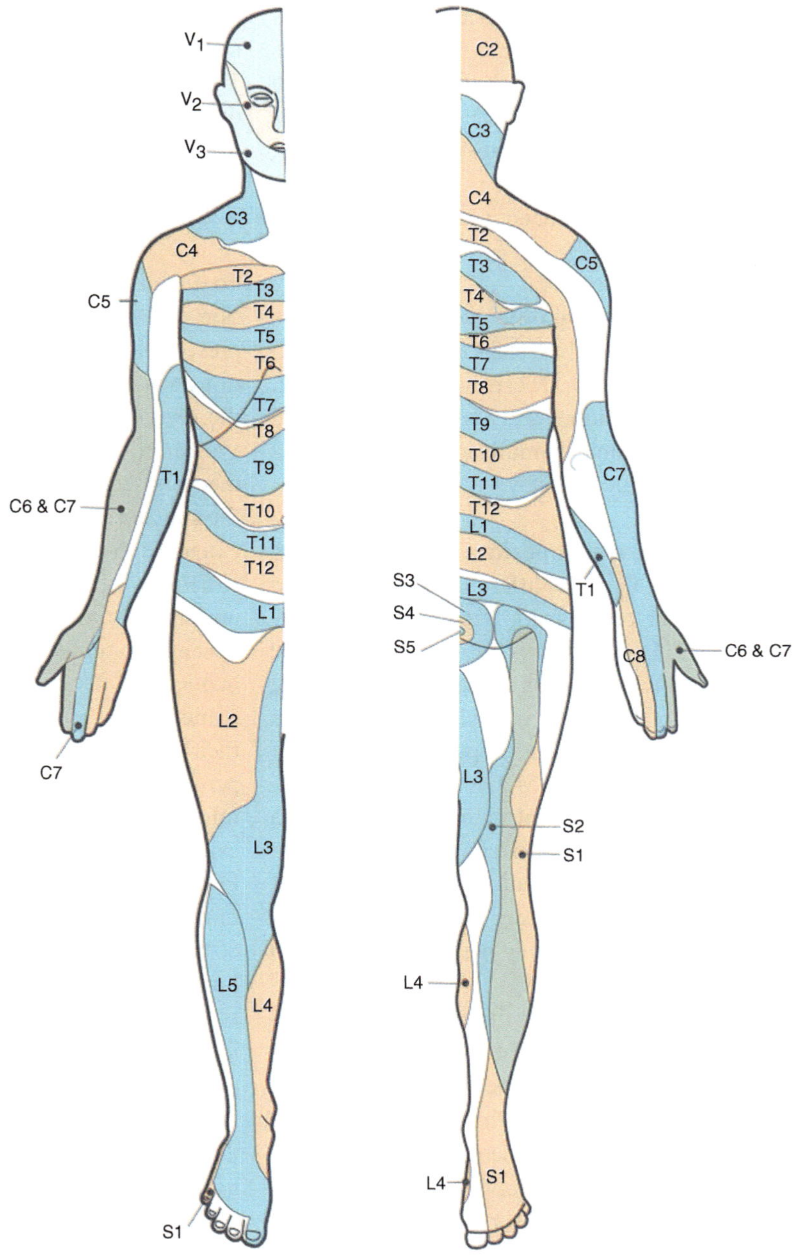

Fig. 2.10 Evidence-based dermatome map according to Lee et al. 2008. A dermatome is a circumscribed skin area whose peripheral neural processes enter the spinal cord through a common dorsal root. The white areas correspond to skin areas with large variability in dermatome membership. (Fig. from Wiesmann and Nikoubashman 2014, p. 70)

2.2.2.2 The Spinothalamic Tract (Protopathic Sensation)

The spinothalamic tract (see Fig. 2.8) is composed of thinly myelinated (Aδ/type III) and nonmyelinated (C/type IV) fibers that form free nerve endings in the periphery and viscera. Thermoreception, nociception, and visceroception signals are transmitted via the spinothalamic pathway.

Spinothalamic afferents synapse with second-order neurons after entering the posterior horn of the spinal cord and cross to the contralateral side of the spinal cord at the level of the entry site.

In the head and face region, the nociceptive Aδ-fibers and C-fibers of the trigeminal nerve are located in the skin of the face and in the mucous membranes of the oral cavity, nasal cavities, and paranasal sinuses. These fibers form the first-order neuron population of trigeminal pain conduction, which, after entering the spinal canal, is connected to second-order neurons and crosses to the opposite side. Subsequently, the spinothalamic and trigeminal afferents travel to the thalamus, where they synapse with third-order neurons, and these connect to the subcortical or cortical areas.

▶ **Definition** **Protopathic sensation** involves the detection of bodily sensations that may pose a threat to the organism. These include pain stimuli, temperature stimuli, and coarse mechanical stimuli. Protopathic stimuli are transmitted via the spinothalamic pathway.

The way in which **positive affective signals** (social touch; C-tactile afferents) are transmitted in the spinal cord is not yet comprehensively understood. Lesion studies indicate that when the spinothalamic pathway is severed, the processing of C-tactile afferents (social touch) remains intact, whereas pain and temperature processing are lost (Marshall and McGlone 2020). In contrast, when the lemniscal pathway is severed, a faint, pleasant sensation of caressing touch is preserved, but the discrimination and localization of touch are lost. Accordingly, both pathways may be involved in transmitting pleasant social touch sensations.

One possible cause for this double representation may be that pleasant touch events never occur independently of mechanosensory events, meaning that it is likely that close associative links exist between these perceptual dimensions. In particular, during development, a person learns that certain mechanosensory events (e.g., slow stroking) are associated with pleasant social situations and positive feelings, and consequently, such mechanosensory events are perceived as particularly pleasant. These learning processes probably take place in early childhood. Indeed, the central role of early childhood experiences in the perception of social touch has been demonstrated by studies on children who experienced little pleasant touch due to experiences of neglect or abuse and were separated from their parents (Devine et al. 2020; Spitoni et al. 2020). In those studies, the children with traumatic experiences rated slow stroking sensations (3 cm/s Sect. 1.1.5) as significantly less pleasant than the children without traumatic experiences.

2.2.3 Cortical Processing

To give a brief overview of the central organization of the haptic system, it requires a simplified presentation of the complex neurobiological relationships between the parts of the system. Given the diversity of the coinciding processes in this system, it would be inappropriate to assume that mechanosensory stimuli are processed only in the somatosensory areas of the brain. Instead, an extensive network of cortical and subcortical structures is involved in the processing of mechanosensory stimuli. The perception of all mechanosensory stimuli (proprioceptive, interoceptive, haptic, and tactile) requires the processing of stimuli from multiple body regions as well as their localization. In addition, mechanosensory perception involves the processing of movement information, motor control processes, emotional evaluations, and multisensory integration. Furthermore, each mechanosensory event is interpreted in relation to other cortical and subcortical processes, such as memory, attention, language, mood, needs, and reward evaluations. If mechanosensory stimuli occur during social interaction, additional complex social evaluation processes are performed, which are based on the individual's social experiences and memories, the reactions of the interaction partner, and social norms.

Despite this complexity, it is necessary to have a general idea of the main cortical structures involved in the haptic system.

2.2.3.1 Cortical and Subcortical Connections

All mechanosensory information (from the body surface and from inside the body) is sent from the brainstem to the thalamus. In the thalamus, primarily the nucleus ventralis posterolateral is and the nucleus ventralis posteromedial is convey mechanosensory information to higher-order areas (Hsiao and Yau 2008; Grunwald 1998). The neurons of these thalamic nuclei project to the contralateral side of the primary somatosensory cortex (SI; postcentral gyrus), the secondary somatosensory cortex (SII), the insula, and subcortical areas (see Fig. 2.11). For example, sensory afferents from the skin and proprioceptive signals from the joints and musculature usually travel directly to the SI. In contrast, sensory afferents from inside the body (e.g., organ activity, interoception) are predominantly projected to subcortical regions and the insula (Critchley and Harrison 2013). In those regions, each interoceptive stimulus is analyzed concerning its significance to the organism. For example, unusual interoceptive sensations may trigger apprehension or fear.

For further cortical processing, afferents from the SI connect to the parietal cortex (mainly posterior regions), as well as to secondary somatosensory regions (SII), the insula, and the frontal and temporal association cortices (Kolb et al. 1993). In addition, the SI receives efferent information from the SII, the association areas, the motor areas, the SI of the contralateral brain hemisphere, and certain subcortical regions, including the thalamus, cerebellum, and basal ganglia. The basal ganglia and cerebellum are involved in measurement and regulation processes to control balance, proprioception, and fine motor skills.

2.2.3.2 Main Functions of Relevant Brain Areas

In the **SI and SII** (postcentral gyrus), predominantly discriminatory mechanical stimuli of the skin, muscles, and joints (exteroception and proprioception) are processed. Specifically, shape and object recognition, the perception of movement direction, and touch localization take place in these cortex areas. The SI is subdivided into four areas (Brodmann areas 1, 2, 3a, and 3b) based on microscopic structural differences (Grefkes and Fink 2007). These four areas differ

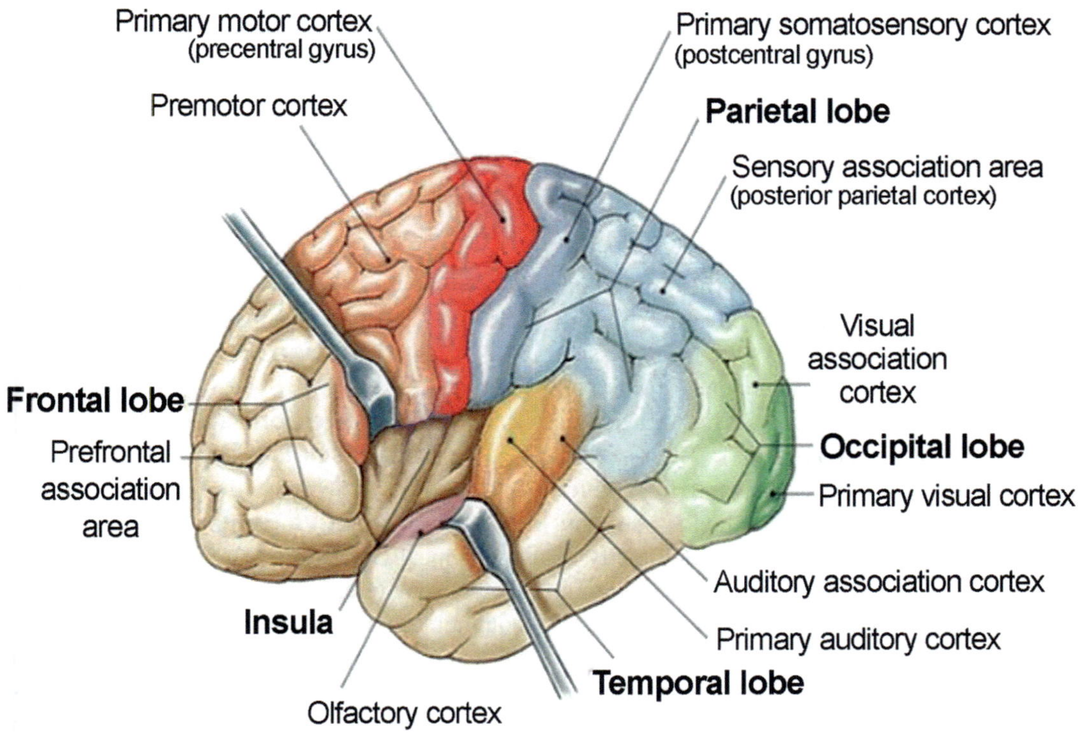

Fig. 2.11 The human brain (left hemisphere). Each cerebral hemisphere is divided into the frontal, temporal, parietal, and occipital cortex, as well as the insular cortex. The neuronal networks of the five brain lobes are associated with various functions. (Fig. adapted from Nacy et al. 2016, p. 140)

not only microscopically but also in their functions. All four areas of the SI are strongly connected via association fibers and exchange information through them. Signals from the mechanoreceptors of the skin first reach areas 3b, 1, and 2 of the SI, and proprioceptive information is mainly sent to areas 3a and 2 (Hsiao and Yau 2008). Area 3b processes sensory information from the body surface. This area is somatotopically organized, meaning it is structured according to the topology of the body surface ("sensory homunculus"). Area 1 mainly processes information about movement and direction of stimuli, area 2 is mainly activated by three-dimensional object properties, such as shape and size, and area 3a processes information from muscle spindles and is closely connected to the motor system. SII is involved in integrating discriminative information from the SI with pain information.

Neurons of the **posterior parietal cortex** (somatosensory association cortex) are involved in multisensory integration (e.g., integrating visual and somatospatial stimuli, and integrating somatosensory and proprioceptive information) and form the basis for cognitive processes. They are crucial for the perception of the body in space and for the representation of one's own body (body schema, cf. Sect. 1.4) (Treede and Baumgärtner 2019; Kolb et al. 1993). Afferents to the temporal lobe likely serve memory processes (Hsiao and Yau 2008).

Connections to the **insula, the amygdala, the orbitofrontal cortex, and the anterior cingulate cortex** are associated with the processing of social and affective components of interpersonal touch (Gordon et al. 2013; Davidovic et al. 2019; Rolls et al. 2003). The C-tactile fibers of the skin (see also Sect. 1.1.5), which are particularly responsive to slow stroking movements, predominantly project directly to the posterior portions of the insula without being processed via the SI or SII (Olausson et al. 2008). Such direct connections to the autonomic brain regions are likely responsible for the fact that even when there are lesions in somatosensory brain areas (SI, SII), interpersonal touch can still be perceived as pleasant. In the insula, a wide network of cortical and subcortical brain regions is brought together by neural connections (Gogolla 2017; Rohkamm and Kermer 2017). The insula is a multisensory hub in which sensory, emotional, motivational, and cognitive functions are integrated. As the insula forms part of the central autonomic nervous system, there are close connections between the insula and the limbic system. The insula is thought to be a control center for the internal state of the body (including heart rate and hunger) because it receives interoceptive afferents from all organ systems and emits autonomic efferents. In this context, the insula is central to linking sensory events with emotional evaluations (Gogolla 2017; Zaki et al. 2012).

Note

Pain stimuli and interoceptive signals project to subcortical regions and the insula. C-tactile fibers are also predominantly connected to the insula. This cortical area is involved in emotional, motivational, and autonomic control processes.

In contrast, discriminatory perceptions of the body surface and proprioceptive information are initially projected mainly to somatosensory cortex areas. From those areas, afferents are sent to other cortical and subcortical brain areas.

2.3 Connective Tissue and Fasciae

2.3.1 What Are Connective Tissue and Fascia?

2.3.1.1 Connective Tissue

Anatomically, a variety of different structures of the body are referred to as connective tissue. The common characteristic between them is that they all emerge from the mesoderm during embryogenesis. In addition to the fibrous connective tissues of the musculoskeletal system (tendons, ligaments, cartilage, and bone), connective tissue also includes the blood, bone marrow, and adipose tissue. In this chapter, the focus is on fibrous connective tissue.

Connective tissue forms the sheaths and suspensions of the organs and separates the tissues, organs, and even cells (van den Berg 2016). It also forms the structural framework of the organs (interstitial connective tissue, or stroma), which determines the organs' shape. Connective tissue fills every body cavity, and every organic subunit, no matter how small (e.g., every single muscle fiber), is surrounded by at least one connective tissue layer. As previously discussed (see Sect. 2.1), most mechanoreceptors and free nerve endings lie embedded in connective tissue structures. Indeed, a large proportion of the mechanosensitive structures in the human body are not located directly in specialized organ tissue but in the connective tissue surrounding the organs or muscle fibers. Similarly, the nerve tracts, blood vessels, and lymph vessels are always well padded with loose connective tissue.

▶ **Definition Connective tissue** is found throughout the body. It is a very heterogeneous tissue consisting of stationary and motile cells surrounded by ground substance. The connective tissue shape and stabilize the organs and are involved in numerous processes, such as the exchange of substances, the storage of fat and water, immune defense, and intero- and proprioception (Junqueira and Carneiro 1991).

2.3.1.2 Fascia

Over the last 20 years, one subset of connective tissue has increasingly become the focus of research interest: the fasciae. The connective tissue structures of the body that are classified as fasciae differ depending on the author, and this classification is a topic of eager discussion (Schleip et al. 2012b). Unfortunately, a strict anatomical definition for the fasciae does not yet exist. This book uses the classification of the first Fascia Research Congress in 2007.

▶ **Definition** Fasciae are fibrous connective tissue structures, both loose and dense, that form a continuous meshwork in the body (Schleip et al. 2012b). The fasciae include ligaments, tendons, aponeuroses, and joint capsules, as well as the periosteum, organ sheaths, and mesentery. In contrast, the following connective tissues are not currently referred to as fascia: cartilage, bone, blood, lymph, and the dermis (the uppermost layer of the skin/cutis).

The fibers of fascia overlap and merge, penetrating and enveloping all the structures of the body. The interconnected fibers are likely the basis for the transmission of force and tension in the body.

In traditional anatomy, the human support and movement system consists of muscles, tendons, joints, ligaments, and bones. Individual muscles are viewed as individual functional units whose force is transmitted via tendons to their associated bones, thus resulting in movement. In this traditional perspective, the fasciae form the holding and filling tissue, which reduces the frictional forces of muscle movement, fills cavities, and protectively envelops nerves, blood vessels, and organs (Wilke et al. 2018). However, for a long time, the fasciae were not considered relevant for the transmission of force and movement (Wilke et al. 2018).

However, research findings from recent years suggest that the fasciae are much more than passive packaging and filling material. Indeed, new findings suggest the following:

- The fasciae are involved in the transmission of muscle forces and tension states to adjacent (and probably even distant) body areas.
- The fasciae are involved in the development of chronic musculoskeletal pain (Langevin 2008).
- The fasciae have the ability to contract independently of muscle contraction (Schleip et al. 2019).

With the newfound interest in this ubiquitous tissue, other properties of connective tissue are coming back into research focus. For example, connective tissues fulfill important functions in supplying nutrients to cells and disposing of pollutants (Hövels 1967); they are the medium of substance and gas exchange, and they play a major role in immune defense (see Sect. 2.3.3). Furthermore, studies on fascia manipulation techniques, stretching exercises (e.g., yoga), and other soft tissue techniques show far-reaching effects on the immune system, hormonal changes, pain, stress, anxiety, and depression, among other aspects. (For more clinical aspects, see Chaps. 6 and 8).

Book Tip

- Stecco, C. (2014). Functional Atlas of the Human Fascial System. Churchill Livingston.
- Myers, T. W. (2020). Anatomy Trains: Myofascial Meridians (for manual therapists and movement professionals). Elsevier, Urban & Fischer Verlag.

2.3.2 Composition of Connective Tissue

Connective tissue consists of both stationary and motile cells (Fig. 2.12). The stationary cells form the structural tissue (the fibers), while the motile cells can actively move between the fiber strands. The motile cells are primarily immune cells. The space between the cells is filled with ground substance (see below).

2.3.2.1 Connective Tissue Cells

Stationary (fixed) cells include the following:

- Fibrocytes/fibroblasts.
- Myofibroblasts.
- Chondrocytes/chondroblasts.
- Fat cells (adipocytes).

Motile (migrating) cells include the following:

- Lymphocytes.
- Mast cells.
- Macrophages.

Important A video of a neutrophil granulocyte (motile cell) chasing and capturing a bacterium can be viewed at https://

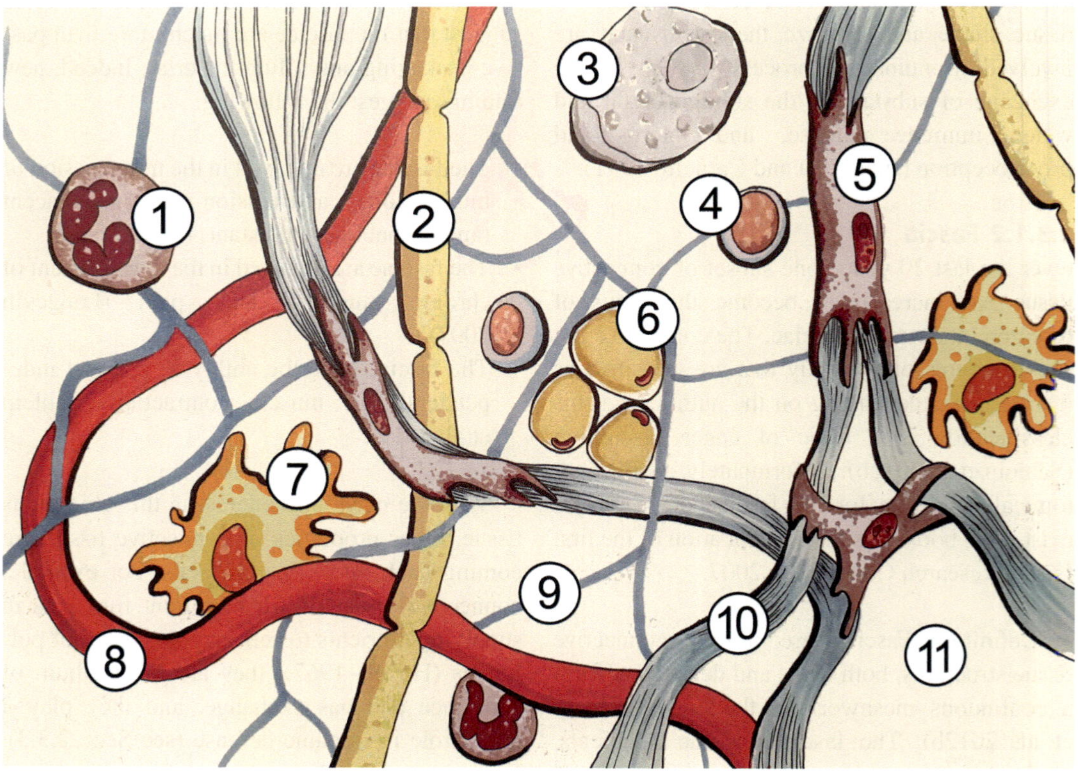

Fig. 2.12 Connective tissue cells and ground substance. 1 Neutrophil granulocyte, 2 Nerve fiber, 3 Mast cell, 4 Lymphocyte, 5 Fibroblast, 6 Adipocyte, 7 Macrophage, 8 Blood vessel, 9 Reticular fiber, 10 Collagen fiber, 11 Ground substance (Illustration: Maria Huettig)

youtu.be/4z8w1jwOVis. (Film recorded by David Rogers, Vanderbilt University, 1950).

2.3.2.2 Ground Substance

The ground substance is a transparent, viscous solution that fills the space between cells in connective tissues and organs, which is why it is also called extracellular fluid. In combination with the fibrous parts of the connective tissue, this substance forms the extracellular matrix. This is the basis for the shape constancy of all tissues and organs.

The main component of ground substance is water, which is bound by hyaluronic acid, thus giving the ground substance its gel-like consistency. Any substance that passes to and from cells must pass through the ground substance. Therefore, it is the transport medium of metabolic products, hormones, vitamins, electrolytes, oxygen, and carbon dioxide, as well as all other substances that are transported between the blood vessels, lymphatic vessels, and organ cells. In addition, the ground substance serves as a medium for the motile cells (immune defense cells) to migrate through tissues (Buddecke 1960).

Furthermore, the hyaluronan in the ground substance ensures the smooth sliding of the fascia and connective tissue layers against each other.

Ground substance consists of the following:

- Water.
- Hyaluronic acid.
- Electrolytes.
- Plasma proteins (which transport, for example, ions, hormones, vitamins, and metabolites).
- Gases (oxygen/carbon dioxide).
- Immune cells.

Note

The ground substance fills the space between tissue cells. In the ground substance, the exchange of metabolic products and gases (oxygen, carbon dioxide) takes place between the blood vessels, the lymphatic system, and the organ cells. Finally, the ground substance also serves as a medium for the motile cells of the immune system to migrate between tissue cells.

2.3.3 Functions of the Connective Tissue

As mentioned before, the fibrous parts of the connective tissue have mechanical and form-giving functions. For example, they determine the shape of organs or give structural support to the musculoskeletal system (cf. Sect. 2.3.1). The entangled network of connective tissue within the body also transmits mechanical tensions and pressures caused by body movements, organ movements, or pathological processes such as space-occupying lesions. These tensions and pressures are registered by the mechanosensitive receptors and free nerve endings embedded in the connective tissue. In this respect, fibrous connective tissues are involved in interoceptive and proprioceptive processes, as well as in the development of visceral pain. Furthermore, changes in the stiffness of connective tissue structures can cause musculoskeletal pain (see Sect. 2.3.4).

Finally, connective tissues are involved in various other processes (Buddecke 1960; Beyer 2001):

- Connective tissues play an essential role in the functioning of the immune system. Since connective tissue structures permeate the entire body, immune cells in the ground substance can penetrate any area of the body, which is essential for both defense against infections and tissue repair (e.g., after injury).
- The connective tissue contributes to maintaining the health of the body's cells by transporting nutrients and metabolites (Weicker et al. 1967). As the medium for substance and gas exchange, the connective tissue is crucial to ensuring an adequate supply of oxygen and nutrients to the cells.

- Furthermore, the connective tissue forms the basis for a stable water and electrolyte balance. The storage and provision of water and electrolytes (including calcium, magnesium, potassium, and sodium) are important physiological functions of the ground substance. Electrolytes are crucial for maintaining the osmotic pressure of the cells, the pH of the blood (acid-base balance), and the reliable functioning of nerve and muscle cells.

2.3.4 Densification and Fibrosis of Connective Tissues: Influence of Stress, Pain, Inflammation, and Stretching

Changes in the stiffness of connective tissue structures (densifications and fibrosis) can be caused by three mechanisms (Wilke et al. 2018; Pavan et al. 2014):

- Remodeling of the connective tissue fibers.
- Changes in the viscosity of the ground substance.
- The contraction of myofibroblasts and fibroblasts (Schleip et al. 2019; Wrobel et al. 2002).

These processes can occur either separately or simultaneously.

▶ **Definition** The development of **fibrosis** is similar to the process of scarring. The increased deposition of connective tissue fibers results in an increasingly stiff and inflexible connective tissue structure, which can impair the function of the affected tissue (Pavan et al. 2014). **Densification** refers to an increase in the density of loose connective tissue, and this is usually caused by an increase in the viscosity or concentration of hyaluronan in the ground substance. Densification can affect the mechanical properties of fasciae without altering their fibrous structure (Pavan et al. 2014).

Collagen fibers have a turnover rate of approximately 300–500 days, meaning it can take several months until connective tissue structurally adapts to changes in physical loading. However, under certain conditions, increased cell proliferation and collagen synthesis occur. These conditions include traumatic or surgical injuries, inflammatory processes, and tissue stretching.

The orientation of the connective tissue fibers depends on the mechanical forces that act upon them. Anatomically appropriate loading of the musculoskeletal structures leads to the optimal distribution of force lines within connective tissue networks. In contrast, incorrect loading, relieving postures, or immobilization can lead to connective tissue linkages that result in a limited range of motion and pain. The ability to adapt to applied forces is based on cellular remodeling. Tissue stretching (e.g., through manual intervention or stretching exercises) results in the release of the enzyme collagenase, which stimulates the breakdown of collagenous fibers and allows for subsequent adaptive remodeling (Langevin et al. 2005; Carano and Siciliani 1996). This process enables, for example, the loosening of existing densifications and fibrosis.

Note
Connective tissues respond to mechanical forces through remodeling processes.

2.3.4.1 Injury, Inflammation, and Immobilization

After injury or surgery, immobilization has a particularly strong effect on fascial elasticity (Bishop et al. 2016). Specifically, the immobilization of a healthy limb causes a smaller decline in facial elasticity compared to immobilization following an injury. This pattern is due to the fact that healing processes stimulate increased cell division in the fibroblasts (Pavan et al. 2014). The **healing process** from an injury consists of four stages:

1. Hemostasis (immediately after an injury): To stop bleeding and drainage, a temporary wound closure is formed through clotting.
2. Inflammation (approximately 5 days): Inflammatory processes mobilize immune

cells and fibroblasts from the surrounding tissues and stimulate them to divide and accumulate in the area of inflammation.
3. Proliferation (approximately 21 days): Fibroblasts form a new provisional extracellular matrix of unstructured collagen fibers with the primary goal of rapidly closing the wound, and the sprouting of new blood vessels occurs.
4. Remodeling (>21 days): The collagen fibers are reorganized and realigned along the tension lines of the mechanical tensile forces acting on the wound and surrounding areas. If the injured area is spared or immobilized, remodeling cannot occur in a physiologically meaningful way. Instead, the random and unstructured deposition of collagen fibers results in a fibrotic scar.

A similar process of unstructured collagen fiber deposition also occurs during other forms of localized or systemic inflammation (e.g., inflammation due to scleroderma, pulmonary fibrosis, or liver cirrhosis), and this process results in the stiffening of the connective tissue structures (Ng et al. 2005).

Inflammatory responses, through the release of lactate, result in a lower tissue pH. Similarly, heavy muscle work (e.g., due to seizures), hypoxia (Pavan et al. 2014), and an acidifying diet (Buclin et al. 2001) lower the tissue pH value. Lactate stimulates the synthesis of collagen (Trabold et al. 2003) and leads to increased contractility of the myofibroblasts (Pipelzadeh and Naylor 1998). In addition, an acidic pH leads to increased viscosity of the hyaluronic acid in the ground substance (Gatej et al. 2005).

Hyaluronan is particularly abundant within and between loose connective tissues (e.g., between deep fasciae and muscles), and both immobility and inflammatory processes lead to an increase in the concentration and viscosity of hyaluronan in the corresponding tissues (Cowman et al. 2015). An increase in the viscosity and concentration of hyaluronan can limit the gliding ability of the fasciae and, thus, be perceived by the affected person as tissue stiffness (Stecco et al. 2013). After strenuous muscle work, for example, the viscosity of hyaluronan may increase by approximately 20% (Gatej et al. 2005).

2.3.4.2 Stress and Pain

An increase in tissue stiffness can lead to the activation of mechanoreceptors and free nerve endings in that area. Current explanatory approaches assume that chronic musculoskeletal pain, such as neck, shoulder, or low back pain, is caused by changes in the elasticity of connective tissues and tension lines (Cowman et al. 2015; Stecco et al. 2013). In addition, inflammatory processes and acidic pH levels in the tissues contribute to the development of pain (Steen et al. 1996).

Preliminary evidence also suggests that the activation of the sympathetic nervous system (e.g., by stress or pain) increases the cell division rate and the contractility of myofibroblasts (Wilke et al. 2018; Bhowmick et al. 2009). Specifically, stress increases the stiffness of fibrous connective tissues. As a result, chronically increased sympathetic nervous system activity due to stress could lead to the sustained contraction of myofibroblasts and, consequently, the development and maintenance of musculoskeletal pain (Wilke et al. 2018).

> **Important** Acute changes in the elasticity of connective tissue are caused mainly by increases in the viscosity of the ground substance.
>
> Long-lasting or chronic stiffening is caused by the deposition of connective tissue fibers and the contraction of myofibroblasts. The consequences of this stiffening include reduced mobility, pain, a poorer cell supply, and the poorer removal of metabolic products.

2.3.4.3 Stretching and Movement

Exercise or massage decreases the viscosity of the intercellular fluid (Dintenfass 1966), thus improving the individual's ability to move because the fibers and layers can slide over each other more easily.

Conversely, stretching (e.g., by manual techniques) can temporarily increase the tissue fluid content, thus making the tissue feel stiff during movement (Schleip et al. 2012a).

Regular stretching and movement (active or passive) can prevent the unstructured accumulation of collagen fibers and stimulate substance transfer in the ground substance (Williams et al. 1988). In this way, the development of densification can be prevented, and densification that has already occurred can be corrected.

However, unlike densification, fibrosis that has already developed is more difficult to influence. The pathological collagen deposits must first be destroyed to stimulate remodeling, but in practice, it is often difficult to distinguish between densification and fibrosis. An experimental study of patients with chronic low back pain (longer than 3 months) indicated that manipulation of the thoracolumbar fascia for an average of 3.5 min was required to reduce the pain intensity by 50% (Borgini et al. 2010).

Active or passive stretching can also positively influence various diseases. For example, in one study, regular active stretching over 4 weeks resulted in significantly **less arterial stiffness** in middle-aged men (Nishiwaki et al. 2015). The participants performed guided, light stretching exercises of the major muscle groups (lower and upper extremities, torso, back, and neck) five times per week for 30 min. Each muscle group was stretched three times for 20 s, followed by 30 s of rest. According to a recent meta-analysis, in addition to reducing arterial stiffness, regular stretching exercises can also reduce heart rate and blood pressure and improve vascular endothelial function (Kato et al. 2020). Furthermore, evening stretching exercises may reduce the frequency and intensity of nocturnal leg cramps (Hallegraeff et al. 2012).

Daily stretching exercises reduce skin thickness and perceived stiffness in **systemic sclerosis** in both animal models and humans, and they also improve tissue elasticity and hand mobility (Xiong et al. 2017; Mugii et al. 2006).

Furthermore, in mouse models, a **reduction in tumor growth** (breast cancer) by 52% could be achieved through daily 10-min light stretching of the chest and back muscles (Berrueta et al. 2018). The authors also reported an increase in cytokines with stretching, which are crucial for maintaining immune defense.

The dynamic plasticity of connective tissues may be the basis for the effects of many physiotherapeutic and complementary medical interventions (Langevin 2008). Many of these methods use mechanical forces (e.g., massage, chiropractic, acupuncture), promote exercise (e.g., rehabilitation sports, walking, gymnastics), or stimulate altered movement patterns (e.g., yoga, QiGong). In the case of acupuncture, anatomical studies have shown that about 80% of all acupuncture points on the upper extremities are located at unique connective tissue structures, namely where two or more connective tissue layers meet (Langevin and Yandow 2002). Anatomical studies from the 1980s and 1990s conducted by Hartmut Heine also indicated that the vast majority of acupuncture points are at points of passage of vascular and nerve bundles through the superficial body fasciae (Heine 2016). Furthermore, it has been shown by microscopy that the rotation of acupuncture needles in the tissue leads to a "winding up" of the superficial connective tissue fibers around the needle tip, which generates tensile forces on the surrounding tissue (Langevin et al. 2002; Langevin and Yandow 2002).

Manual or movement-based methods used to treat pain caused by densifications or fibrotic connective tissues have the advantage of not causing any of the typical side effects associated with pain medication, such as gastritis or sedation (Langevin 2008). Nevertheless, some caution should be exercised when performing manipulations, as the applied forces can create micro-injuries and inflammation, which can increase densification and pain. Consequently, the force applied during treatments must be appropriately dosed and adapted to each patient.

2.4 Physiological Effects of Pleasant Touch (on Hormones, Neurotransmitters, and the Immune System)

Psychological stress can promote the development of various diseases and the spread of various types of cancer. In addition, there is evidence that negative life events and stress can trigger or worsen the symptoms of autoimmune diseases (Birbaumer and Schmidt 2006).

Conversely, positive emotions and psychosocial support should have a beneficial effect on health (see also Sect. 5.5). Currently, an increasing number of studies are focused on examining the health-promoting and protective effects of positive emotions and relaxation. Based on these studies, it seems social support and pleasant physical contact play a central role in health. To date, the physiological, hormonal, and immunological consequences of pleasant touch have been studied predominantly using massage studies, whereas only a few experimental studies have examined the effects of holding hands, exchanging hugs, or interacting with pets (see also Sect. 5.5.2). These studies show that any pleasant physical contact can help reduce anxiety, stress, and pain, reduce negative moods and depression, and have beneficial effects on sleep and the immune system. The effects of pleasant physical contact are so versatile that physical contact has already been referred to in popular science as a "home pharmacy" (Grunwald 2017).

▶ **Important** In principle, positive effects only arise from touching if the person *touched* perceives the touch as pleasant and appropriate. Forced or painful touches, as well as touches carried out by a person or in a situation perceived as inappropriate, are always stress-triggering (for more details, see Sect. 5.1).

The following sections (Sects. 2.4.1 and 2.4.5) describe the physiological effects of pleasant touch and massage on hormones, neurotransmitters, and the immune system. Additionally, the health-promoting effects of pleasant touch on specific diseases are described in Chaps. 6 and 8.

▶ **Definition** Neurotransmitters and hormones are chemical messengers.

Neurotransmitters play a key role in signal transmission or blockade in the central and peripheral nervous systems. Specifically, when an electrical signal reaches a synapse, neurotransmitters are released into the synaptic cleft, and the neurotransmitters cause an electrical signal to be formed in the subsequent nerve cell. The nerve cells of the autonomic nervous system can also transmit their information directly to the target organ through neurotransmitters.

Conversely, **hormones** are transported to their target sites via the bloodstream, and they transmit their information by docking to specific receptors on cells.

2.4.1 Oxytocin

Oxytocin (ancient Greek *for "swift childbirth"*) is a neuropeptide that is produced in the hypothalamus and stored in the pituitary gland. From there, oxytocin is released when needed. Oxytocin acts as both a hormone and a neurotransmitter. After its discovery in 1906 by Henry Dale, the effects of oxytocin were initially associated with the birth process (contraction of the uterus) and the **secretion of breast milk** (Ott and Scott 1910; Dale 1906). Today, it is used as a chemical agent to induce labor, increase **labor activity** during birth, and accelerate the birth process (Oláh and Steer 2015). However, some medical experts are critical of the artificial administration of oxytocin, as overdoses are suspected to cause oxygen deficiency in the child during birth (Oláh and Steer 2015). Natural increases in oxytocin can be achieved through physical interaction with one's partner (back massage, caress, kissing, or stimulation of the nipples).

After birth, oxytocin is used to prevent bleeding and accelerate the detachment and expulsion of the placenta. This process is initiated during breastfeeding by natural oxytocin release, which causes contractions of the uterine wall (Moir 1964). In addition, oxytocin stimulates milk production and triggers maternal caring behavior (Richard et al. 1991). Between parents and their newborn children, the release of oxytocin contributes to psychological bonding. The release of oxytocin also leads to a **sense of connection and well being** between individuals of all ages, thus promoting social behavior and pair bonding. It is now known that oxytocin is released during any pleasant physical contact between people; indeed, this is true for relaxing massages, pleasant touching, caressing, and erotic stimulation for both women and men (Li et al. 2019; Carter 1992). Particularly high levels of oxytocin are released during stimulation of the genitals and the nipples and during orgasm.

However, oxytocin is not just associated with social touch in humans. Oxytocin is also released in other mammals and even during cross-species physical contact. For example, in a previous study, in both dogs and their owners, higher levels of oxytocin were measured when the dogs were petted more often (Handlin et al. 2012). These and similar findings indicate that physical interaction with a pet also leads to the release of oxytocin in humans. (For more details, Sect. 5.5).

> ▶ **Important** Oxytocin is released during childbirth, breastfeeding, and pleasant physical contact both between humans and between humans and animals. It influences social behavior, anxiety, well-being, and stress.

As a neurotransmitter in the brain, oxytocin is involved in several regulatory mechanisms (Uvnäs-Moberg et al. 2014). Oxytocin reaches brain areas that regulate social behaviors, anxiety, aggression, pain perception, and well-being through neuronal connections. It is assumed that oxytocin regulates the activity of the hypothalamic-pituitary-adrenocortical axis, thereby contributing to stress reduction (Uvnäs-Moberg et al. 2014). Oxytocin is also associated with the autonomic nervous system, as it causes increased activity in the parasympathetic nervous system and decreased activity in the sympathetic nervous system.

The influence of oxytocin on the autonomic nervous system and its interactions with other neurotransmitter systems trigger several processes in the human body. These include anxiety- and stress-reducing effects that are accompanied by a reduction in cortisol levels, physical relaxation, a reduction in blood pressure, and potentially altered pain perception. However, to date, it has not been conclusively clarified whether oxytocin has an analgesic effect in humans or merely influences pain evaluations. The results of studies examining the effects of oxytocin administration are contradictory, and the mechanisms of these effects remain unclear. Currently, it is a matter of discussion whether, in humans, oxytocin induces changes in the emotional and cognitive aspects of pain perception (e.g., by enhancing social support effects) (Kreuder et al. 2019; Boll et al. 2018). (For touch and social support, see in-depth Sect. 5.5).

2.4.2 Serotonin/Dopamine

2.4.2.1 Serotonin

The majority (about 95%) of the body's serotonin is produced by the enterochromaffin cells of the intestinal mucosa. In addition, serotonin is produced by serotonergic cells in the central nervous system (CNS; mainly in the raphe nuclei of the brainstem) (Gröll 2020b).

In the CNS, serotonin is an important neurotransmitter that has modulating effects on many brain functions. For example, it is involved in regulating body temperature, emotional processes, mood, pain perception, eating, and sexual behavior. It is believed that serotonin in sufficient amounts leads to a positive mood and a balanced mind. Conversely, serotonin deficiencies or excesses can play a role in the development of psychiatric disorders (including anxiety disorders, depression, hallucinations, and euphoria).

The hallucinogenic and euphoric effects of lysergic acid diethylamide (LSD) are also related to serotonin. Indeed, this psychoactive substance enhances the effect of serotonin at certain receptors in the brain.

Furthermore, some serotonin in the brain is converted into melatonin. This hormone is mainly released during darkness, has a sleep-promoting effect, and, thus, controls the day-night rhythm of the human body.

Serotonin likely has a constricting effect on blood vessels in the brain. This effect of serotonin is utilized in the treatment of migraines through the administration of triptans. In particular, triptans enhance the vasoconstrictive effect of serotonin in the brain, which can improve migraine symptoms.

Outside the CNS, serotonin also influences various processes. In the gastrointestinal tract, for example, it influences intestinal peristalsis and stimulates bowel activity. In the peripheral bloodstream, it can have both vasodilatory (e.g., skeletal muscle) and vasoconstrictive (e.g., lung and kidney) effects, depending on the area of the body and the situation.

▶ **Important** Serotonin is involved in the regulation of body temperature, emotional processes, pain perception, eating, and sexual behavior. In addition, some serotonin in the brain is converted into melatonin, which has a sleep-promoting effect.

2.4.2.2 Dopamine

Dopamine is mainly produced in the substantia nigra in the midbrain. From there, neuronal connections project to the cortex, the basal ganglia, and the limbic system. As a neurotransmitter, dopamine is involved in both the control of emotional reactions and movements. Dopamine is the most important neurotransmitter in the human **reward and reinforcement system**. Indeed, feelings of happiness, satisfaction, and joy are closely related to the level of dopamine in the brain, and actions, experiences, and rewards that are perceived as pleasant lead to an increased release of dopamine. This release of dopamine initiates learning processes, which later lead to dopamine release at the mere expectation of a pleasant event or a reward. This effect, in turn, reinforces behaviors and action patterns.

In the motor system, dopamine promotes movement and influences the intensity of movements. In the case of dopamine deficiency in the basal ganglia (e.g., in the context of Parkinson's disease), movements can no longer be performed appropriately or cannot even be started (Gröll 2020a).

In addition, dopamine plays a vital role in the regulation of the immune system by binding to the dopaminergic receptors of immune cells (leukocytes, see Sect. 2.4.5) and, thus, influencing their activity (Sarkar et al. 2010).

The results of a previous study showed that, after massages, there was an increase in serotonin and dopamine in the urine, and positive effects on mood and well-being were identified (Field et al. 2004). In addition, positive effects of massage on motor symptoms in Parkinson's disease have also been reported, which may be indicative of the dopaminergic effects of massage (Angelopoulou et al. 2020).

▶ **Important** Dopamine is the most important messenger in the human reward and reinforcement system.

2.4.3 Stress Hormones

Psychological stress and stressful experiences lead to the release of catecholamines (adrenaline and noradrenaline) and glucocorticoids (cortisol and cortisone). These substances put the body in a state that enables a **fight-or-flight response.** In this state, resources are activated to provide additional energy to the cardiovascular system and musculature for physical defense or running. Concurrently, "unnecessary" processes (including the immune system and digestion) are inhibited to conserve energy. However, prolonged psychological strain and stress are associated with adverse health effects.

2.4.3.1 Adrenaline and Noradrenaline

Adrenaline and norepinephrine (also called noradrenaline) are released during stress, anxiety, and pain, which can be either real or imagined (e.g., during an exciting movie, nocturnal ruminations, or the memory of an experience). Both substances take effect very quickly but only work for a short time and are broken down again just a few minutes after they are released. Adrenaline acts primarily as a hormone, while noradrenaline functions primarily as a neurotransmitter in the central and sympathetic nervous systems. Adrenaline and noradrenaline play a major role in activating resources for a fight-or-flight response. This response includes an accelerated pulse, increased blood pressure, dilation of the bronchi, and the activation of fat and sugar reserves as a source of energy. Concurrently, gastrointestinal activity and immune system functions are inhibited to conserve energy.

Stress and relaxation are opposite reactions that are mutually exclusive. In moments of relaxation and well-being, parasympathetic functions are activated, thus promoting normal digestion, recovery, and healing. Therefore, any activity that promotes relaxation and well-being, such as an embrace or a relaxing massage, helps to reduce stress reactions and the effects of adrenaline/norepinephrine.

2.4.3.2 Cortisol, Antidiuretic Hormone, and Adrenocorticotropic Hormone

Antidiuretic hormone (ADH) and adrenocorticotropic hormone (ATCH) are produced in the hypothalamus and stored in the pituitary gland. ADH is also known as vasopressin and, among many other processes in the body, is involved in stress regulation. One of the main functions of ADH is to trigger vasoconstriction, which increases blood pressure. Moreover, it also causes the release of ATCH, which, in turn, controls the release of cortisol and its precursor, cortisone, from the adrenal gland.

Cortisol promotes gluconeogenesis, which refers to glucose being produced from the body's proteins and fats to provide the necessary energy during a stress reaction. The glucose produced through this process is transported via the bloodstream to its target sites, which increases blood glucose levels. To prevent the glucose from being broken down unused, **cortisol inhibits the release of insulin**. Furthermore, cortisol has an inhibitory effect on the immune system, which saves further energy for the stress response. Specifically, cortisol **blocks inflammatory and immunological processes,** which is why it is also used as a drug to reduce inflammatory reactions in the body, for example, in autoimmune diseases. However, prolonged high concentrations of cortisol lead to wound healing disorders, susceptibility to infections, inhibition of bone formation (which can lead to osteoporosis), impaired secretion of sex hormones, and impaired carbohydrate and fat metabolism. Due to the inhibiting effect of cortisol on insulin, chronically high cortisol levels can also contribute to the development of type 2 diabetes.

Consequently, it is desirable that high concentrations of stress hormones only occur in the body for minimal periods of time.

The direct effects of touch on stress hormones have been demonstrated using Swedish massage, among other methods. In this context, lower ADH, ATCH, and cortisol levels have been measured in massaged individuals compared to control groups (Rapaport et al. 2012; Morhenn et al. 2012) (for further health benefits of massage, see Chap. 8).

► **Important** Stress hormones put the body in an optimal state for a fight-or-flight response. However, prolonged stress is linked to adverse health effects, including the development of type 2 diabetes.

2.4.4 Immune System

Psychosocial interactions can influence immune responses and, thus, affect an individual's state of health in terms of both disease-causing and health-promoting effects. However, thus far, most research has focused on the relationship between psychosocial stress, the immune system, and disease rather than the health-promoting effects of psychosocial interactions. Stressful life events, negative emotions, stress, anxiety, and depression increase the release of pro-inflammatory cytokines. Prolonged high levels of pro-inflammatory cytokines are suspected of promoting various diseases and functional impairments (Kiecolt-Glaser et al. 2002). Specifically, they are associated with premature aging, cardiovascular disease, type 2 diabetes, and some lymphoproliferative cancers (Birbaumer and Schmidt 2006).

Evidence for the association between psychosocial stress and disease is provided by studies of individuals who have been victims of abuse (physical or sexual abuse). In particular, these individuals tend to show more medical symptoms, functional disorders, somatic complaints, and psychiatric disorders, visit the doctor more often, are more likely to experience pain, and require surgery more often than individuals who have not experienced abuse. There is evidence that the intensity of the traumatic experience correlates with the severity of the health consequences. Indeed, life-threatening physical or sexual violence entails more substantial negative health consequences than less significant assaults (Leserman et al. 1996, 1997; Talbot et al. 2009).

In addition, it is known that catecholamines and glucocorticoids (stress hormones, see Sect. 2.4.3) reduce the impact of natural killer (NK) cells and the lymphocyte count in tissues. These immune cells are crucial for slowing down metastatic oncological processes. As a result, stress and anxiety (such as that triggered by surgery) can lead to renewed or increased tumor metastasis (Birbaumer and Schmidt 2006). In this context, more stressful and painful operations and experiencing less social support are related to a higher probability of tumor growth and spread.

In contrast, increasing numbers of studies indicate that pleasant touch and massage can positively affect the immune system in terms of the number and activity of immune cells, as well as the messenger substances of the immune system and immunoglobulins. (For the effects of massage/touch on cancer and other diseases, see Sect. 8.1)

> ▶ **Important** Stress and anxiety have adverse effects on the immune system and promote inflammation. Conversely, relaxation can have immune-regulatory and anti-inflammatory effects.

2.4.4.1 Vagus Nerve and Cytokines

Cytokines are messenger substances in the immune system that enable immune cells to communicate with each other. They are relevant for the regulation of the immune system by controlling the differentiation and growth processes of immune cells. Five main groups of cytokines can be distinguished: interferons, interleukins (ILs), chemokines, growth factors, and tumor necrosis factors (TNFs; Blaeschke et al. 2020). Cytokines fulfill multiple functions. Essentially, they direct the inflammatory response to the site of infection or injury, thus promoting healing processes (Johnston and Webster 2009). Cytokines can be divided into those that are primarily pro-inflammatory and those that are primarily anti-inflammatory. Pro-inflammatory cytokines include TNF-α, IL-1, and IL-6 (Blaeschke et al. 2020). The anti-inflammatory cytokines include IL-10, IL-13, and proteins that bind TNF-α, thereby terminating its pro-inflammatory effect (Johnston and Webster 2009).

Experiments have shown that the efferent arm of the vagus nerve (that is, the descending pathway of the parasympathetic nervous system) is related to anti-inflammatory processes. Therefore, the activation of the efferent vagus nerve is associated with the production of *fewer* pro-inflammatory cytokines. This descending neuronal connection between the central nervous system and the immune system prevents an overshooting of inflammatory reactions (Johnston and Webster 2009; Pavlov et al. 2003), and this applies to both local and systemic inflammatory processes.

The targeted electrical stimulation of the efferent arm of the vagus nerve can elicit these **immune-regulatory and anti-inflammatory effects**. In addition, there is evidence that various complementary medicine techniques can also trigger these immunomodulatory effects. For example, Swedish massages, as well as light touch, lead to altered concentrations of cytokines in the blood (Rapaport et al. 2010). Furthermore, relaxation techniques, meditation, biofeedback, acupuncture, and massages can **increase heart rate variability** (Johnston and Webster 2009; Diego and Field 2009; Meier et al. 2020), which indicates an increase in parasympathetic activity and, especially, efferent vagus nerve activity. Accordingly, pleasant massage and touch seem to promote anti-inflammatory and immune-regulatory effects (Rapaport et al. 2010). (cf. association of loneliness and illness due to a cold virus, Sect. 5.1).

2.4.4.2 Immune Cells

The cells of the immune system are also called white blood cells (leukocytes), and these cells can be divided into six groups: granulocytes, monocytes, macrophages, mast cells, dendritic cells, and lymphocytes (Blaeschke et al. 2020). Lymphocytes, in turn, are divided into three types: T-lymphocytes, B-lymphocytes, and NK cells. B-cells and T-cells are essential for specific immune defense, whereas all the other cell types are involved in non-specific defense.

Although immune cells are referred to as "white blood cells", they are not exclusively present in the blood vessels. For example, macrophages, mast cells, and dendritic cells, which arise from precursor cells in the blood, are found in body tissues (Blaeschke et al. 2020).

Immune cells perform a variety of tasks to protect the organism from disease. Some neutralize invading germs or parasites, whereas others have cytotoxic capabilities (i.e., they kill virus-infected cells and tumor cells). Another type of immune cell disposes of dead cells and cell debris. Specific immune defense cells recognize and remember antigens, after which specific antibodies can be released in defense against invading bacteria, viruses, fungi, parasites, or other foreign substances. In addition, immune cells and their precursor cells produce cytokines (see previous section: Vagus Nerve and Cytokines). These regulate the immune response by influencing inflammatory reactions and stimulating the growth, differentiation, and division of other immune cells.

The number of immune cells and their cytotoxicity increase during an immune response to allow the immune system to respond to infection, injury, or disease. However, psychosocial stress, some drugs (e.g., chemotherapy), and certain viruses (e.g., human immunodeficiency virus) can reduce the cell count and cytotoxicity. Various studies have shown a beneficial effect of Swedish massage on immune markers (Khiewkhern et al. 2013; Hernandez-Reif et al. 2005; Rapaport et al. 2010; Groer et al. 1994). However, for this effect, it is a prerequisite that the person has a positive attitude toward massages and that the massage is perceived as pleasant and relaxing (Fernández-Lao et al. 2012).

2.4.5 Relieving Pain Through Touch

The pain-relieving effects of touch and massage cannot be attributed to specific hormones or messenger substances. Instead, a complex interplay of physiological and cognitive processes contributes to pain processes and their perception (see also bio-psycho-social pain model in Sect. 1.1.7). Direct and indirect effects of touch on pain can be distinguished, and these effects also influence each other. Firstly, the **indirect effects of touch on pain** are triggered by social support (Sect. 5.5) and placebo effects that occur due to positive expectations and the setting. Accordingly, a person's psychological well-being and mood influence their perception of pain. Therefore, sympathy and comfort conveyed by social touch can change a person's mood and have analgesic effects. Furthermore, social interactions and physical contact can divert attention from pain, thereby reducing the perceived intensity of the pain. Additionally, placebo effects can reduce stress, reinforce health-promoting behaviors, and activate self-healing processes (placebo effects, see Sect. 5.3).

Secondly, the **direct effects of touch on pain** are mediated by touch-induced changes in hormone and neurotransmitter levels (oxytocin, serotonin, dopamine, stress hormones, and cytokines). Additionally, local changes in the skin, muscles, and connective tissue can also be induced by touch, which has positive effects on pain processes. For example, both light stroking touches (lymphatic drainage) and more intensive massage strokes can stimulate increased lymphatic and metabolic transport. As a result, metabolic waste products and pain-causing substances can be flushed out more effectively. Massages of the muscles and connective tissue also stimulate increased blood flow and can lead to local increases in temperature. Moreover, loosening connective tissue adhesions can also improve muscle flexibility and elasticity, thus reducing pain during movements.

Therefore, the direct effects of touch and massage on pain perception depend on the form of the touch, the cause of the pain, and on the indirect effects caused by the people involved and the setting (cf. Chap. 5).

Conclusion
Pleasant interpersonal touch (e.g., hugs or relaxation massages) can trigger various health-promoting physiological processes by reducing stress and stress hormones, which can have a positive effect on immune functions, digestion, blood sugar levels, and the cardiovascular system. In addition, other hormonal and psychophysiological effects are triggered by pleasant touch, such as the release of oxytocin, dopamine, and serotonin, which positively affect mood and sleep, improve well-being, and reduce pain. Furthermore, touch triggers psychological processes that can reduce loneliness and strengthen social bonds between people (see also Sect. 5.5).

References

Abraham J, Mathew S. Merkel cells: a collective review of current concepts. Int J Appl Basic Med Res. 2019;9(1):9–13. https://doi.org/10.4103/ijabmr.IJABMR_34_18.

Amunts K, Bechmann I, Nitsch R, Paulsen F, Schmitt O, Wree A, Zilles K. Nervensystem und Sinnesorgane. In: Zilles K, Tillmann BN, editors. Anatomie. Berlin, Heidelberg: Springer; 2010. p. 599–764.

Angelopoulou E, Anagnostouli M, Chrousos GP, Bougea A. Massage therapy as a complementary treatment for Parkinson's disease: a systematic literature review. Complement Ther Med. 2020;49:102340. https://doi.org/10.1016/j.ctim.2020.102340.

Baumann KI, Halata Z, Moll I. The Merkel cell. Structure-development-function-cancerogenesis. Berlin, London: Springer; 2011.

Bear MF, Connors BW, Paradiso MA. Neurowissenschaften. In: Engel AK, editor. Ein grundlegendes Lehrbuch für Biologie, Medizin und Psychologie. 4th ed. Berlin, Heidelberg: Springer; 2018.

Bergua A, editor. Das menschliche Auge in Zahlen. Berlin, Heidelberg: Springer; 2017.

Berrueta L, Bergholz J, Munoz D, Muskaj I, Badger GJ, Shukla A, et al. Stretching reduces tumor growth in a mouse breast cancer model. Sci Rep. 2018;8(1):7864. https://doi.org/10.1038/s41598-018-26198-7.

Beyer L. Die Bedeutung des Bindegewebes für die diagnostischen und therapeutischen Anstze der manuellen Medizin. Man Med. 2001;2(39):56–7.

Bhowmick S, Singh A, Flavell RA, Clark RB, O'Rourke J, Cone RE. The sympathetic nervous system modulates CD4(+)FoxP3(+) regulatory T cells via a TGF-beta-dependent mechanism. J Leukoc Biol. 2009;86(6):1275–83. https://doi.org/10.1189/jlb.0209107.

Birbaumer NP, Schmidt RF. Biologische Psychologie. 6, vollst. überarb. und erg. Aufl. Heidelberg: Springer Medizin; 2006.

Bishop JH, Fox JR, Maple R, Loretan C, Badger GJ, Henry SM, et al. Ultrasound evaluation of the combined effects of thoracolumbar fascia injury and movement restriction in a porcine model. PloS One. 2016;11(1):e0147393. https://doi.org/10.1371/journal.pone.0147393.

Blaeschke F, Otte B, Schneider N. Das Immunsystem. In: Horn F, editor. Biochemie des Menschen. 8. überarbeitete underweiterte Auflage. Stuttgart: Georg Thieme Verlag; 2020. p. 700–27.

Boll S, Almeida de Minas AC, Raftogianni A, Herpertz SC, Grinevich V. Oxytocin and pain perception: from animal models to human research. Neuroscience. 2018;387:149–61. https://doi.org/10.1016/j.neuroscience.2017.09.041.

Borgini E, Stecco A, Day JA, Stecco C. How much time is required to modify a fascial fibrosis? J Bodyw Mov Ther. 2010;14(4):318–25. https://doi.org/10.1016/j.jbmt.2010.04.006.

Briner RP, Carlton SM, Coggeshall RE, Chung KS. Evidence for unmyelinated sensory fibres in the posterior columns in man. Brain. 1988;111(5):999–1007. https://doi.org/10.1093/brain/111.5.999.

Buclin T, Cosma M, Appenzeller M, Jacquet AF, Décosterd LA, Biollaz J, Burckhardt P. Diet acids and alkalis influence calcium retention in bone. Osteoporos Int. 2001;12(6):493–9. https://doi.org/10.1007/s001980170095.

Buddecke E. Biochemie des Bindegewebes. Angew Chem. 1960;72(18):663–77. https://doi.org/10.1002/ange.19600721804.

Carano A, Siciliani G. Effect of continuous and intermittent forces on human fibroblasts in vitro. Eur J Orthodont. 1996;18(1):19–26.

Carter CS. Oxytocin and sexual behavior. Neurosci Biobehav Rev. 1992;16(2):131–44. https://doi.org/10.1016/s0149-7634(05)80176-9.

Cauna N. Fine morphological characteristics and microtopography of the free nerve endings of the human digital skin. Anat Rec. 1980;198(4):643–56. https://doi.org/10.1002/ar.1091980409.

Cowman MK, Schmidt TA, Raghavan P, Stecco A. Viscoelastic properties of Hyaluronan in physiological conditions. F1000Research. 2015;4:622. https://doi.org/10.12688/f1000research.6885.1.

Critchley HD, Harrison NA. Visceral influences on brain and behavior. Neuron. 2013;77(4):624–38. https://doi.org/10.1016/j.neuron.2013.02.008.

Dale HH. On some physiological actions of ergot. J Physiol. 1906;34(3):163–206. https://doi.org/10.1113/jphysiol.1906.sp001148.

Davidovic M, Starck G, Olausson H. Processing of affective and emotionally neutral tactile stimuli in the insular cortex. Dev Cogn Neurosci. 2019;35:94–103. https://doi.org/10.1016/j.dcn.2017.12.006.

Devine SL, Walker SC, Makdani A, Stockton ER, McFarquhar MJ, Mcglone FP, Trotter PD. Childhood adversity and affective touch perception: a comparison of United Kingdom care leavers and non-care leavers. Front Psychol. 2020;11:557171. https://doi.org/10.3389/fpsyg.2020.557171.

Diego MA, Field T. Moderate pressure massage elicits a parasympathetic nervous system response. Int J Neurosci. 2009;119(5):630–8. https://doi.org/10.1080/00207450802329605.

Dintenfass L. Rheology of complex fluids and some observations on joint lubrication. Fed Proc. 1966;25(3):1054–60.

Fernández-Lao C, Cantarero-Villanueva I, Díaz-Rodríguez L, Fernández-de-las-Peñas C, Sánchez-Salado C, Arroyo-Morales M. The influence of patient attitude toward massage on pressure pain sensitivity and immune system after application of myofascial release in breast cancer survivors: a randomized, controlled crossover study. J Manipulative Physiol Ther. 2012;35(2):94–100. https://doi.org/10.1016/j.jmpt.2011.09.011.

Field T, Diego MA, Hernandez-Reif M, Schanberg S, Kuhn C. Massage therapy effects on depressed pregnant women. J Psychosom Obstet Gynaecol. 2004;25(2):115–22. https://doi.org/10.1080/01674820412331282231.

Fradette J, Larouche D, Fugère C, Guignard R, Beauparlant A, Couture V, et al. Normal human Merkel cells are present in epidermal cell populations isolated and cultured from glabrous and hairy skin sites. J Investig Dermatol. 2003;120(2):313–7. https://doi.org/10.1046/j.1523-1747.2003.12024.x.

Gatej I, Popa M, Rinaudo M. Role of the pH on hyaluronan behavior in aqueous solution. Biomacromolecules. 2005;6(1):61–7. https://doi.org/10.1021/bm040050m.

Gogolla N. The insular cortex. Curr Biol. 2017;27(12):R580–6. https://doi.org/10.1016/j.cub.2017.05.010.

Gohlke F, Janßen E, Leidel J, Heppelmann B, Eulert J. Histomorphologische Befunde zur Propriozeption am Schultergelenk. Der Orthopade. 1998;27(8):510–7. https://doi.org/10.1007/PL00003524.

Goodwin AW, Wheat HE. Physiological mechanisms of the receptor system. In: Grunwald M, editor. Human haptic perception: basics and applications. Basel: Birkhäuser; 2008. p. 93–102.

Gordon I, Voos AC, Bennett RH, Bolling DZ, Pelphrey KA, Kaiser MD. Brain mechanisms for processing affective touch. Hum Brain Mapp. 2013;34(4):914–22. https://doi.org/10.1002/hbm.21480.

Grefkes C, Fink GR. Somatosensorisches System. In: Schneider F, Fink GR, editors. Funktionelle MRT in Psychiatrie und Neurologie. Berlin, Heidelberg: Springer; 2007. p. 279–96.

Griffin MJ. Handbook of human vibration. Reprinted ed. London: Elsevier; 2004.

Groer M, Mozingo J, Droppleman P, Davis M, Jolly ML, Boynton M, et al. Measures of salivary secretory immunoglobulin A and state anxiety after a nursing back rub. Appl Nurs Res. 1994;7(1):2–6. https://doi.org/10.1016/0897-1897(94)90013-2.

Gröll M. Dopamin. In: Horn F, editor. Biochemie des Menschen. 8. überarbeitete und erweiterte Auflage. Stuttgart: Georg Thieme Verlag; 2020a. p. 544–6.

Gröll M. Serotonin. In: Horn F, editor. Biochemie des Menschen. 8. überarbeitete underweiterte Auflage. Stuttgart: Georg Thieme Verlag; 2020b. p. 547–9.

Grunwald M. Haptische Reizverarbeitung und EEG-Veränderungen. Unveröffentlichte Dissertation. Jena; 1998.

Grunwald M. Homo hapticus. Warum wir ohne Tastsinn nicht leben können. München: DroemerKnaur; 2017.

Grunwald M. Haut als sensorisches System. Der Schmerzpatient. 2019;2(02):76–83. https://doi.org/10.1055/a-0823-0732.

Grunwald M, Mueller SM. Scientific principles of palpation. In: Mayer J, Standen C, Barral J-P, editors. Osteopathic medicine textbook. 1st ed. München: Elsevier; 2017. p. 251–65.

Halata Z, Baumann KI. Anatomy of receptors. In: Grunwald M, editor. Human haptic perception: basics and applications. Basel: Birkhäuser; 2008. p. 85–92.

Hallegraeff JM, van der Schans CP, de Ruiter R, de Greef MHG. Stretching before sleep reduces the frequency and severity of nocturnal leg cramps in older adults: a randomised trial. J Physiother. 2012;58(1):17–22. https://doi.org/10.1016/s1836-9553(12)70068-1.

Handlin L, Nilsson A, Ejdebäck M, Hydbring-Sandberg E, Uvnäs-Moberg K. Associations between the psychological characteristics of the human–dog relationship and oxytocin and cortisol levels. Anthrozoös. 2012;25(2):215–28. https://doi.org/10.2752/175303712x13316289505468.

Heine H. Zur Morphologie der Akupunkturpunkte. Deutsche Zeitschrift für Akupunktur. 2016;59(3):49–51. https://doi.org/10.1016/S0415-6412(16)30095-9.

Hernandez-Reif M, Field T, Ironson G, Beutler J, Vera Y, Hurley J, et al. Natural killer cells and lymphocytes increase in women with breast cancer following mas-

sage therapy. Int J Neurosci. 2005;115(4):495–510. https://doi.org/10.1080/00207450590523080.
Hövels O. Stoffwechsel im Bindegewebe. In: Weicker H, Althoff H, Baumgartner G, Beckmann R, Betke K, Bettex M, et al., editors. Erkrankungen der Stützgewebe Erkrankungen des Blutes und der Blutbildenden Organe. (Handbuch der Kinderheilkunde 6). Berlin, Heidelberg: Springer; 1967. p. 41–2.
Hsiao S, Yau J. Neural basis of haptic perception. In: Grunwald M, editor. Human haptic perception: basics and applications. Basel: Birkhäuser; 2008. p. 103–12.
Jabonero V. Die Bedeutung der Varikositäten postganglionärer Nervenfasern und die lichtoptische Identifizierung der Aktivzonen im Bereich der Neuroeffektoren-Synapse. Acta Neuroveg. 1967;30(1):372–82. https://doi.org/10.1007/bf01239915.
Johnston GR, Webster NR. Cytokines and the immunomodulatory function of the vagus nerve. Br J Anaesth. 2009;102(4):453–62. https://doi.org/10.1093/bja/aep037.
Junqueira LC, Carneiro J. Bindegewebe. In: Junqueira LC, Carneiro J, editors. Histologie. 3rd ed. Berlin, Heidelberg: Springer; 1991. p. 140–71.
Kato M, Nihei Green F, Hotta K, Tsukamoto T, Kurita Y, Kubo A, Takagi H. The efficacy of stretching exercises on arterial stiffness in middle-aged and older adults: a meta-analysis of randomized and non-randomized controlled trials. Int J Environ Res Public Health. 2020;17(16):5643. https://doi.org/10.3390/ijerph17165643.
Khiewkhern S, Promthet S, Sukprasert A, Eunhpinitpong W, Bradshaw P. Effectiveness of aromatherapy with light thai massage for cellular immunity improvement in colorectal cancer patients receiving chemotherapy. Asian Pac J Cancer Prev. 2013;14(6):3903–7. https://doi.org/10.7314/apjcp.2013.14.6.3903.
Kiecolt-Glaser JK, McGuire L, Robles TF, Glaser R. Psychoneuroimmunology and psychosomatic medicine: Back to the future. Psychosom Med. 2002;64(1):15.
Knoche H. Über die feinere Innervation der Niere des Menschen. Z Zellforsch Mikrosk Anat. 1951;36(5):448–75.
Kolb B, Whishaw IQ, Pritzel M. Neuropsychologie. Heidelberg: Spektrum Akad. Verl; 1993.
Kreuder A-K, Wassermann L, Wollseifer M, Ditzen B, Eckstein M, Stoffel-Wagner B, et al. Oxytocin enhances the pain-relieving effects of social support in romantic couples. Hum Brain Mapp. 2019;40(1):242–51. https://doi.org/10.1002/hbm.24368.
Krückmann E. Ueber die Sensibilität der Hornhaut. Graefes Arhiv für Ophthalmol. 1895;41(4):21–41. https://doi.org/10.1007/bf01694395.
Langevin HM. Potential role of fascia in chronic musculoskeletal pain. In: Audette JF, Bailey A, editors. Integrative pain medicine. Totowa, NJ: Humana Press; 2008. p. 123–32.
Langevin HM, Yandow JA. Relationship of acupuncture points and meridians to connective tissue planes. Anat Rec. 2002;269(6):257–65. https://doi.org/10.1002/ar.10185.
Langevin HM, Churchill DL, Wu J, Badger GJ, Yandow JA, Fox JR, Krag MH. Evidence of connective tissue involvement in acupuncture. FASEB J. 2002;16(8):872–4. https://doi.org/10.1096/fj.01-0925fje.
Langevin HM, Bouffard NA, Badger GJ, Iatridis JC, Howe AK. Dynamic fibroblast cytoskeletal response to subcutaneous tissue stretch ex vivo and in vivo. Am J Physiol Cell Physiol. 2005;288(3):C747–56. https://doi.org/10.1152/ajpcell.00420.2004.
Lee MWL, McPhee RW, Stringer MD. An evidence-based approach to human dermatomes. Clin Anat. 2008;21(5):363–73. https://doi.org/10.1002/ca.20636.
Lehmann-Horn F. Motorische Systeme. In: Schmidt RF, Lang F, Heckmann M, editors. Physiologie des Menschen. Mit Pathophysiologie. Sonderausgabe der 31. Auflage. Berlin: Springer; 2017. p. 127–62.
Leserman J, Drossman DA, Li Z, Toomey TC, Nachman G, Glogau L. Sexual and physical abuse history in gastroenterology practice: how types of abuse impact health status. Psychosom Med. 1996;58(1):4–15.
Leserman J, Li Z, Drossman DA, Toomey TC, Nachman G, Glogau L. Impact of sexual and physical abuse dimensions on health status: development of an abuse severity measure. Psychosom Med. 1997;59(2):152–60. https://doi.org/10.1097/00006842-199703000-00007.
Li Q, Becker B, Wernicke J, Chen Y, Zhang Y, Li R, et al. Foot massage evokes oxytocin release and activation of orbitofrontal cortex and superior temporal sulcus. Psychoneuroendocrinology. 2019;101:193–203. https://doi.org/10.1016/j.psyneuen.2018.11.016.
Löken LS, Wessberg J, Morrison I, McGlone F, Olausson H. Coding of pleasant touch by unmyelinated afferents in humans. Nat Neurosci. 2009;12(5):547–8. https://doi.org/10.1038/nn.2312.
Marshall AG, Mcglone FP. Affective touch: the enigmatic spinal pathway of the C-tactile afferent. J Exp Neurosci. 2020;15:2633105520925072. https://doi.org/10.1177/2633105520925072.
Meier M, Unternaehrer E, Dimitroff SJ, Benz ABE, Bentele UU, Schorpp SM, et al. Standardized massage interventions as protocols for the induction of psychophysiological relaxation in the laboratory: a block randomized, controlled trial. Sci Rep. 2020;10(1):14774. https://doi.org/10.1038/s41598-020-71173-w.
Michailow S. Über die sensiblen Nervenendigungen in der Harnblase der Säugetiere. Archiv Mikrosk Anat. 1907;71(1):254–83. https://doi.org/10.1007/bf02979917.
Mitchell JH, Schmidt RF. Cardiovascular reflex control by afferent fibers from skeletal muscle receptors. Compr Physiol. 2011:623–58. https://doi.org/10.1002/cphy.cp020317.
Moir JC. The obstetrician bids, and the uterus contracts. Br Med J. 1964;2(5416):1025–9. https://doi.org/10.1136/bmj.2.5416.1025.

Morhenn V, Beavin LE, Zak PJ. Massage increases oxytocin and reduces adrenocorticotropin hormone in humans. Altern Ther Health Med. 2012;18(6):11–8.

Mugii N, Hasegawa M, Matsushita T, Kondo M, Orito H, Yanaba K, et al. The efficacy of self-administered stretching for finger joint motion in Japanese patients with systemic sclerosis. J Rheumatol. 2006;33(8):1586–92.

Nacy SM, Kbah SN, Jafer HA, Al-Shaalan I. Controlling a servo motor using EEG signals from the primary motor cortex. Am J Biomed Eng. 2016;6(5):139–46. https://doi.org/10.5923/j.ajbe.20160605.02.

Ng CP, Hinz B, Swartz MA. Interstitial fluid flow induces myofibroblast differentiation and collagen alignment in vitro. J Cell Sci. 2005;118(20):4731–9. https://doi.org/10.1242/jcs.02605.

Nishiwaki M, Yonemura H, Kurobe K, Matsumoto N. Four weeks of regular static stretching reduces arterial stiffness in middle-aged men. SpringerPlus. 2015;4(1):1–11. https://doi.org/10.1186/s40064-015-1337-4.

Nordin M. Low-threshold mechanoreceptive and nociceptive units with unmyelinated (C) fibres in the human supraorbital nerve. J Physiol. 1990;426:229–40. https://doi.org/10.1113/jphysiol.1990.sp018135.

Oláh KSJ, Steer PJ. The use and abuse of oxytocin. Obstet Gynecol. 2015;17(4):265–71. https://doi.org/10.1111/tog.12222.

Olausson HW, Cole J, Vallbo A, McGlone F, Elam M, Krämer HH, et al. Unmyelinated tactile afferents have opposite effects on insular and somatosensory cortical processing. Neurosci Lett. 2008;436(2):128–32. https://doi.org/10.1016/j.neulet.2008.03.015.

Ott I, Scott JC. The action of infundibulin upon the mammary secretion. Exp Biol Med. 1910;8(2):48–9. https://doi.org/10.3181/00379727-8-27.

Pavan PG, Stecco A, Stern R, Stecco C. Painful connections: densification versus fibrosis of fascia. Curr Pain Headache Rep. 2014;18(8):441. https://doi.org/10.1007/s11916-014-0441-4.

Pavlov VA, Wang H, Czura CJ, Friedman SG, Tracey KJ. The cholinergic anti-inflammatory pathway: a missing link in neuroimmunomodulation. Mol Med. 2003;9(5–8):125–34. https://doi.org/10.1007/bf03402177.

Peck D, Buxton DF, Nitz A. A comparison of spindle concentrations in large and small muscles acting in parallel combinations. J Morphol. 1984;180(3):243–52. https://doi.org/10.1002/jmor.1051800307.

Phillips JR, Johansson RS, Johnson KO. Representation of braille characters in human nerve fibres. Exp Brain Res. 1990;81(3):589–92. https://doi.org/10.1007/BF02423508.

Pipelzadeh MH, Naylor IL. The in vitro enhancement of rat myofibroblast contractility by alterations to the pH of the physiological solution. Eur J Pharmacol. 1998;357(2–3):257–9. https://doi.org/10.1016/s0014-2999(98)00588-3.

Rapaport MH, Schettler P, Breese C. A preliminary study of the effects of a single session of Swedish massage on hypothalamic-pituitary-adrenal and immune function in normal individuals. J Altern Complement Med. 2010;16(10):1079–88. https://doi.org/10.1089/acm.2009.0634.

Rapaport MH, Schettler P, Bresee C. A preliminary study of the effects of repeated massage on hypothalamic-pituitary-adrenal and immune function in healthy individuals: a study of mechanisms of action and dosage. J Altern Complement Med. 2012;18(8):789–97. https://doi.org/10.1089/acm.2011.0071.

Richard P, Moos F, Freund-Mercier MJ. Central effects of oxytocin. Physiol Rev. 1991;71(2):331–70. https://doi.org/10.1152/physrev.1991.71.2.331.

Rohkamm R, Kermer P, editors. Taschenatlas Neurologie. 4th ed. Stuttgart: Georg Thieme Verlag; 2017.

Rolls ET, O'Doherty J, Kringelbach ML, Francis S, Bowtell R, McGlone F. Representations of pleasant and painful touch in the human orbitofrontal and cingulate cortices. Cereb Cortex. 2003;13(3):308–17. https://doi.org/10.1093/cercor/13.3.308.

Sarkar C, Basu B, Chakroborty D, Dasgupta PS, Basu S. The immunoregulatory role of dopamine: an update. Brain Behav Immun. 2010;24(4):525–8. https://doi.org/10.1016/j.bbi.2009.10.015.

Schiebler TH, Schmidt W, Zilles K. Haut und Hautanhangsorgane. In: Schiebler TH, Schmidt W, Zilles K, editors. Anatomie. Berlin, Heidelberg: Springer; 1995. p. 205–18.

Schleip R, Duerselen L, Vleeming A, Naylor IL, Lehmann-Horn F, Zorn A, et al. Strain hardening of fascia: static stretching of dense fibrous connective tissues can induce a temporary stiffness increase accompanied by enhanced matrix hydration. J Bodyw Mov Ther. 2012a;16(1):94–100. https://doi.org/10.1016/j.jbmt.2011.09.003.

Schleip R, Jäger H, Klingler W. What is 'fascia'? A review of different nomenclatures. J Bodyw Mov Ther. 2012b;16(4):496–502. https://doi.org/10.1016/j.jbmt.2012.08.001.

Schleip R, Gabbiani G, Wilke J, Naylor I, Hinz B, Zorn A, et al. Fascia is able to actively contract and may thereby influence musculoskeletal dynamics: a histochemical and mechanographic investigation. Front Physiol. 2019;10:336. https://doi.org/10.3389/fphys.2019.00336.

Spitoni GF, Pietro Z, Guido G, Antonucci G, Gaspare G, Lingiardi V, et al. Disorganized attachment pattern affects the perception of affective touch. Sci Rep. 2020;10(1):9658. https://doi.org/10.1038/s41598-020-66606-5.

Stecco A, Gesi M, Stecco C, Stern R. Fascial components of the myofascial pain syndrome. Curr Pain Headache Rep. 2013;17(8):352. https://doi.org/10.1007/s11916-013-0352-9.

Steen KH, Steen AE, Kreysel H-W, Reeh PW. Inflammatory mediators potentiate pain induced by experimental tissue acidosis. Pain. 1996;66(2):163–70. https://doi.org/10.1016/0304-3959(96)03034-5.

Stopford JS. The protective and discriminative divisions of sensation. J Anat. 1929;63(3):285–90.

Talbot WH, Darian-Smith I, Kornhuber HH, Mountcastle VB. The sense of flutter-vibration: comparison of the human capacity with response patterns of mechanoreceptive afferents from the monkey hand. J Neurophysiol. 1968;31(2):301–34. https://doi.org/10.1152/jn.1968.31.2.301.

Talbot NL, Chapman B, Conwell Y, McCollumn K, Franus N, Cotescu S, Duberstein PR. Childhood sexual abuse is associated with physical illness burden and functioning in psychiatric patients 50 years of age and older. Psychosom Med. 2009;71(4):417–22. https://doi.org/10.1097/PSY.0b013e318199d31b.

Thoma R. Bemerkung über die Vater-Pacini'schen Körperchen der Gefässwand. Archiv Pathol Anat. 1889;116(3):542–3. https://doi.org/10.1007/bf02282095.

Trabold O, Wagner S, Wicke C, Scheuenstuhl H, Hussain MZ, Rosen N, et al. Lactate and oxygen constitute a fundamental regulatory mechanism in wound healing. Wound Repair Regen. 2003;11(6):504–9. https://doi.org/10.1046/j.1524-475x.2003.11621.x.

Treede RD, Baumgärtner U. Das somatosensorische system. In: Brandes R, Lang F, Schmidt RF, editors. Physiologie des Menschen. Mit Pathophysiologie. 32rd ed. Berlin: Springer (Springer-Lehrbuch); 2019. p. 644–65.

Uvnäs-Moberg K, Handlin L, Petersson M. Self-soothing behaviors with particular reference to oxytocin release induced by non-noxious sensory stimulation. Front Psychol. 2014;5:1529. https://doi.org/10.3389/fpsyg.2014.01529.

van den Berg F, editor. Angewandte Physiologie. Das Bindegewebe des Bewegungsapparates verstehen und beeinflussen. Unter Mitarbeit von Jan Cabri. 4th ed. Stuttgart, NY: Georg Thieme Verlag KG; 2016.

Vega-Bermudez F, Johnson KO. SA1 and RA receptive fields, response variability, and population responses mapped with a probe array. J Neurophysiol. 1999;81(6):2701–10. https://doi.org/10.1152/jn.1999.81.6.2701.

Vogt PM. Praxis der Plastischen Chirurgie. In: Plastisch-rekonstruktive Operationen - Plastisch-ästhetische Operationen - Handchirurgie - Verbrennungschirurgie. Berlin, Heidelberg: Springer-Verlag; 2012. Online verfügbar unter http://gbv.eblib.com/patron/FullRecord.aspx?p=884738.

Walker SC, Trotter PD, Swaney WT, Marshall A, Mcglone FP. C-tactile afferents: cutaneous mediators of oxytocin release during affiliative tactile interactions? Neuropeptides. 2017;64:27–38. https://doi.org/10.1016/j.npep.2017.01.001.

Watanabe N, Hotta H. Heart rate changes in response to mechanical pressure stimulation of skeletal muscles are mediated by cardiac sympathetic nerve activity. Front Neurosci. 2016;10:614. https://doi.org/10.3389/fnins.2016.00614.

Weicker H, Althoff H, Baumgartner G, Beckmann R, Betke K, Bettex M, et al. Erkrankungen der Stützgewebe Erkrankungen des Blutes und der Blutbildenden Organe (Handbuch der Kinderheilkunde, 6). Berlin, Heidelberg: Springer; 1967.

Wiesmann M, Nikoubashman O. Dermatome und Kennmuskeln. In: Wiesmann M, Linn J, Brückmann H, editors. Atlas Klinische Neuroradiologie. Wirbelsäule und Spinalkanal. Berlin: Springer; 2014. p. 69–71.

Wilke J, Schleip R, Yucesoy CA, Banzer W. Not merely a protective packing organ? A review of fascia and its force transmission capacity. J Appl Physiol. 2018;124(1):234–44. https://doi.org/10.1152/japplphysiol.00565.2017.

Williams PE, Catanese T, Lucey EG, Goldspink G. The importance of stretch and contractile activity in the prevention of connective tissue accumulation in muscle. J Anat. 1988;158:109–14.

Wrobel LK, Fray TR, Molloy JE, Adams JJ, Armitage MP, Sparrow JC. Contractility of single human dermal myofibroblasts and fibroblasts. Cell Motil Cytoskeleton. 2002;52(2):82–90. https://doi.org/10.1002/cm.10034.

Xiong Y, Berrueta L, Urso K, Olenich S, Muskaj I, Badger GJ, et al. Stretching reduces skin thickness and improves subcutaneous tissue mobility in a murine model of systemic sclerosis. Front Immunol. 2017;8:124. https://doi.org/10.3389/fimmu.2017.00124.

Zaki J, Davis JI, Ochsner KN. Overlapping activity in anterior insula during interoception and emotional experience. Neuroimage. 2012;62(1):493–9. https://doi.org/10.1016/j.neuroimage.2012.05.012.

Perceptual Thresholds and Disorders of the Haptic System

3

Stephanie Margarete Mueller and Martin Grunwald

Contents

S. M. Mueller (✉) · M. Grunwald
Haptic Research Lab, Paul-Flechsig-Institute for Brain Research, Leipzig University, Leipzig, Germany
e-mail: s.mueller@medizin.uni-leipzig.de; mgrun@medizin.uni-leipzig.de

S. M. Mueller et al., *Human Touch in Healthcare*, https://doi.org/10.1007/978-3-662-67860-2_3

3.1 The Haptic System over the Life Course

3.1.1 In Utero

3.1.1.1 Ontogenesis of Mechanosensation

Studies aimed at exploring the sensory capabilities of human fetuses *in utero* are limited by two factors (Hepper 2008):

(a) The observation of the fetus is methodologically limited and is only possible for short intervals (e.g., by ultrasound).

(b) To determine whether a fetus detects a stimulus, only reactive behavioral changes can be observed (e.g., a full-body movement following a loud sound or touch). If a fetus reliably shows the expected response, the fetus has likely detected the stimulus. Conversely, the absence of a response is not evidence of a lack of sensory capabilities in relation to that stimulus. Instead, the fetus may have the sensory capabilities to detect the stimulus but lack the ability to respond to it. A response requires both the presence of motor pathways and the linkage between sensory and motor functions.

As early as 6 weeks after fertilization, the **first spontaneous movements** of intrauterine embryos become visible via ultrasound (van Dongen and Goudie 1980). These movements are uncoordinated and twitching. Anatomical studies of extrauterine embryos have shown that from the seventh week of gestation, fine nerve fibers (free nerve endings) reach the skin of the face, shoulders, axilla, and thighs (Bradley and Mistretta 1975). At this time, extrauterine embryos can already respond to tactile stimulation of the lips with nonspecific movements (Hepper 2008; Hooker 1942). Consequently, the **sense of touch is the first sensory system** to develop in human ontogeny (Fig. 3.1). In the following weeks, other body areas become sensitive to touch. Indeed, by the 14th week of gestation (GA), tactile stimuli in

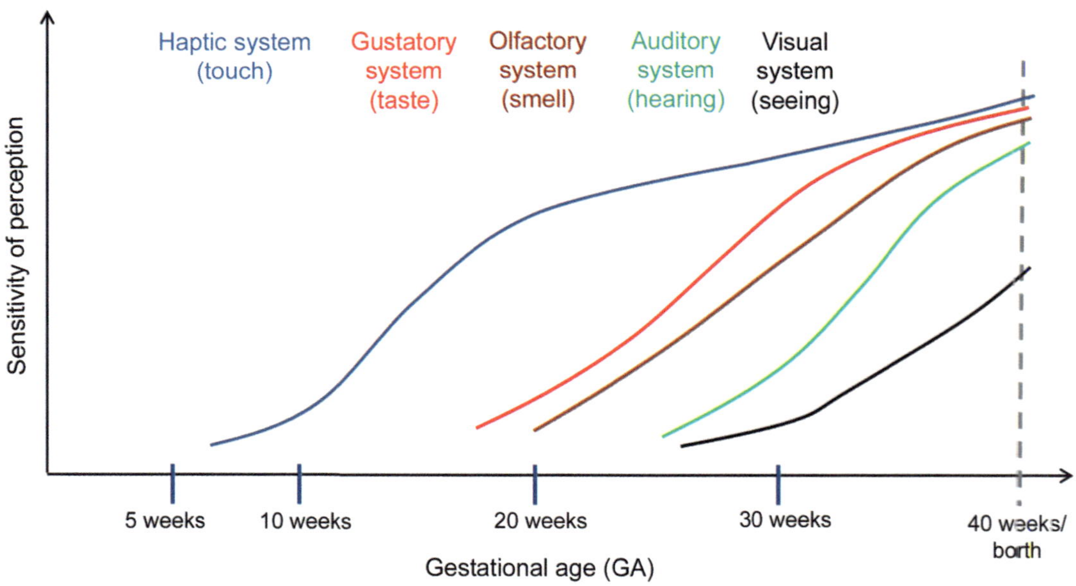

Fig. 3.1 Maturation of the sensory systems. Schematic representation of the maturation phases of the sensory systems. (Graphic: Haptic Research Lab, University of Leipzig)

almost all areas of the body lead to fetal movement responses. During this period, the encapsulated mechanoreceptors (including Pacinian, Merkel, and Meissner corpuscles; Sect. 2.1) develop gradually, and they are fully developed by the fifth month of pregnancy (Bradley and Mistretta 1975). In parallel, the vestibular organ develops in the inner ear, and becomes morphologically mature by the 14th week of gestation and registers changes in the body's position from the 24th week of gestation onward (Hepper 2008).

► **Definition** Up to 6 weeks gestation, the organism is called an **embryo**. From 6 weeks gestation up to 40 weeks gestation, the organism is called a **fetus**.

Since embryos show spontaneous movements and reactive movements to stimuli very early during development, it is assumed that their sensory and motor functions develop simultaneously. The biological purpose of the **parallelism of sensory and motor development** is to ensure that targeted movements can be executed, which is only possible if movements are controlled and adapted by sensors (Grunwald 2017). Up until the eighth week of gestation, the movements of the fetus remain uncoordinated, twitching, and usually involve the entire body. However, from the ninth week isolated arm movements can be observed via ultrasound, and from the tenth week, isolated leg movements occur (de Vries et al. 1985). Furthermore, as early as the ninth week of gestation, one-handed hand-head contacts are observable. Gradually, from the 12th week, it becomes possible for the fetus to move its individual fingers and open and close the hand.

Up to the tenth week, touching of the body and environment tends to occur accidentally through spontaneous movements. However, between the tenth and 12th week of gestation, the fetus begins **actively touching** its body and its environment, as well as sucking on the thumb (Reissland et al. 2015, 2014; Zoia et al. 2007). At the latest, **sensory integration processes of haptic and proprioceptive stimuli** begin to take place when the fetus starts producing active movements, as these integration processes are essential for coordinated movements. At this stage, most of the touches performed by the fetus occur on the face. Indeed, the repeated simultaneous stimulation of the hand and face is probably the cause of the close neural connection in the cortex between these two body regions.

The fetus' exploration of the body through touch generates unique sensory impressions. Specifically, touching one's own body produces haptic sensations on the body part performing the touch as well as on the body part receiving the touch. Moreover, such sensory events promote **discrimination between one's own body and the environment**, and this ability to distinguish between the body and the environment is ultimately the basis for the development of a **self-concept** (see also Sect. 1.4).

Approximately up to the 14th week of gestation, the haptic system is the only sense available to the fetus (see Fig. 3.1). First reactions to olfactory or gustatory stimuli have been observed from the 15th week onwards. And reactions to sounds have been observed from the 24th week onwards (Hepper 2008).

By the 20th week of gestation, the fetus' entire repertoire of movements has matured. The head, hands, feet, trunk, and facial musculature can move individually and in a relatively coordinated manner within the confined space of the uterus. By the 24th week of gestation, neural connections and synapses between the thalamus and cortex have matured (Nevalainen et al. 2014; Tau and Peterson 2010), meaning that the neuronal basis for **multisensory and pain perception** will be in place by this time at the latest. From the 35th week of gestation, pain and tactile stimuli are processed separately in the brain. Before that time, both types of stimuli trigger nonspecific cortical responses (Fabrizi et al. 2011).

Conclusion

In summary, fetuses show a variety of movements from a very early stage of development. They also perceive their body and environment through touch stimuli.

These sensorimotor experiences are a critical prerequisite for the healthy development of the neural and motor systems (Khazipov et al. 2004; Milh et al. 2007; Fagard et al. 2018).

3.1.1.2 Role of Lanugo Hair

Between the 13th and 17th weeks of gestation, lanugo hair develops on the entire body of the fetus (except on the soles of hands and feet). These hairs are 5 to 7-mm long, which is a considerable length compared to the body size of the fetus, which is approximately 10 cm. As with the body hair that develops later in life (cf. Sect. 1.1.4), each of these lanugo hairs is surrounded by several mechanoreceptors, meaning every slight movement of a hair can be registered. In the amniotic sac, the fetus floats in amniotic fluid. Every movement of the mother or the fetus causes the amniotic fluid to move, which, in turn, causes the lanugo hairs on the fetus' body to move. In this way, sensations are constantly triggered on the surface of the fetus' body and transmitted to the brain. Without the lanugo hairs functioning like antennae to amplify each stimulus, the fetus would experience few sensory stimuli during this period (Grunwald 2017). In fact, the fetus' other sensory systems are not yet sufficiently developed, and the fetus is protected from light, sound, temperature changes, and mechanical stimuli by the uterus and maternal abdominal wall. Some scientists have suggested that fetal development is directly dependent on the **permanent physical stimulation** of the mechanoreceptors and the lanugo hairs (Bystrova 2009; Irmak et al. 2004). They assume that already *in utero*, coupling occurs between skin contact and the release of the hormone oxytocin (Sect. 2.4.1). Accordingly, the action potentials from the skin and lanugo hairs activate those brain regions (hypothalamus, insula) that are also connected with social and emotional evaluation processes after birth and in adults. Both oxytocin and the insula play a central role in infants' social, cognitive, and physical development after birth. In addition, pleasant bodily touches lead to the secretion of oxytocin in adult humans and the activation of the insula (cf. Sect. 2.2.3).

▶ **Important** The lanugo hair increases sensitivity to mechanical stimuli, meaning that movements provide stimulation of the haptic system and, thus, neural stimulation, which is essential for the growth of the fetus.

3.1.1.3 Concept of Closeness

For humans and many other mammals, "warm and soft" are usually associated with well-being and comfort. This is true both metaphorically ("to warm someone's heart") and in terms of the use of physical contact to find rest or comfort. The concept of "closeness" is also used in language to describe both spatial distance and to describe the characteristics of an emotional relationship (being close to someone). Importantly, the physical conditions warm, soft, and close are precisely the qualities that best describe the uterine environment of the fetus. Especially in the last weeks of pregnancy, the fetus is permanently in contact with the soft wall of the uterus, the ambient temperature is ideally adapted to the body temperature of the fetus, and in the course of a healthy pregnancy, the fetus is protected from all unpleasant stimuli. Through the mother's movements (and voice), the fetus also experiences that it is not alone in the world. Therefore, in fetuses, **physical closeness** to something else is experienced even if no other sensory systems except the haptic system have developed (Grunwald 2017). In particular, even if a fetus is deaf or blind, it will develop a concept of closeness because of the uterine physical contact. The neuronal representation of physical proximity is, thus, one of the first results of the fetus' engagement with the properties of its environment (Grunwald 2017).

In fetuses, these physical experiences are likely linked to positive emotions via the release of oxytocin and the activation of the insula.

Similar associations likely occur through the stimulation of the vestibular organ during maternal whole-body movements. These neuronal associations in fetuses may explain why holding, carrying, and rocking have a calming effect on infants (Cascio et al. 2019; Grunwald 2017).

Conclusion
The concept of closeness refers to a set of environmental conditions that are universally perceived as pleasant and positive. The perception of closeness *in utero* forms the basis for infants to react positively to large-scale physical contact with another person immediately after birth.

3.1.2 Neonatal Period and First Year of Life

Infants respond to skin stimuli all over the body. Especially in the first months of life, physical contact is essential as a means of communication with infants. In addition, physical contact with primary caregivers is crucial for all of the postnatal growth and developmental processes in infants (Grunwald 2017; Montagu 1986).

3.1.2.1 Perceptual Dimensions

Following birth, the environmental characteristics experienced by the infant change substantially. During the postnatal period, a spectrum of new body stimulations replaces the hitherto full-body contact they experienced. Specifically, until birth, the fetus was always in direct physical contact with the mother's womb, both during the sleeping and waking phases. After birth, physical contact changes in quality and intensity and is limited to localized body regions. In addition, the newborn experiences significantly lower temperatures outside the mother's womb compared to inside.

The high somatosensory sensitivity of fetuses and their existing body schema (Sect. 1.4) make it very likely that newborns can perceive the loss of full-body contact after birth, as well as all the other physical changes. Additionally, further to the changes in the physical environment registered by the newborn, even the familiar movement sequences of its limbs can no longer be performed because of the body being subject to gravitational forces that the musculature cannot yet oppose. For example, instead of the mother's womb holding the head in a stable position, gravity now acts on all the newborn's limbs. The newborn's clumsy movements may appear to the observer as reflecting physical helplessness in the first week after birth. However, this motor limitation should not obscure the existing abilities: all dimensions of the haptic system (i.e., exteroception, interoception, and proprioception) develop during pregnancy and are **already functional at birth**. During the first year of life, the infant learns to actively use these perceptual dimensions to explore and interpret their body and environment. As the infant's muscle strength increases, the associations between movement, proprioception, balance, and the vestibular system are practiced and developed. Moreover, through sensations such as hunger, cold, fear, and pleasure, infants learn to interpret stimuli from within the body, thereby training their interoception. Through active exploration and increasingly complex physical interactions with the environment, the infant can encounter different materials and explore various motor functions. These experiences are fundamental prerequisites for healthy physical and mental development (see also Sect. 3.4.2. and Chap. 7).

▶ **Important** All dimensions of the haptic system (i.e., exteroception, interoception, and proprioception) develop during pregnancy and are already functional at birth. The ability to actively explore the environment develops and is refined during the first year of life.

3.1.2.2 Explorative Skills

The postnatal development of the haptic system is characterized by **considerable developmental advances**. In human children, perceptual differentiation of tactile sensing and haptic exploration increases very quickly in the first year of life. In addition, **multisensory integration processes** increasingly encompass a variety of sensory channels, meaning that perceptual information from other sensory channels is increasingly associated with tactile-haptic stimuli. Postnatal development is based on motor and cognitive maturation processes as well as on the child's naturally occurring, consistent exploration of materials and objects.

Mouth exploration is the first haptic manipulation observed in postnatal life, and it involves putting parts of the body or objects into the mouth and exploring them. At this point of development, the mouth and tongue are the areas of the body with the best fine-motor skills and are apt exploration tools. Over time, as the child develops increasing dexterity, other exploration strategies are added. For example, 2–3-month-old infants can already hold objects with one or both hands and press their hands on or stroke surfaces. Furthermore, 6–12-month-old infants actively manipulate objects by repeatedly lifting them, dropping them, and rotating them in their hands and exhibit other rhythmic stereotypies, such as hitting, scratching, pressing, and swiveling. These actions provide experiences of texture properties, weight, and hardness. From about 9 months of age, children can hold an object with one hand and touch it exploratively with the other. At this stage, the first differences in weight are recognized when comparing objects. By 2 years of age, mouth exploration has usually ceased, and the fingers are preferred for object manipulation.

3.1.2.3 Consequences of a Lack of Physical Contact

One indispensable prerequisite for physical and cognitive maturation processes is loving physical contact and touch by the primary caregivers (For more details, see Chap. 7). Physical contact is one of the most fundamental needs of an infant, along with the need for food and sleep (Grunwald 2017). If a newborn is only provided with basic care for extended periods of time and does not experience any closeness in the form of physical affection, the vital functions of the infant can fail, and it may die. If the infant should remain alive under such circumstances, **mental and physical damage** occurs beyond repair. In fact, children who have endured such neglect and deprivation are highly impaired in all dimensions of their behavior. For example, language development, as well as all other cognitive and social aspects of behavior, are pathologically altered, these children show significant growth retardation and severe impairments in motor function, and impairments of organ functions, including the skin, are regularly observed. The Viennese psychiatrist Rene Spitz was one of the first to systematically observe such effects in children in orphanages (van Rosmalen et al. 2012). Further insights were provided by the isolation experiments of Harry Harlow, who raised baby monkeys with mother models made of wire and cloth (Harlow 1959; Ainsworth 1962). Moreover, recent studies of Romanian orphans who survived under extreme conditions of isolation have fully illustrated the irreparable psychological and physical consequences of lack of physical contact in early childhood (Bos et al. 2011, 2009; Ghera et al. 2009; Humphreys et al. 2015; McGoron et al. 2012; Nelson et al. 2014).

Conversely, adequate physical contact can promote cognitive, emotional, and physical growth and development processes, alleviate stress, and prevent mental illness. Adequate physical contact is also required for the formation of healthy bonds between the child and their primary caregivers (For more details, see Chap. 7).

▶ **Important** Depending on the duration of deprivation, a lack of social touch in infancy and toddlerhood can cause impairments in cognitive and emotional development and physical growth. Complete deprivation of physical contact or even isolation cause irreparable psychological and physical damage and can lead to the death of the child.

▶ **Book Tip**

- Deborah Blum (2002). Love at Goon Park: Harry Harlow and the Science of Affection.

3.1.3 Childhood and Youth

3.1.3.1 Haptic and Tactile Perception

Across child development, manual exploration becomes increasingly active and accurate. By the age of 7 years old, children's behavior changes from simply holding objects to more active exploration (Cronin 1977). During childhood and adolescence, age-related improvement continues due to the maturation processes of the CNS and the training of motor skills. For example, young adults are more adept than first graders at recognizing objects through **active haptic exploration** with the palm of the hand, as well as objects that are moved passively on the palm of their hand. Children's ability to complete haptic matching tasks (finding a target object in a group of comparison objects) is also subject to developmental improvements (Kleinman 1979); specifically, preschoolers give correct answers randomly, whereas second graders perform significantly better. After that, increases in improvement slow down; for example, in group comparisons of fourth graders versus young adults, the young adults show only slightly better performances in haptic matching tasks.

The development of haptic exploration competence occurs in two stages (Kleinman 1979):

- Young children collect information mainly unsystematically. However, as cognitive development progresses, the number of information units that can be held in working memory increases.
- Later, increasingly orderly exploration strategies are used, involving critically reviewing and comparing information.

The most significant developmental advances in haptic exploration strategies occur between kindergarten and second grade (Kleinman 1979). Further improvements in haptic perceptual performance into adulthood are likely due to increasing differentiation abilities and attentional focus (Cronin 1977).

The development of haptic recognition contrasts with the development of **the tactile recognition of objects** through static-passive touch. First and fifth graders do not differ; however, young adults show slightly better performance than younger persons (Cronin 1977). Conflicting findings exist regarding the development of the tactile **two-point threshold** (Sect. 1.1.1). Indeed, some studies show declining performance with increasing age, beginning in childhood (Peters and Goldreich 2013; Stevens and Choo 1996), whereas another study reported significantly better tactile-spatial discrimination performance in 10–16 year olds than in 6–9 year olds (Sect. 4.2.2 Grating Domes) (Bleyenheuft et al. 2006). Therefore, an increase in finger size during infancy worsens tactile-spatial resolution (by increasing the distance between receptors), whereas the tactile discrimination ability improves due to cognitive maturation processes (cf. Fig. 3.4 in Sect. 3.2.1).

Unequivocally, superior performance in childhood (compared to older individuals) has been documented for the **perception of vibration.** Accordingly, the highest sensitivity to vibratory stimuli occurs around 10 years of age and then continuously deteriorates with increasing age (cf. Fig. 3.2).

> ▶ **Important** Both passive-tactile stimulus recognition (two-point threshold) and active-haptic shape exploration improve from early childhood to young adulthood. This development is based on cortical maturation processes and improved attentional focus. The developmental maximum of the haptic system is usually reached in early adulthood.

3.1.3.2 Body Contact

Interpersonal physical contact continues to play a central role in the development of emotional, motor, and social brain functions through childhood and youth. Physical contact forms the **basis for physical growth and maturation processes** (Chap. 7) and has positive effects on various health processes (including stress reduction, emotion regulation, and immune function Sect. 5.5 and Chap. 8). Additionally, for younger people, there is a greater connection between healthy psychological and physical development and sufficient interpersonal contact (Grunwald 2017). In this respect, the postnatal and infant phases require the most physical stimulation and contact. Indeed, an infant's ability to move is related to them developing a healthy curiosity to explore their environment. As the ability to perform targeted and coordinated movements increases, periods of spatial distance from the primary care-

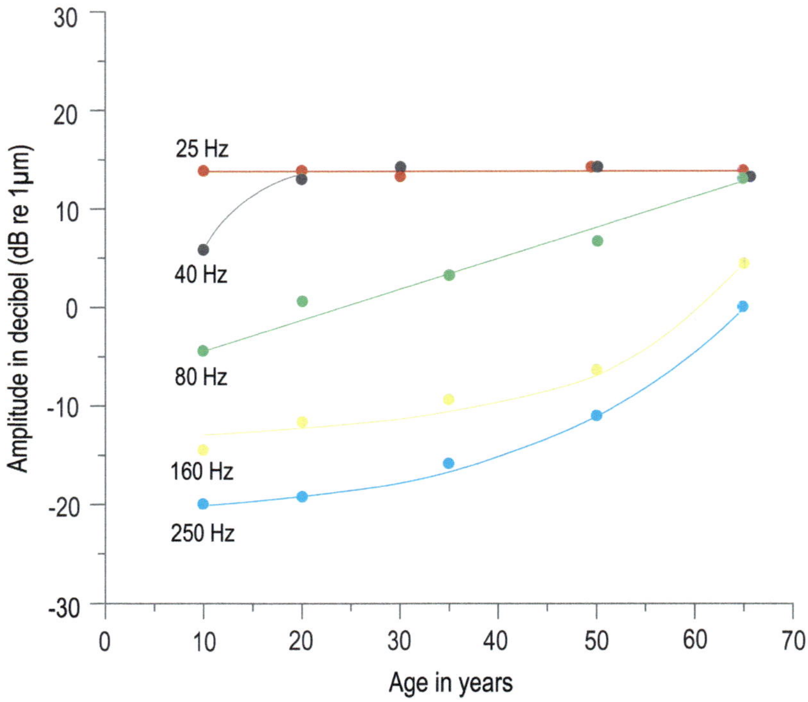

Fig. 3.2 Vibration perception as a function of age. Sensitivity to vibration stimuli is at a maximum in childhood, around the age of 10. For high frequencies, perceptual thresholds increase progressively with age. The perception thresholds for low frequencies are independent of age. (Reproduced from Verrillo 1980)

takers will automatically arise, and these periods are just as important for healthy development as time spent with their caregivers. Therefore, walking toddlers require different contact phases than infants, who cannot yet move freely in space on their own.

As a child's movement autonomy and language develop, their need for cognitive and social stimuli also changes. Specifically, infants in direct proximity to their mothers are still fully occupied with the stimulus conditions resulting from this situation. However, when the spectrum of their perceptual abilities gradually expands, their interest in other environmental stimuli expands with it. If a child capable of walking feels the need for physical closeness, they will seek the closeness of a caregiver of their own accord, provided that the social environment does not prevent this reaction. A healthy child's physical and psychological autonomy culminate during puberty with the accompanying physical affection for romantic partners. The **need for physical closeness** remains constant in this phase. However, social and physical contact are now predominantly sought outside the family.

Children continuously express their needs for adequate body stimulation across the developmental stages, both linguistically and nonlinguistically. The parental task consists of nothing less than deciphering these signals and transforming them into appropriate actions. Without a doubt, these processes also require learning and developmental efforts on the part of the parents, who constitute the child's social environment, especially when the parents did not grow up in adequate social contexts themselves. Additionally, each child sets its own standards in terms of the level of body stimulation required, and, thus, instructions and rules about the extent and duration of child-related physical contact are counterproductive. However, persistently too much or too little should be avoided.

Although the biological consequences of prolonged deprivation of contact are far more severe, it must be highlighted that *too much* bodily stimulation can also be problematic. When an infant or toddler signals that they require rest and withdrawal, not meeting this need constitutes an inadequate response from the social environment. When parents merely implement their own need for contact in the face of clear defensive signals from a child in need of rest and withdrawal, this behavior does not promote the child's well-being or development. Instead, with repeated inadequate bodily interactions, the child may learn that parental needs are more important than their own. During their future development, the child may experience difficulties distinguishing their own needs from those of others. In the worst case, the child's ability to perceive their own needs may not develop properly or may only develop insufficiently. Such undesirable developmental outcomes can have severe consequences for the mental and physical health of those affected.

> **Important** Younger children have a greater need for physical contact. However, both persistently too little and too much physical contact should be avoided.
>
> Sustained contact aversion in childhood may indicate the presence of a neurodevelopmental disorder.

3.1.4 Adulthood and Old Age

3.1.4.1 Tactile Perception

With increasing age, tactile perceptual ability steadily declines. For example, perception thresholds for tactile stimuli can double to quadruple from ages 20 to 80 (Stevens and Choo 1996; Thornbury and Mistretta 1981). Some body regions are more affected than others by reductions in tactile perceptual abilities. Interestingly, hands and feet seem more susceptible than proximal body regions (upper arm, abdomen, tongue, and lip) to these reductions. For both simultaneous two-point threshold and point localization (successive spatial threshold Sect. 1.1.2), substantial age-related differences have been found in the feet (sole and big toe) and fingertips (Stevens and Choo 1996; Corso 1971). For example, while 18–28 year olds have a two-point threshold on the foot of approximately 4 mm, individuals aged over 65 years show, on average, a 400% increase in the two-point threshold of the foot, with a threshold of 16 mm. For the fingertips, the threshold values have been shown to double or even triple from 1.1 mm in young adults to 2.8 or 3.5 mm in older adults, depending on the study (Stevens and Choo 1996; Libouton et al. 2010). The effects are similar for males and females.

To a similar extent, the detection threshold for light pressure stimuli (Semmes-Weinstein monofilaments Sect. 1.1.1) also decreases with age (Thornbury and Mistretta 1981).

Despite this general trend, a subset of individuals exhibit tactile perceptual abilities in old age that are comparable to those of younger individuals (Mueller et al. 2014b; Stevens and Patterson 1995; Thornbury and Mistretta 1981). This means there are large individual differences in tactile sensitivity across all ages, and that older individuals are not a homogeneous group with similar limitations.

The **causes for declining tactile sensitivity** and spatial resolution are primarily associated with the age-related decrease in the number of Meissner and Merkel corpuscles (Thornbury and Mistretta 1981; Bolton et al. 1966; Bruce 1980; García-Piqueras et al. 2019). Additional losses in sensitivity can be caused by diseases that cause peripheral neuropathies (e.g., diabetes mellitus, multiple sclerosis, and diseases of the kidneys, thyroid gland, and liver) (Mueller et al. 2014b) (see also Sect. 3.3).

> **Important** Tactile perception abilities (localization, spatial discrimination, pressure sensation, and the two-point threshold) decrease with age. Distal body regions (hands, feet) are more affected than proximal ones (e.g., lip, abdomen) by these reductions in perceptual abilities. However, some older individuals do not differ from younger individuals in their tactile sensitivity.

3.1.4.2 Vibration

The perception of vibratory stimuli is also associated with age, and this association is stronger for high frequencies compared to lower frequencies (Gescheider et al. 1994; Verrillo 1980; Humes et al. 2009). For high frequencies, perception thresholds increase progressively with age, with an accelerated increase observed in individuals older than 65 years (Gescheider et al. 1994). Conversely, low-frequency vibrations (<40 Hz) appear to be perceived by adults of all ages in a consistent way (Verrillo 1980) (Fig. 3.2).

At a constant frequency, the perceptibility of a stimulus can be improved by increasing the amplitude (intensity) of the vibration. For example, in childhood, at a frequency of 100 Hz, an average amplitude of 5 μm is sufficient for perceptible stimulation on the feet. However, for individuals aged over 70 years, a 10-fold higher amplitude (on average 52 μm) is required (Corso 1971; Cosh 1953). Similarly, at the fingertip, the perception threshold for a frequency of 100 Hz is, on average, 1 μm in young adults and 3–6 μm in individuals aged over 60 years (Lautenbacher et al. 2005).

Causes: There are two predominant influencing factors for the age-associated changes in vibration perception. Firstly, as Pacinian corpuscles mainly register high frequencies, the age-related decrease in sensitivity to high frequencies is hypothesized to be caused by changes in this receptor type. However, histological studies show only minor changes in the number and anatomical structure of the Pacinian corpuscles in older age (García-Piqueras et al. 2019; Cauna and Mannan 1958). Second, changes in vibration perception could occur due to the age-dependent decrease in neuronal conduction and processing speed.

3.1.4.3 Haptic Perception

Haptic perceptual ability also declines with age. However, the deterioration usually occurs later (after age 65, see Fig. 3.3) and less clearly than for tactile perception. For instance, in a study using **haptic comparison tasks**, participants of different ages had to explore several haptic figures and find the one that corresponded to the sample figure, and no differences in accuracy were found between young adults ($M = 18$ years) and middle-aged adults ($M = 41$ years) (Kleinman and Brodzinsky 1978). However, older adults ($M = 76$ years) made more errors than the two younger groups. Similar results have been reported for intermodal comparison tasks, in which a haptically explored figure has to be recognized within visual images (Mueller 2011; Thompson et al. 1965; Kalisch et al. 2012b).

Comparatively, the influence of aging processes on **haptic thresholds** has been much less studied than for haptic comparison tasks. Currently, it is known that haptic sensitivity (**roughness discrimination**) can be largely preserved despite a deterioration in the *tactile* perception threshold (two-point discrimination or

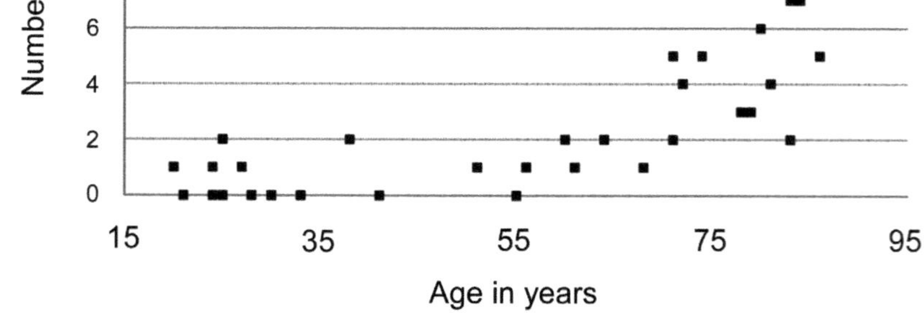

Fig. 3.3 Decline in the recognition of complex haptic figures with age. The number of errors in the Haptic Figures Test increases abruptly from about age 70. These results are based on healthy participants. The age is indicated in years on the *x*-axis. (Graphic: Haptic Research Lab, University of Leipzig)

Grating Orientation Task) (Sathian et al. 1997; Libouton et al. 2010). Roughness discrimination tests are usually performed with sandpaper of different grain sizes. The participants' task consists of actively stroking the fingertip over two pieces of sandpaper and indicating which is rougher and which is smoother.

Two studies examined the absolute haptic threshold (**detection threshold**) in adults between 18 and 50 years of age using the Haptic Threshold Test (Sect. 4.2.3), which measures the limits of haptic detection. It was shown that the age-related changes in the haptic threshold depended on how much the fingertips were used by the individual for exploration in everyday life (Mueller et al. 2014b, 2019). In individuals whose everyday lives did *not* place particular demands on their haptic sensitivity, the haptic perception threshold increased from an average of 8 µm at age 18 to 23 µm at age 50. In contrast, the haptic perception threshold remained stable until at least age 50 in individuals with regular intensive use of the fingertips for haptic perception. (For more on training effects, see Sect. 4.1.1). Regrettably, to date, there are no systematic studies on changes in the absolute haptic threshold in older age groups.

Causes of age-effects on haptic perception: As already described in previous chapters (Sect. 1.1.3), haptic perception places higher demands on cognitive processes than tactile perception because, for haptic perception, the information from receptors of several body areas has to be processed and interpreted. Haptic perception always includes touch information from skin receptors, as well as movement, force, and position information (proprioception) from receptors located in deeper tissues (Halata and Baumann 2008; Symmons et al. 2008). The complex processing required for haptic perception can both compensate and enhance ageing effects. For example, some perceptual processes can be compensated for by proprioceptive information when skin sensitivity declines (due to a decrease in the number of skin receptors). However, declining cognitive abilities due to aging or dementia are the dominant cause for declining haptic perception abilities (Kalisch et al. 2012b) (Sect. 3.3.3). Specifically, older individuals use less systematic search strategies and can hold fewer units of information in their working memory, which makes the haptic recognition of figures and objects more difficult. Further influencing factors on haptic perception include limitations in selective attention, concentration, or motivation (Kleinman and Brodzinsky 1978).

> **Important** Age-related or dementia-related declines in cognitive abilities are the primary cause of declining haptic perceptual abilities.

3.1.4.4 Proprioception

With increasing age, the accuracy of the perception of joint positions decreases, and the perception threshold for movement increases. The intensity of these changes differs between different body regions. Proprioceptive abilities in older age are usually investigated in the legs and feet or the arms and hands.

In the **upper extremities**, older people show limitations in both passive motion detection and joint position perception compared to younger adults. For example, when a wrist is passively and slowly moved, older adults only detect the movement on average after twice the distance compared to younger adults (Wright et al. 2011). Therefore, the threshold for motion detection in the wrist is approximately doubled in older adults. Similar changes have been found for the perception of static joint positions. For example, when participants are asked to place their hand without movement on balls of different sizes, older participants find it more difficult to detect differences in size than younger people (Kalisch et al. 2012a; Norman et al. 2013). In contrast, when exploring balls through active movements of the fingers and hands, older and younger people show no significant differences in ball size perception (Norman et al. 2013). Overall, the proprioceptive ability of the fingers and hands is subject to minimal age-related changes compared to the dramatic changes in tactile thresholds (Kalisch et al. 2012a). That means, the proprioception of actively moved fingers and metacarpals is widely preserved in older adults unless it is limited by musculoskeletal degeneration (e.g., osteoarthritis) (Ferrell et al. 1992; Kokmen et al. 1978).

Age-related changes in upper extremity proprioception are particularly dependent on how much **physical activity** a person engages in during their daily life. For example, older individuals who perform neither whole-body motor activities (e.g., swimming, walking, and dancing) nor fine-motor-demanding hobbies (e.g., model making, needlework, playing a musical instrument) tend to show the poorest performance in proprioceptive tasks. In contrast, physically active older adults with arm-specific hobbies tend to demonstrate similar passive motion detection, precision, and smoothness of active movements as younger people (Adamo et al. 2009).

Another determining factor of older people's proprioception abilities is whether the proprioceptive tasks require **cognitive resources (e.g., memory)**. The relationship between sensory and cognitive performance increases with age. Specifically, declining cognitive resources with age negatively affect sensory processing, and, furthermore, impaired sensory functions (e.g., hearing and vision) complicate cognitive processes. Experiments have shown that older adults find it more difficult than younger people to compensate for limited perceptual abilities. Declining cognitive functions (including processing speed, cognitive flexibility, and sensory integration) especially affect those proprioceptive tasks that require matching different body parts. Therefore, tasks such as "Put the right hand in the same position as the left" or "Please remember and repeat the movement/arm position" are particularly strongly affected by cognitive degeneration (Kalisch et al. 2012b; Adamo et al. 2007).

Balance, stance, and the movement stability of the **lower extremities** require the interplay of visual, vestibular, haptic, and proprioceptive processes. If one or more of these systems is impaired, gait and stance insecurity occurs, which increases the risk of falls. Each of these systems is affected by age-related changes in sensitivity.

With increasing age, the perception of static joint position deteriorates, as does the perception of the motion of the hips (Wingert et al. 2014), knees, and ankles (Petrella et al. 1997; Pai et al. 1997; Kaplan et al. 1985; Ribeiro and Oliveira 2007). The perceptual accuracy of joint position is about 50% lower in older adults (older than 65 years) than in young adults (younger than 30 years). While young adults can perceive joint position deviations of approximately 3.5°, the mean perceived deviation in older adults is approximately 6.5° (Petrella et al. 1997; Kaplan et al. 1985). For these older adults, diseases such as arthritis can additionally contribute to impaired proprioception (Pai et al. 1997).

People who are regularly physically active in old age show fewer propriceptive limitations than inactive older adults (Ribeiro and Oliveira 2007; Pickard et al. 2003). In fact, studies show that the proprioceptive performance of active older adults is significantly better than that of inactive older adults. These findings not only reflect the proverbial phrase "If you don't use it, you lose it" but also highlight the trainability and rehabilitation potential of motor and sensory processes into old age (Sect. 4.1.3).

▶ **Important** Age-related changes in proprioception are mainly dependent on three factors:

- Movement (the perception of static joint positions is usually more impaired than movement perception).
- Cognitive resources (with increasing age, proprioceptive tasks requiring cognitive resources, e.g., memory, are more impaired than other proprioceptive tasks).
- Physical activity (inactive individuals show the most severe proprioceptive impairments).

3.1.4.5 Need for Interpersonal Touch

The need for touch remains unchanged as individuals' age (Routasalo and Isola 1996). Older people appreciate the same forms of touch as younger ones. Accordingly, gentle stroking movements with speeds of 1–10 cm/s (cf. Sect. 1.1.5) are rated as the most pleasant by persons of all ages (Sehlstedt et al. 2016). Furthermore, a perceived lack of touch can lead to a feeling of "skin hunger" at any age. When an individual experiences skin hunger, this means that they begin to value touch more and develop a longing for touch. Prolonged periods of touch deprivation in adulthood and old age can foster feelings of loneliness, isolation, depression, and anxiety which can, in turn, affect sleep and increase drug or alcohol intake. The affected individual may feel stressed, underappreciated, or dissatisfied with personal relationships, while they may not necessarily be aware that they are, in fact, touch deprived.

Particularly in older age, the opportunities for casual touch can be reduced, since family members often live far away (Seilbeck and Langmeyer 2018), and limited physical mobility restricts the individual's daily routine (Hogstel 1985). Social touch from health care professionals that goes beyond nursing or therapeutic indications, can improve physical and psychological well-being, especially in old age. In addition to positive effects on feelings of loneliness, depression, and anxiety, studies have shown that touch is associated with improvements in food intake and medication adherence, as well as a reduction in agitation and aggressive behavior in the context of dementia (For more details, see Sect. 5.5.2).

> **Important** The need for social touch remains the same throughout adulthood but differs between individuals. Young and old people perceive the same types of touch as positive. A perceived lack of touch leads to an increased need for physical contact.

3.1.4.6 Pain

In order to assess the age dependence of pain perception, both the pain threshold (the intensity at which a stimulus is perceived as painful) and pain tolerance (the maximum pain intensity that can be tolerated) can be examined. Through these examinations, studies have observed a continuous increase in the pain threshold to heat from young to older adulthood (Chapman and Jones 1944; Gibson et al. 2003), analogous to changes in other haptic system dimensions. However, pressure and electrical stimuli produce similar pain thresholds in people over 60 years of age as in younger persons.

In contrast, some findings suggest that pain tolerance may be lower in older age. In other words: while sensitivity to mild pain stimuli decreases, higher-intensity pain is less tolerated by older individuals (Lautenbacher et al. 2017). Three age-related factors, which probably influence each other, have been discussed as the cause of lower pain tolerance in older adults:

1. Summation effects (more frequent and prolonged pain in more body sites)
2. Poorer neural filters (declining inhibitory mechanisms) (Cole et al. 2010)
3. Stronger emotional-motivational component (pain is used to attract social and emotional attention) (Lautenbacher 2012)

To date, age-related changes have been studied primarily with pain stimuli that act on the body from the outside (exteroception). In contrast, age-related changes in visceral pain stimuli have been less well studied. However, initial studies suggest that visceral pain sensations may be altered in older individuals (Moore and Clinch 2004). Altered perception of pain stimuli in the internal organs would explain the altered presentation of some medical conditions (e.g., myocardial infarction, gastroduodenal ulcer, and pneumothorax), which can present with little or no pain symptoms in old age (Moore and Clinch 2004). Pain is the most important signal for the detection of pathological processes, meaning that a lack of visceral pain perception can lead to life-threatening clinical consequences. The underlying causes of altered visceral pain perception are unknown to date (Moore and Clinch 2004).

> **Important** With increasing age, more intense stimuli are required to trigger a pain sensation (increase in the pain threshold). However, pain tolerance tends to decrease with age (high-intensity pain is less tolerated). The perception of visceral pain stimuli is also possibly altered in old age.

3.2 Causes of Interindividual Differences in Perceptual Thresholds

The sensitivity of the dimensions of the haptic system varies across individuals. Many of these differences can be explained by age-dependent changes in skin moisture, mechanoreceptor density, nerve conduction velocity, and cognitive maturation and degeneration processes. Nevertheless, even young individuals and individuals within an age group differ greatly in their exteroceptive, interoceptive, and proprioceptive abilities.

Studies examining the haptic system show, without exception, large variance in the haptic abilities across individuals (Mueller and Grunwald 2013). However, the causes of these differences have not yet been conclusively clarified. It is likely that both predisposition (skin characteristics, intelligence, and finger size) and environmental factors (early childhood stimulation, everyday activities, and targeted training) influence haptic, tactile and proprioceptice abilities.

▶ **Important** Human exteroception, proprioception, and interoception are characterized by significant interindividual differences in sensitivity. These differences are caused by predisposition, environmental factors, and aging.

3.2.1 Predisposition

3.2.1.1 Skin Properties

Individuals differ in the properties of their skin. In terms of **tactile perception**, the skin's flexibility and malleability to spatial surfaces and object details play a central role. Specifically, the **skin's flexibility** describes the extent to which the skin penetrates small spaces and the steepness of the skin crater that occurs when a pointed object touches the skin. The skin is more deformable along (parallel to) the papillary grooves than across the grooves.

One previous study reported that, in young adults, up to 50% of the individual variance in tactile thresholds (Grating Domes Sect. 4.2.2) could be explained by the skin's malleability (Vega-Bermudez and Johnson 2004), as individuals with more malleable skin achieved better tactile thresholds. However, in another study, no such effects were found in young adults (Peters et al. 2009).

Interestingly, the skin flexibility is the same in younger and older adults (Vega-Bermudez and Johnson 2004).

The extent to which the skin's flexibility affects **haptic perception** has not yet been investigated. However, skin flexibility likely has only minor relevance for haptic perception. Indeed, during the active exploration of surfaces and object details, stimulus changes, vibration, and acceleration (Meissner and Pacinian corpuscles) are triggered, and receptors with small receptive fields (Merkel cells) are activated. Surface features and object details are, thus, perceived as stimulus changes during a haptic exploration process (e.g., when stroking over a surface). In contrast, *tactile* discrimination requires that surface details deform the skin sufficiently relative to the surrounding surface in order for them to be discriminable as static pressure stimuli.

Comparisons of the flexibility of men's and women's skin have yielded contradictory results (Peters et al. 2009; Woodward 1993). Consequently, it is unclear whether systematic sex differences exist in skin flexibility.

▶ **Important** Skin adaptability to surfaces and object details may explain up to 50% of individual differences in tactile sensitivity. Conversely, haptic sensitivity is much less affected by skin malleability.

3.2.1.2 Finger Size

Another factor that influences tactile sensitivity is the size of the fingertip. A group of researchers showed that a relationship exists between the **finger size and tactile discrimination ability** (Peters et al. 2009; Peters and Goldreich 2013). Accordingly, individuals (both adults and children) with relatively small fingertips show better tactile discrimination performance than individuals with large fingertips. According to the studies' authors, the mechanoreceptors in small fingertips are closer together, allowing for the finer spatial resolution of tactile structures.

Interestingly, for the age range from 6 to 24 years old, opposite effects of finger size and age have been identified. In particular, tactile discrimination ability has been shown to improve from childhood to young adulthood. This is surprising, as finger size also increases with age during childhood, but individuals with larger fingertips show poorer discrimination performance regardless of age (Fig. 3.4). Indeed, the distance between the mechanoreceptors increases with increasing finger size, which worsens the tactile discrimination ability. However, during childhood, while the finger size increases, the maturation processes of the neural system lead to an improvement in the efficiency of the CNS in processing tactile stimuli.

Accordingly, two processes act on tactile perceptual ability in the course of child development into young adulthood, and therefore, only slight improvements in tactile thresholds are usually measured during childhood and adolescence. The two processes are (Peters and Goldreich 2013):

- A continuous deterioration in tactile perceptual ability with increasing finger size
- An improvement in this ability due to cognitive maturation processes

Therefore, to evaluate the effects of finger size on tactile perception, individuals of the same age must be compared.

In contrast to tactile perception, active exploration processes (**haptic perception**) are **most likely not influenced by finger size**. This is because exploratory movements activate several receptors both simultaneously and sequentially. Therefore, the distribution density of mechanoreceptors is less relevant for haptic sensitivity. For this reason, tactile test results should not be used to infer haptic sensitivity (cf. Sect. 1.1.3).

▶ **Important** Due to the smaller distance between mechanoreceptors, individuals with smaller fingertips show better tactile thresholds than individuals with larger fingertips. In contrast, active haptic perception is not influenced by the distribution density of the mechanoreceptors.

3.2.1.3 Intelligence and Education

Fluid intelligence is largely innate and forms the basis of an individual's cognitive capabilities.

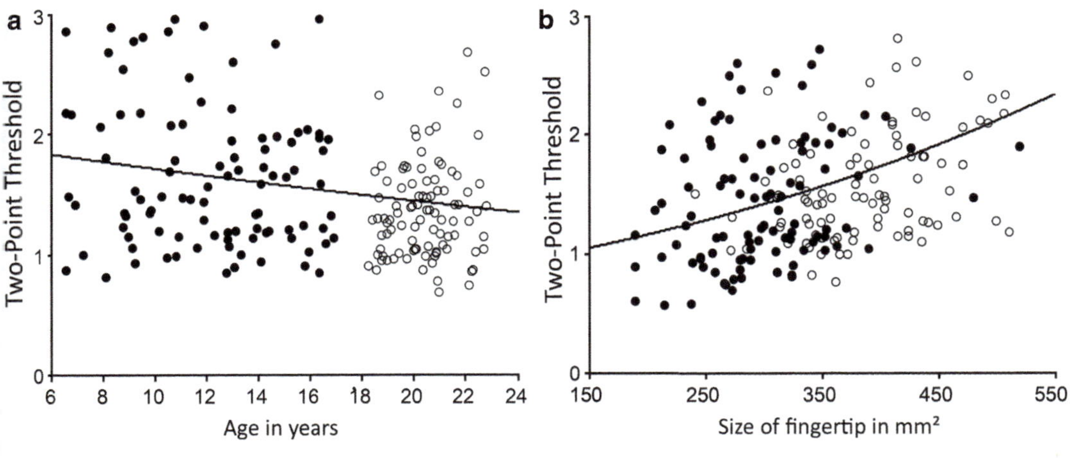

Fig. 3.4 (**a**, **b**) Two-point threshold, age, and finger size. (**a**) The two-point threshold improves from childhood to young adulthood. (**b**) Individuals with larger fingertips show poorer two-point thresholds. On average, both processes (age-related cognitive development and increasing fingertip size) overlap during child development. Therefore, only slight improvements in tactile thresholds are detected during childhood and adolescence. (Figure from Peters and Goldreich 2013)

This type of intelligence comprises information processing speed, reasoning, memory, and concentration skills, and it contributes between 50 and 70% to an individual's performance on intelligence tests. Based on fluid intelligence, crystallized and social intelligence develop through knowledge acquisition and experience, increase with age, and are highly dependent on culture and education.

As mentioned in previous chapters, haptic exploration and recognition tasks require cognitive resources in the form of concentration, working memory, cognitive flexibility, and sensory integration (Sects. 1.1.2 and 3.1.4). Children who show poorer performance in tactile and haptic tasks also tend to show poorer performance in several other skill areas, including language acquisition, memory, learning, reading, visuospatial tasks, and concept formation and categorization tasks (Boll and Berent 1977; Finlayson and Reitan 1976). There is also a strong relationship between tactile and haptic performance and academic achievement (Boll et al. 1978). Consequently, individuals of the same age with different educational achievement levels tend to show significantly different mean haptic thresholds (Mueller and Grunwald 2013; Mueller et al. 2014).

Study results from various tactile, haptic, and proprioceptive tasks indicate a positive correlation between sensory perception and performance in intelligence tests. Accordingly, differences in cognitive ability explain approximately 20% of the interindividual differences in perceptual sensitivity (Li et al. 1998; Stankov et al. 2001).

► **Important** Approximately 20% of individual differences in complex sensory tasks are explained by differences in fluid intelligence (*g*-factor).

3.2.2 Environmental Factors

The development, maturation, and maintenance of human sensory and motor abilities are strongly influenced by the frequency and intensity of the use of these abilities. This process begins in the womb (Sect. 3.1.1) and continues into old age. Consequently, differences in the amount of early childhood stimulation with tactile and haptic stimuli may cause individual differences in sensitivity in adulthood. In addition, individuals differ significantly in the haptic perception demands and opportunities in their daily lives. A frequently cited example for causes of individual differences in haptic perception is the better tactile performance of visually impaired and blind individuals who have learned to read Braille (Grant et al. 2000). Accordingly, the tactile performance of blind individuals is not inherently better than that of sighted individuals. Indeed, blind individuals outperform sighted individuals only in those haptic abilities that they have specifically trained (Heller and Ballesteros 2006; Heller 1991). For example, if sighted individuals practice reading Braille, they can acquire the same tactile discrimination ability as blind Braille readers (Grant et al. 2000). Similar training effects have been shown in professional pianists, whose tactile discrimination ability is superior to that of nonmusical control individuals (Ragert et al. 2004).

Therefore, it can be assumed that individual differences in haptic perception (beyond those explained by age, receptor density, intelligence, or neural disorders; see also Sect. 3.3) are caused by differences in the everyday use of the haptic system (Wong et al. 2013; Mueller et al. 2014b).

These findings of use-dependent changes in haptic performance describe the causes of individual differences but also demonstrate that there is an opportunity for the training and rehabilitation of haptic perception skills. Consequently, individual differences in haptic performance do not have to be accepted as unchangeable. For example, studies have shown that individuals with lower baseline scores can achieve particularly large improvements in haptic perception through training (Wong et al. 2013). Other results show that regular training can reduce the age-related deterioration in haptic sensitivity (Mueller et al. 2014b). (For more details on training, see Sect. 4.1.)

> **Important** Individual differences in haptic sensitivity are influenced by the extent of early childhood stimulation, everyday activities, and targeted training. In addition, several physical diseases, injuries, and disorders can affect the haptic system.

3.3 Disorders of the Haptic System Caused by Lesions and Nervous System Degenerative Diseases

Disturbances in mechanosensation occur when one or more aspects of the haptic system malfunction, fail, or are damaged. Haptic processing disturbances can occur at any point of processing and can have various causes. For example, stimulus detection, information processing, or signal conduction can be impaired, as well as their central integration or the required cognitive resources to process the incoming information. In addition, there may be temporary disturbances in the haptic system, such as due to a lack of attention.

3.3.1 Damage to the Peripheral Nervous System

3.3.1.1 Mechanoreceptors

Changes in tactile and haptic perception, both temporary and permanent, may occur due to lesions of the skin layers. Skin layer lesions may cause the mechanoreceptors in the skin to be destroyed, or the skin's structure, elasticity, or moisture may be altered. For example, calluses, scars, eczema, cuts, or burns can cause local sensory loss. Furthermore, peripheral circulatory disorders and inflammatory processes can lead to (poly)neuropathies. The subsequent changes in the free nerve endings and encapsulated receptors can impair or prevent stimulus detection. These processes can occur in the context of scleroderma (Poncelet and Connolly 2003), Raynaud's syndrome, and rheumatoid arthritis (Puéchal et al. 1995). In addition to haptic and tactile sensitivity limitations, these diseases can lead to declining proprioceptive abilities. For example, patients with rheumatoid arthritis or osteoarthritis may experience decreased proprioceptive sensitivity in the fingers, knees, or hip joints.

3.3.1.2 Peripheral Nerves

Touch sensitivity may also decrease due to degeneration, injury, or compression of peripheral nerves (Masuhr and Neumann 2007). In the upper limbs, carpal tunnel syndrome (CTS) is frequently responsible for such nerve compression injuries. Specifically, CTS is characterized by pressure damage to the median nerve (N. medianus) in the carpal tunnel, which provides sensitive innervation to the radial fingers (thumb, index, middle finger, and half of the ring finger). The pressure damage causes sensory deficits in these areas and reduced nerve conduction velocity.

Stab and cut injuries or transections of the median nerve or the ulnar nerve can also cause sensory and motor deficits in the hands. Similarly, nerve damage in the area of the pelvic girdle or the legs leads to motor, sensory, or vegetative dysfunctions of the genitals and the lower extremities.

In addition, circulatory disturbances can cause ischemic nerve lesions. For example, poor perfusion of the brachial artery can lead to a lesion of the median nerve, which causes sensory deficits in the fingers (Masuhr and Neumann 2007).

If several peripheral nerves are damaged simultaneously, this is called polyneuropathy (PNP). PNP conditions can be hereditary or acquired and are classified as metabolic, toxic, and immunological according to their cause. Different PNPs affect the sensory, motor, and autonomic nerves to different degrees. The symptoms of *sensory PNP* include pain, tingling paresthesias, and spasms. In particular, diabetes mellitus, chronic renal insufficiency, thyroid disorders (hyper- and hypothyroidism), hepatitides, liver cirrhosis, and alcohol dependence are frequently associated with sensory neuropathies. Furthermore, sensory neuropathys can also occur in amyotrophic lateral sclerosis (ALS) (Riancho et al. 2021).

3.3.2 Damage to the Central Nervous System

3.3.2.1 Spinal Cord

The signals from all the mechanoreceptors of the muscles, connective tissues, joints, and skin are projected through the long afferent sensory pathways of the spinal cord via the thalamus to the cortex (Hsiao and Yau 2008). Spinal nerve injuries and compressions may cause distal sensory and motor deficits of the arms, legs, and trunk, depending on the level of spinal cord injury. In addition to lesions caused by trauma, other possible causes include degenerative changes in the spine (e.g., spinal stenosis) and herniated discs.

3.3.2.2 Brain

Damage to any brain regions associated with mechanosensory or touch processing can lead to changes or failures in perception (For details on cortical processing of the haptic system, see Sect. 2.2). Such anatomical or functional impairments may be caused by an aneurysm, inflammation, a tumor, an infarct, or a traumatic injury. Lesions may occur in both cortical and subcortical brain regions. In addition to lesions, degenerative diseases of the central nervous system (e.g., multiple sclerosis, Alzheimer's disease, or Parkinson's disease) and neurodevelopmental disorders (e.g., ADHD, autism spectrum disorder) can lead to impairments of the haptic system. Furthermore, various psychiatric disorders are associated with changes in extero-, intero-, and proprioception, which may be caused by functional processing deficits in the CNS (cf. Sect. 3.4).

Studies with patients who have suffered cortical lesions provide insights into the associated impairments in extero-, intero-, and proprioception:

Lesions of the **primary somatosensory cortex** (SI; postcentral gyrus) caused, for example, by circulatory disorders of the brain (stroke) are usually accompanied by severely altered sensory thresholds in the contralateral side of the body (Capasso et al. 2009; Kolb et al. 1993). As a result, disturbances in vibration detection, temperature perception, and the perception of tactile, haptic, proprioceptive, and pain stimuli may occur. Due to the somatotopic organization of the SI (sensory homunculus, cf. Sect. 2.2.3), sensory impairments of individual body parts (e.g., the hand) may occur, depending on which part of the SI is injured. Sensory deficits caused by lesions in the SI can be similar to the deficits caused by spinal nerve injuries (Capasso et al. 2009).

Lesions of the **parietal cortex** (PC) frequently lead to impairments in the recognition of complex haptic structures. These impairments can affect object recognition, sensory integration processes, as well as the individual's perception of their own body (Kolb et al. 1993). Patients with PC injuries (BA 5 and BA 7) may find it difficult to bring their limbs into the desired position, especially without visual support. These problems most likely result from deficits in integrating the information from the muscles, skin, and joints with the neural body representation (body schema).

Relatedly, PC injuries can also cause a phenomenon called **akinesthesia**, which refers to deficits in the ability to perceive movement and the spatial position of one's limbs. Another group of disorders resulting from PC lesions is **somatosensory agnosia** (e.g., astereognosis/tactile agnosia or asomatognosia). Patients with **astereognosis** are unable to identify objects by touch and active exploration without visual information. This disorder is accompanied by increased perception thresholds and deficits in sensory integration. **Asomatognosia** is the loss of awareness of a body part, and this disorder includes impairments such as the inability to recognize body parts as one's own. The inability to locate and label body parts of one's body is called **autotopagnosia**. Specifically, autotopagnosia is considered a form of body schema disorder and usually occurs in association with dementia or disorientation (Peters 2007). Furthermore, denial of or the inability to perceive one's illness (**anosognosia**) is associated with right ventral parietal lobe dysfunction. Anosognosia often occurs after right-sided strokes in combination with left-sided hemiparesis and neglect.

The characteristic somatosensory deficits associated with parietal cortex injuries are also known as Verger-Dejerine syndrome, which is named after the two French physicians who first described the symptoms at the beginning of the twentieth century (Kolb et al. 1993). Accordingly, parietal lesions usually lead to at least one of three disorder patterns, which may occur independently of each other:

- Elevated perceptual thresholds for tactile, haptic, warmth, and pain stimuli
- Impaired haptic recognition of everyday objects (astereognosis)
- Impairments in spatial orientation and proprioceptive information processing

The effects of lesions are not necessarily permanent, as cortical neurons have considerable functional and morphological plasticity. Damaged functions can also be partially taken over by the other hemisphere.

3.3.3 Advanced Topic: Degenerative Diseases of the CNS (Using the Example of Alzheimer's Dementia and Parkinson's Syndrome)

Degenerative diseases of the nervous system are often accompanied by changes in sensory perception processes. Depending on the neural areas affected, patients show different limitations and perceptual symptoms. For example, some patients with multiple sclerosis show neuropathic pain symptoms in the hands and feet or increased thresholds for vibration stimuli (Khan et al. 2018).

Parkinson's disease and Alzheimer's dementia are discussed below as examples of the perceptual changes that may occur due to degenerative disorders of the CNS.

3.3.3.1 Parkinson's Disease (PD)

Limitations in proprioception, haptic perception, and tactile perception manifest in the early stages of Parkinson's disease (Konczak et al. 2009). Compared to healthy controls, patients show significantly poorer limb position and joint angle perception, passive and active motion perception, tactile-spatial thresholds (grating domes; two-point threshold), roughness discrimination (various textures), and vibration perception (Li et al. 2010; Shin et al. 2005; Konczak et al. 2007; Prätorius et al. 2003; Zia et al. 2000). It is likely that sensory deficits exist many years before the onset of the typical motor symptoms of Parkinson's disease (Hawkes et al. 2010). Therefore, sensory deficits could serve as early diagnostic markers of this disease (Li et al. 2010). However, currently, no reliable test exists to distinguish disease-related from aging-related somatosensory declines due to the large variability in perceptual thresholds between healthy individuals (cf. Sect. 3.1.4).

Of particular interest to research is the declining proprioceptive acuity that occurs due to Parkinson's disease because of the association between proprioceptive acuity with motor changes (Konczak et al. 2009). According to the current research, the deficits experienced by patients with Parkinson's disease in proprioception and haptic sensitivity are caused by deficits in the adequate processing of movement and force information (Konczak et al. 2008; Li et al. 2010). Signals from the motor cortex (descending via the motor pathways) interfere with the ascending sensory signals and cause sensory gating. Specifically, ascending signals from the skin are inhibited by cortical commands, such as movements (e.g., tremors) (Sathian et al. 1997). The inhibition of the signals from the skin causes the brain to interpret them as less intense, resulting in sensory deficits. Another pathological gate-control mechanism occurs in the formatio reticularis (brainstem) (Hawkes et al. 2010). In fact, degenerative processes in the brainstem may be responsible for the deficits in the early stages of Parkinson's disease (i.e., before the motor symptoms appear). The sensory deficits are amplified by the later degeneration of the basal ganglia (Konczak et al. 2012). Currently, it is thought that altered gating, as well as altered multisensory integration, are among the primary pathological mechanisms of Parkinson's disease. Accordingly, the faulty stimulus processing and gating processes in patients could be the cause of many of the observable motor and sensory symptoms (Konczak et al. 2009).

Based on these insights, interventions that train proprioceptive and haptic perception are increasingly used to improve motor processes in patients with Parkinson's disease (Sect. 4.1.3).

A standard therapy for Parkinson's disease is dopamine replacement therapy (DRT), but study findings regarding the effects of DRT on proprioception are contradictory. Some studies suggest that medication elicits an improvement in proprioceptive and haptic perception (Li et al. 2010; Shin et al. 2005). In contrast, other studies have shown that DRT might have adverse effects on proprioception (O'Suilleabhain et al. 2001; Wolpe et al. 2018). For example, in one study, joint position and motion perception were more impaired in the drug ON status compared to the OFF status (O'Suilleabhain et al. 2001).

Whether the implantation of a pulse generator into the brain (deep brain stimulation) to improve motor symptoms also affects sensory perception requires further study. Preliminary findings suggest that detection thresholds for temperature and mechanical skin stimuli may be improved after deep brain stimulation electrode implantation (Cury et al. 2016; Sabourin et al. 2020), and it is also possible that deep brain stimulation may have a positive effect on some proprioceptive processes. Studies suggest that deep brain stimulation is associated with improvements in goal-directed arm movements, reductions in postural sway, and increased postural stability (Lee et al. 2013; Rocchi et al. 2002; Vaugoyeau et al. 2020).

3.3.3.2 Mild Cognitive Impairment and Alzheimer's Dementia

All patients with mild cognitive impairment (MCI), Alzheimer's dementia (AD), or other forms of dementia show deficits in perceptual processes. Current studies aim at finding characteristics and assessment criteria by which patients with different types of dementia can be distinguished from each other and patients with mild cognitive impairment can be distinguished from persons with age-related changes.

For example, static and dynamic balance are more impaired in patients with AD than in healthy controls of the same age (Suttanon et al. 2012; Chong et al. 1999). This likely explains the increased tendency to fall in patients with AD. Distracting stimuli and thoughts further increase the risk of falling due to the impaired cognitive processes in patients with AD.

Furthermore, haptic and tactile perceptual processes are impaired in patients with AD and MCI. In a recent study, healthy elderly controls and patients with MCI (mean age 79.25 years) could be distinuguished through a haptic exploration task and concurrent EEG (brain wave) recordings. The haptic task consisted of exploring deep reliefs and subsequently drawing them (Grunwald et al. 2002a) (cf. Fig. 3.5). During these complex haptic exploration tasks, the theta EEG activity differed between patients with MCI and the healthy control group. Theta activity decreased more in occipital areas in MCI patients than in healthy controls. The authors interpreted this effect to indicate compensatory processes for low cognitive capacity in patients with MCI. During the haptic tasks, patients with MCI required longer mean exploration times and showed lower reproduction quality of deep reliefs than healthy controls. The authors concluded that EEG patterns during complex perceptual (haptic) tests could be used to distinguish between healthy controls and patients with MCI and that this could be used to make a diagnosis.

In a study on tactile perception, participants judged the relative size of angular shapes (bold-reliefs) that were passively pressed against their fingertips (Yang et al. 2010). The participants had to indicate which of two consecutive angles was more acute. Patients with AD showed significantly worse results than patients with MCI. Both patient groups scored significantly worse than healthy controls. The authors assumed that impaired working memory functions are the leading cause of these effects.

In another study, patients and controls successively explored a total of ten simple geometric deep reliefs (e.g., circle, triangle, open and closed squares, and three parallel lines) with one hand and, following each exploration, drew the

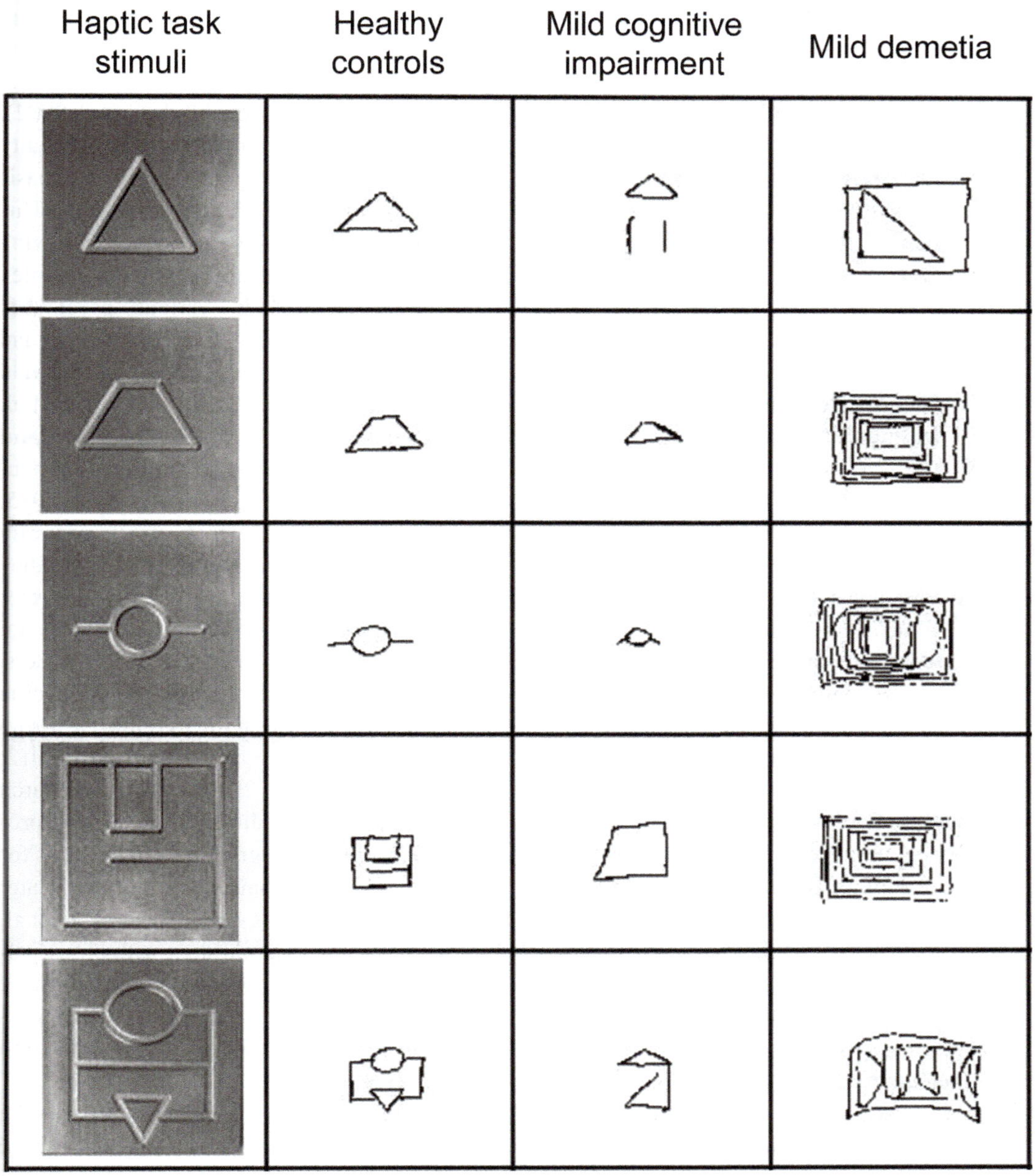

Fig. 3.5 Reproductions of haptically explored deep reliefs. Representative examples of the drawings of one person per group: control group, patients with mild cognitive impairment, and patients with mild dementia. (Figure from Grunwald et al. 2002a)

explored figure with the other hand (Müller et al. 1992). Compared to patients with vascular dementia and healthy controls, AD patients required more time to process each stimulus and made significantly more errors. Especially complex stimuli (three parallel lines, plus signs, and open squares) caused considerable difficulties for both dementia groups (AD and vascular dementia) with more than 60% error rate.

Recognition of haptically explored everyday objects is also deficient in patients with AD (Ballesteros and Reales 2004). Similar to other haptic tasks, impaired object recognition is most likely due to **deficits in memory functions** in patients with AD.

3.4 Disorders of the Haptic System in Psychiatric and Neurodevelopmental Disorders

3.4.1 Impairments of Proprioception, Sensory Integration, and Body Schema in Psychiatric Disorders

Few studies investigate the association between psychiatric disorders and the haptic system; both in clinical practice and research. The existing neuropsychological tests, that assess mechanosensory dimensions (Sect. 4.2), are predominantly used for the assessment of psychomotor development and intelligence assessment; in neurology and neurorehabilitation, these tests are used for status diagnostics and follow-up assessment.

However, for some psychiatric diseases, studies exist on proprioceptive, tactile, and haptic perceptual abilitie; in recent years, psychiatric studies on social touch and interoceptive processes (see Sect. 3.4.3) have also gained attention.

Compered to many other sensory tasks, proprioceptive and haptic exploration tasks are more complex. When touching objects or relief surfaces, sensory information from the skin of the fingertips but also from muscles, joints, and connective tissue must be processed (for more details, see Sect. 1.1.3). Furthermore, to recognize an object, it has to be explored piece by piece, the pieces have to be remembered and subsequently put together into a meaningful whole. This process is called **sensory integration**; which describes the ability to combine sensory information meaningfully. Recently, studies investigate the association between deficits in sensory integration ability and neural body representation with the development and maintenance of neuropsychiatric disorders (including ADHD, schizophrenia, and autism spectrum disorders) (Sheffield et al. 2009; Gadsby 2016, 2017; Yaryura-Tobias et al. 2002). We go a step further and postulate that faulty sensory integration processes may be the basis of most, if not all, psychiatric disorders. This assumption is based on the steadily growing number of studies that show deficits in complex perceptual processes in various psychiatric patient groups (including anorexia nervosa and obsessive-compulsive disorder) (Grunwald et al. 2001a; Mueller et al. 2014a; Shaffer et al. 1985; Karadag et al. 2011). Such **sensory and motor impairments** are also referred to as neurological soft signs (NSS) (Shaffer et al. 1985; Karadag et al. 2011), which occur primarily during multisensory tasks, suggesting that they are based on disturbed sensory integration processes. Strikingly, the occurrence of NSS is not related to specific neurological disorders. Instead, they are likely causing a nonspecific **vulnerability** in children **for psychiatric disorders** (Levit-Binnun and Golland 2012; Ghassemzadeh et al. 2012). Recent research suggests that abnormalities in perceptual processes and sensory integration form the basis for motor and social impairments that may later develop into psychiatric disorders (Hornix et al. 2019). For example, in children with obsessive-compulsive disorder, deficits in visual-motor and fine-motor skills are indicators of the persistence of obsessive-compulsive disorder into adulthood (Bloch et al. 2011).

Sensory integration is not only a prerequisite for successful perceptual processes but also for an adequate **body representation (body schema**; see Sect. 1.4). Like other neuro-cognitive processes, the neural representation of one's body can be disturbed. As a result, affected individuals experience the physical dimensions of their body or its parts distorted or feel body parts do not belong to them (e.g., body dysmorphic disorder, body integrity identity disorder). It is currently unknown whether disorders of sensory integration processes are always accompanied by altered body representation.

> **Important** Studying the body and its haptic/proprioceptive functions can contribute significantly to understanding and treating psychiatric disorders.

Impaired (multi-)sensory integration is currently investigated as a maintaining mechanism for the eating disorder anorexia nervosa. The deficits in sensory processing seem to affect both the perception of the body (e.g., estimation of the size of body parts) and actions performed with the body (e.g., movement sequences, haptic and proprioceptive tasks).

3.4.1.1 Impairments of the Haptic System in Anorexia Nervosa

Anorexia nervosa (AN) is characterized by a refusal to maintain a healthy weight, a fear of gaining weight, and an inability to correctly perceive one's body size (DSM-5, American Psychiatric Association 2018). Generally, 85% of the average weight for the corresponding height is considered clinically relevant (Body Mass Index cut-off value: 17.5). According to current theory, AN is associated with a disturbance of the body schema as well as the body image. (For more information on body schema and body image, see Sects. 1.4 and 1.5 or Grunwald and Mueller 2020). Functional disturbances of the **right parietal cortex** are likely the neurophysiological basis for the impairment of the body schema in anorexia nervosa (Grunwald et al. 2001a; Bär et al. 2015; Pietrini et al. 2011; Mohr et al. 2010). The right posterior parietal cortex (pPC) is associated with multisensory integration processes and spatial perception. The first evidence for an impairment of right parieto-occipital brain regions in anorexia nervosa was provided by EEG-measurements during haptic exploration tasks (Grunwald et al. 2001a, b), thus confirming the hypothesis that the pPC plays a central role in the impaired processing of the body schema. The researchers showed that test procedures that posed particular demands on the right parietal cortex were impaired in the patients with AN but not healthy controls. Tasks that place demands on haptic dimensions are particularly likely to tax the parietal cortex. Accordingly, patients with anorexia nervosa show impaired performance in proprioceptive (Grunwald et al. 2002b) and haptic tasks (Grunwald et al. 2001b; Nico et al. 2010; Gadsby 2017) as well as in the execution of movement sequences and action control (Guardia et al. 2012; Keizer et al. 2013; Metral et al. 2014). In EEG studies, patients with AN had lower theta activity over right parietal areas than healthy controls (Grunwald et al. 2001a, 2004b). The altered theta activity persisted after weight gain and discharge from the hospital.

The tasks of the studies included exploring unknown geometric deep reliefs and a proprioceptive test (angle paradigm: Haptimeter Sect. 4.2.4). During the processing of the deep reliefs (haptic exploration and subsequent drawing of the figure), AN showed significantly worse reproductions than healthy controls (Grunwald et al. 2001b). Reproductions remained poor even **after weight gain and normalization of body mass index** (BMI). The authors highlight the heterogeneity in the quality of the reproductions among AN patients and call for more in-depth analyses to determine the prognostic value of this heterogeneity for disease progression and treatment outcome. A recent study found similar deficits in haptic perception of deep reliefs in individuals with **obesity** compared with normal-weight individuals (Gambino et al. 2020). This finding raises the question if impairments in sensory integration and parietal brain regions may be involved in the development of obesity.

The inadequate body perception remains unchanged in patients with AN even after repeated psychotherapeutic interventions (Grunwald 2008; Grunwald et al. 2004a). Therefore, it can be assumed that body schema disturbances are a central factor for the chronification and maintenance of anorexia nervosa (Grunwald and Mueller 2020).

Based on their findings, Grunwald and his colleagues developed a therapeutic approach, which is currently tested in various clinics. In this approach, patients with AN wear customized neoprene suits, that stimulate the body's surface with each movement. This may increase the patients' body awareness and help them integrate their actual spatial dimensions (details in Grunwald and Weiss 2005). Replications of the case study are pending.

3.4.2 Tactile Defensiveness and the Haptic System in Neurodevelopmental Disorders

Neurodevelopmental disorders comprise a group of syndromes (DSM-5, American Psychiatric Association 2018) in which the development of the central nervous system is impaired (Cascio 2010). The term is used for developmental brain disorders that are genetic (e.g., fragile X syndrome) or acquired (e.g., fetal alcohol syndrome; infantile cerebral palsy). In addition, the term includes disorders in which only individual aspects of neurocognitive development are impaired, resulting in neuropsychiatric disorders, motor disorders, language or learning difficulties (e.g., ADHD, autism spectrum disorders, dyslexia) (Bishop 2010).

▶ **Definition** According to the definition in DSM 5 (American Psychiatric Association 2018), **neurodevelopmental disorders** include:
- Intellectual Impairment
- Communication Disorders
- Autism Spectrum Disorder
- Attention Deficit/Hyperactivity Disorder
- Specific Learning Disorders
- Motor Disorders
- Tic Disorders

3.4.2.1 Somatosensory Processing

Perceptual abilities have rarely been analyzed in past studies of neurodevelopmental disorders (Cascio 2010). However, an increasing number of recent studies suggest **both altered perceptual abilities and altered behavioral responses to sensory input** in individuals with neurodevelopmental disorders. Among the most commonly reported difficulties are haptic/tactile recognition and unusual affective responses to mechanosensory stimuli, which vary in severity among different patient groups.

In practice, the diagnostic focus has been primarily on motor, language, and social skills. However, it must be kept in mind that these skills develop during early childhood, while the brain abnormalities that underlie neurodevelopmental disorders usually develop much earlier, usually during embryonic and fetal development. Therefore, current research efforts seek to evaluate in how far impairments in perceptual processes (including sensory integration, cortical inhibition/filtering, and emotional appraisal) are associated with the development of motor, language, and social disorders (Thye et al. 2018). Such considerations are based on modern advancements of sensory integration theory introduced by Jean Ayres (Ayres and Marr 1998; Karch and Freitag 2017) and on the findings of animal or human deprivation studies (Harlow 1958; Spitz 1949). Social touch and somatosensory perceptual processes are critical for the healthy **psychomotor development** of a child (cf. Chap. 7), including the development of social, cognitive, communication (verbal and nonverbal), and motor skills (Grunwald 2017; Harlow 1958; Spitz 1949). Therefore, impaired somatosensory processing is likely to hinder psychomotor development.

In the case of severe impairments, these are usually diagnosed during regular examinations in infancy or toddlerhood and subsequently treated with early childhood special education and occupational therapy. However, mild or moderate impairments may be overlooked in the early years of life and remain undiagnosed. Therefore, in order to detect mild and moderate impairments as early as possible, somatosensory processing should be tested in infancy.

▶ **Important** Young children with impaired sensory processing typically show developmental delays in fine and gross motor skills, impaired balance and coordination. Furthermore, these children are often highly distractible, show tactile defensiveness, and have language and visuospatial difficulties (Eeles et al. 2013).

Reliable detection of sensorimotor disorders in infancy and early childhood requires standardized assessment of both motor and sensory abilities. Several procedures are available to assess psychomotor skills in early childhood, but these generally do *not* include sensory skills (Eeles et al. 2013). That means, as of yet, the **sensitivity of the haptic system and somatosensory processing** are not part of standard early childhood assessments.

Because very young children are not capable of following instructions, measuring perceptual abilities is difficult, and, therefore, only the children's reactions to certain stimuli can be observed. **Sensory reactivity differences** are particularly indicative of developmental disorders an can be tested in early childhood. Unusual responses to tactile, haptic, and touch stimuli are reported by parents of children with a wide variety of neurodevelopmental disorders, including Autism Spectrum Disorder, ADHD, Fragile X Syndrome, Infantile Cerebral Palsy, and Early Childhood Sensory Deprivation (Rogers et al. 2003; Tomchek and Dunn 2007; Mangeot et al. 2001). **Sensory reactivity differences** are characterized by Baranek et al. (1997):

- **Hyperreactivity:** Very strong reaction to stimuli of low intensity, hardly any habituation to persistent stimuli. Avoidant and rejecting behaviors may occur (see tactile defensiveness).
- **Hyporeactivity:** Low or absent response to strong stimuli, e.g., heat, cold, pain stimuli.
- **Sensation Seeking:** Unusual stimuli are perceived as pleasant, are brought about, and constantly repeated, e.g., rubbing against or tapping on textures, intense squeezing or hugging (see weighted vests/blankets Sect. 8.3.8).

To assess sensory reactivity one standardized test (Test of Sensory Functions in Infants) (DeGangi and Greenspan 1989) is available and two questionnaires (Sensory Profile) that have to be filled out by primary caregivers (Dunn 2017; Provost and Oetter 1994):

The **Test of Sensory Functions in Infants** consists of 24 items to be administered in interaction with the infant (DeGangi and Greenspan 1989). Visual-haptic integration exercises, vestibular stimulation, oculomotor control, and touch of various materials are performed with the child. While performing the tests, the medical professional observes if any unusual behaviors occur. Expectably, the retest reliability of the test is medium, and the test's objectivity is weak, as the assessment depends on the subjective evaluation of the person performing the test. Assessment results should therefore be interpreted with caution and not used as the sole diagnostic criterion (Jirikowic et al. 1997).

Sensory processing disorders in infants, young children, and elementary school children can also be assessed by interviewing parents or caregivers (Sensory Profile questionnaire) (Dunn 2017). (A self-assessment questionnaire exists for adults.) The "**sensory profile**" records the extent to which sensory processing disorders occur in everyday life and whether everyday activities and social contacts are impaired. It has to be considered that only the behavior—a person's reactions—can be recorded through interviews or self-assessments but not their perceptual abilities or sensory threholds (see later in this chapter: 'sensory perception ability' and Sect. 4.2.1. Clinical diagnostic test procedures).

3.4.2.2 Tactile Defensiveness

One commonly reported behavior in children with neurodevelopmental disorders is tactile defensiveness.

▶ **Definition Tactile defensiveness** describes an unusual hypersensitivity, hyperreactivity, and aversion to non-harmful social touch or other tactile events (e.g., certain clothing or materials), or rejection of food because of its texture (Smith et al. 2020). In practice, children who are hypersensitive to tactile-haptic stimuli often also show aversive behavior to other sensory stimuli (including visual and auditory).

As described in the definition, tactile defensiveness is closely associated with **hyperreactivity**. Studies indicate that there is also a close association with feelings of anxiety, as well as stereotypic and oppositional behaviors. In other words, these children not just react to unpleasant stimuli but also try to prevent or avoid them by exhibiting stereotypic behaviors (e.g., preference for certain clothing or food). In a study on children with autism spectrum disorders (ASD) and other neurodevelopmental disorders, those children who responded with strong tactile defensiveness also exhibited more inflexible and repetitive behaviors, such as repetitive speech acts, evasive eye movements, and preference for certain clothing (Baranek et al. 1997).

Other studies indicate that motor stereotypies are also related to **sensory hypersensitivity** and strong avoidance behaviors (Joosten et al. 2009; Joosten and Bundy 2010). In these studies, children with autism and intellectual impairment used stereotypic behaviors to **relieve feelings of anxiety and fear**. The results provide empirical evidence to support the notion that anxiety, fear, and challenging behaviors in children with developmental disabilities may be explained in part by sensory hypersensitivity.

Similarly, in children with ADHD, hyperreactivity may be related to the severity of **hyperactivity.** Tactile defensiveness in individuals with ADHD may also be related to genetic factors, comorbid anxiety disorder (Cascio 2010), or comorbid **oppositional defiant disorder** (Ghanizadeh 2008, 2011). Accordingly, the frequency of oppositional behaviors in children with ADHD is related to tactile hypersensitivity. Tactile hypersensitivity is *not* related to sex or ADHD subtypes.

> ▶ **Important** Severe sensory processing disorders are associated with anxiety disorders and challenging behaviors (e.g., tactile defensiveness, motor stereotypies, and oppositional behavior disorder) in children with neurodevelopmental disorders. Sensory hypersensitivity and the resulting sensory overload are likely the cause of challenging behaviors.

Rejection behavior toward tactile stimuli and touch can occur as early as infancy (Mammen et al. 2015). Studies suggest that infants' responses to tactile stimuli may provide important clues to identify children at high risk for neurodevelopmental disorders. For example, in one study, the extent of tactile defensiveness at 9 months of age predicted the **severity of impairment in social and communication skills** at 18 months of age (Mammen et al. 2015).

The link between sensory processing disorders and developmental impairments is likely determined by a self-perpetuating cycle (Thye et al. 2018). For instance, children's defensive behavior may lead to insecurity in primary caregivers, resulting in less social touch and impeding the development of secure attachment. Lack of touch and **insecure attachment** are, in turn, related to behavioral problems, anxiety, depression, and impaired self-esteem. Additionally, there is evidence of **decreased oxytocin levels** in individuals with autism spectrum disorders (ASD) (Gregory et al. 2009; Modahl et al. 1998). Oxytocin promotes that touch is perceived as pleasant and that individuals seek physical contact (cf. Sect. 2.4.1). If oxytocin is lacking, these processes do not occur, and children seek less physical contact. Consequently, it is more difficult to build social bonds, and fewer social situations occur in which the affected children can practice social and communicative skills. (For touch intervention in ASD, see Sect. 8.3.8.)

3.4.2.3 Sensory Thresholds of Persons with Hypo- or Hyperreactivity

In everyday life, it may seem like individuals with hyperreactivity and tactile defensiveness have superior perceptual abilities. Conversely, hyporeactivity is often assumed to be associated with lower sensitivity (Güçlü et al. 2007). As mentioned earlier in this chapter (Sect. 3.4.2), the majority of studies on "sensory processing disorder" are based on parental interviews about the children or self-assessments in adults. These data do not allow any conclusions about the sensory abilities of the individuals concerned. Furthermore, standard tests for children that measure sensory perception are normed for children from 3 to 4 years of age (SIPT and TAKIWA, cf. Sect. 4.2.1). Testing younger children's perceptual abilities is not feasible because children younger than 3 years old are not mature enough to follow the instructions due to the complexity of the tests.

Scientific studies on touch perception in children and adults with neurodevelopmental disorders show contradictory results. For example, no difference in vibrotactile perception thresholds was found in boys (ages 8–12 years) with **autism spectrum disorder (ASD)** compared to boys without ASD (Güçlü et al. 2007). However, adults with ASD show a significantly lower detection threshold for vibrotactile stimuli (33 Hz) at the forearm than adults without ASD (Cascio et al. 2008). In contrast, stimulus detection on the hand, was the same in adults with and without ASD. In another study, adults with Asperger syndrome had a significantly lower detection threshold than neurotypical adults at high frequencies (200 Hz) at the fingertip but not at low frequencies (30 Hz) (Blakemore et al. 2006).

The roughness of sandpaper and the light pressure stimuli provided by von Frey filaments (cf. Sect. 1.1.1) can be perceived equally by children with and without ASD (O'Riordan and Passetti 2006). Adults with and without ASD also showed no differences in the detection of light pressure stimuli (von-Frey filaments), temperature changes (punctual warm-cold stimuli), or adaptation to tactile stimuli (Cascio et al. 2008).

Other studies found higher sensitivity (von-Frey monofilament) on the face but not the hand in children with ASD, but impaired proprioception (Riquelme et al. 2016).

During painful heat and cold stimuli, adults with ASD showed significantly lower pain thresholds (heat: 43.6 °C; cold: 16.7 °C) than adults without ASD (heat: 46.6 °C; cold: 9.0 °C) (Cascio et al. 2008). Similarly, children with ASD showed lower pain thresholds to pressure stimuli (Riquelme et al. 2016).

On **complex tactile and haptic tests**, such as Sensory Integration and Practice Test (Siaperas et al. 2012; Roley et al. 2015), Luria-Nebraska Tactile Scale (Abu-Dahab et al. 2013) and Halstead-Reitan Neuropsychological Test Battery (cf. Sect. 4.2.1), individuals with ASD usually score lower than controls (Minshew and Hobson 2008). There was no association between the test performance of individuals with ASD and their self-rated or externally rated hyper- or hyposensitivity (Minshew and Hobson 2008). Another study found that individuals with ASD who rated themselves highly sensitive performed *worse* in proprioceptive tests (e.g., lower precision in adopting a specific angle with the elbow) than neurotypical controls (Fuentes et al. 2011).

To date, it is unclear what mechanisms underlie these effects. Some authors argue that contradictory effects could be explained by the heterogeneity of ASD subtypes, as well as deficits in motor functions and reaction speed (Zetler et al. 2019). In addition, the hyper- and hyposensitivity could be related to an altered emotional or cognitive evaluation of the stimuli (Cascio 2010; Smirni et al. 2019). That is, pain stimuli, for example, may be evaluated more emotionally/anxiously by individuals with ASD than by neurotypical individuals.

Imaging studies also suggest that individuals with ASD show lower activation in brain regions involved in processing social-emotional information than neurotypical individuals. This has previously been shown for visual, auditory, and C-tactile stimuli (Kaiser et al. 2016; Yang et al. 2015). For example, when individuals with ASD are stroked on the forearm with a soft brush, the insula on both sides, right amygdala, and ventrolateral prefrontal cortex are less active than in individuals without ASD. The authors interpreted the findings as evidence that stroking stimulates fewer social associations in individuals with ASD than in participants without ASD. However, despite the difference in brain activation, individuals with and without ASD rated the stroking stimuli equally pleasurable (Kaiser et al. 2016).

Children with **attention deficit hyperactivity disorder (ADHD)** predominantly perform worse on tactile tests than children without ADHD. This is true both for simple detection thresholds (He et al. 2021; Puts et al. 2017) and for more complex tasks such as subtests of the Sensory Integration and Practice Test (SIPT) (Parush et al. 1997, 2007). For example, in one study, children with ADHD scored worse than the control group without ADHD on all subtests of the SIPT: Impaired were proprioception (finger is passively moved, thereupon actively repeat the movement), graphesthesia (letters or digits are 'written' on palm and are to be named), point localization (show place that was touched), finger identification (show which finger was touched), shape recognition I (palpated 3D figure must be identified on visual display), shape recognition II (twin of a palpated 3D figure must be palpated from a selection) (Parush et al. 2007). However, children with ADHD who scored high in **hyperreactivity and tactile defensiveness** did not differ in SIPT performance from children with ADHD without tactile defensiveness (Parush et al. 2007). Nevertheless, the group with high scores in hyperreactivity and tactile defensiveness showed increased somatosensory evoked potentials (EEG measurement) over frontal and parieto-central areas (somatosensory cortex). These results suggest that tactile hyperreactivity is related to the cortical processing of somatosensory information but not to impaired sensory perception (Parush et al. 2007; Cascio 2010). That is, tactile hyperreactivity likely arises from **cognitive or affective evaluations**—similar to patients with ASD. In contrast, impaired sensory perception can occur both in ADHD with and without tactile hyperreactivity.

Compared to individuals without ADHD, individuals with ADHD also have reduced pain threshold and pain tolerance (Treister et al. 2015). Interestingly, this effect is partially reversed by Ritalin use: with Ritalin, pain threshold and pain tolerance increased significantly in patients with ADHD but remained lower than that of the control group.

> **Important** To date, there is no evidence that hyper- or hyporeactivity reflect the actual sensory sensitivity of an indivisual. Instead, hyperreactivity and tactile defensiveness are likely caused by cognitive and affective evaluation processes. That means, hyperreactivity is not an indication of increased sensory abilities; on the contrary, "high sensitivity" in neurodevelopmental disorders is often accompanied by impaired sensory performance (impaired perceptual processes).

3.4.3 Interoception (Psychosomatics)

Processes inside the body (e.g., heartbeat, respiration, digestion, and hunger) cause sensory afferents that may be consciously perceived (see also Sect. 1.2). Two aspects of perception can be considered (Cameron 2001):

- The sensory detection (awareness)
- The accuracy of perception (accuracy)

Individuals differ significantly in their interoception ability. These differences are due to the individual's characteristics, the situation, conditioning and training effects, and the measurement method. The interoceptive process most commonly used to study interoceptive ability is the heartbeat. This can produce very different results depending on the **method of investigation**. For example, some individuals may be able to perceive that their heart is beating stronger or weaker depending on the situation (awareness) but are unable to distinguish or count individual heartbeats with confidence (accuracy). In most recent studies, therefore, an attempt is made to objectively measure the accuracy of the detection ability by measuring the pulse and having the person press a button for each alleged heartbeat (Schandry and Weitkunat 1990).

Person characteristics that may influence the ability to correctly perceive heartbeats are age, BMI, and fitness (Cameron 2001). Leaner and more physically fit individuals, as well as younger individuals, tend to show better heartbeat detection ability. The effect of age may be conditioned by BMI and fitness, as increasing age is often associated with decreasing fitness and higher body weight. Accordingly, due to a higher proportion of body fat, the transmission of the vibration triggered by heartbeats may be attenuated (Cameron 2001). On the other hand, it has been found that not only extremely overweight but also severely underweight (anorexia nervosa) persons show impaired interoception (see later in this chapter) (Herbert and Pollatos 2014; Pollatos et al. 2008).

In addition, **situational influences** can alter detection ability, such as body position, emotional states, and physical activity. For example, most individuals perceive their heartbeat best when lying down, moderately well when sitting, and least well when standing. Physical activity can substantially increase cardiac interoception. Emotional states (e.g., anxiety) can also increase awareness of the heartbeat.

> **Important** Interoception ability varies from individual to individual and can be altered by situational influences. It depends on both physical and psychological factors.

However, training and conditioning effects generate the most interesting individual differences in interoception. They can influence both the organ functions themselves and their detection ability. Through classical conditioning, organ functions can be coupled to stimuli that typically do not affect visceral functions. Pavlov's typical example of classical conditioning (salivation in a dog is triggered by a bell that was previously sounded coupled with food) testifies to this possibility very clearly. Such conditioning effects can contribute to the **emergence and maintenance of various psychosomatic disorders** (e.g., chronic pain, see Sect. 1.2.4). In contrast, conditioning of health-promoting processes is also possible (Gannon 1977; Miller 1969), for example in the form of biofeedback training (e.g., lowering blood pressure utilizing biofeedback).

In addition, interoceptive skills can be trained, for example, repeatedly focusing attention on visceral processes can improve the accuracy of detection skills. Feedback can further enhance the effects (Schandry and Weitkunat 1990; Meyerholz et al. 2019). If interoceptive skills are impaired, interoception training can reduce symptoms of various disorders in the short term (e.g., somatoform disorder) (Schaefer et al. 2014). Interoceptive ability may also improve through repeatedly adopting certain postures ("power posing"; cf. Sect. 5.4). In a study with healthy participants, after 1 week of daily "power posing" interoceptive detection and accuracy improved (Weineck et al. 2019). However, it is currently unclear whether this can affect preexisting psychological or psychosomatic illnesses (see below).

3.4.3.1 Increased vs. Impaired Interoceptive Ability

Interoceptive processes are closely related to cortical evaluation processes (emotion, cognition; cf. Sect. 2.2.3). I.e., every stimulus that arises inside the body can influence behavior. For example, a full bladder may trigger going to the toilet, breathlessness may trigger taking a break during sports, and unfamiliar sensations can trigger concern or even fear. For this reason, the relevance of interoception for the development of psychosomatic disorders is increasingly studied (Cameron 2001).

The origins of the study of interoception go back to writings by William James in the late nineteenth century on the emergence of emotions (James 1884). According to his writings, emotions are directly tied to the presence and perception of physical states (Schandry 1981). According to this hypothesis, visceral (e.g., heart rate) and physical changes (e.g., posture, facial expression) need to occur and need to be perceived in order for a person to feel emotions. Therefore, if the visceral or bodily expression were prevented or if the perception of the processes (i.e., interoception) were impaired, no emotion or only attenuated emotion should occur. On the other hand, people with stronger interoception should feel emotions more intensely.

Accordingly, studies investigated whether individuals who differ in their natural emotionality also differ in their interoceptive ability. Studies on the accuracy of heart rate perception support this assumption: higher accuracy of perception goes hand in hand with **stronger emotional lability and situational anxiety** (state anxiety) (Schandry 1981). Beyond the natural variance in emotionality, the interoceptive ability is associated with various psychiatric, psychosomatic, and developmental disorders.

For example, the development and maintenance of somatic symptom disorder (formerly known as "somatization disorder" or "somatoform disorder") is closely related to the perception and evaluation of physical processes (Schaefer et al. 2014). However, findings on interoception in patients with somatic symptom disorder are contradictory: While some studies report high interoceptive accuracy, other studies show impaired interoceptive abilities. Meanwhile, heterogeneous patient groups are thought to have led to the contradictory results: until 2018, **hypochondria** (fear of suffering from a severe illness) was classified as part of somatoform disorders (ICD 10). Therefore, older studies on interoception in somatoform disorders often include patients with hypochondriasis. This is relevant because individuals with hypochondriasis perceive interoceptive processes *more* accurately than individuals with other somatoform disorders (e.g., Pollatos et al. 2007; Domschke et al. 2010). In the current ICD-11 classification guidelines, hypochondriasis is classified as an anxiety disorder or obsessive-compulsive disorder. Increased interoception accuracy is also reported for patients with **anxiety and panic disorders** (Ehlers and Breuer 1992; Schandry 1981). In contrast, patients with a specific phobia seem to have normal interoception.

On the other hand, individuals with **somatic symptom disorders** (without illness anxiety) tend to have *impaired* interoception. There is evidence that more severe disorder manifestation is associated with more impaired heartbeat detection (Schaefer et al. 2012).

Patients with **depression** have also been repeatedly found to have lower interoceptive accuracy (Pollatos et al. 2009; Eggart et al. 2019).

Impairments in interoception have also been reported for patients with various **eating disorders**. Accordingly, in overweight or obese individuals, the BMI level correlates with interoception impairment (Herbert and Pollatos 2014). Also, in patients with anorexia nervosa (AN), impairments in both sensory detection (awareness) (Fassino et al. 2004) and perception accuracy have been reported (Pollatos et al. 2008). The accuracy of perception may be explained by comorbid depression or anxiety disorder. In a sample of AN patients without depression or anxiety, no differences in interoceptive accuracy were found compared to the healthy control group (Kinnaird et al. 2020). Similarly, in patients with bulimia nervosa (BN), detection seems to be impaired, but not the accuracy of perception (Pollatos and Georgiou 2016). Therefore, impairments in interoceptive accuracy could be explained by BMI, comorbid depression, and anxiety disorders in patients with BN.

► **Important** Interoception is increased in anxiety disorders, panic disorders, and hypochondria; but impaired in somatic symptom disorders, depression, and eating disorders.

References

Abu-Dahab SMN, Skidmore ER, Holm MB, Rogers JC, Minshew NJ. Motor and tactile-perceptual skill differences between individuals with high-functioning autism and typically developing individuals ages 5-21. J Autism Dev Disord. 2013;43(10):2241–8. https://doi.org/10.1007/s10803-011-1439-y.

Adamo DE, Martin BJ, Brown SH. Age-related differences in upper limb proprioceptive acuity. Perceptual Motor Skills. 2007;104(3 Pt 2):1297–309. https://doi.org/10.2466/pms.104.4.1297-1309.

Adamo DE, Alexander NB, Brown SH. The influence of age and physical activity on upper limb proprioceptive ability. J Aging Phys Act. 2009;17(3):272–93. https://doi.org/10.1123/japa.17.3.272.

Ainsworth MDS. Deprivation of maternal care. A reassessment of its effects. Geneva: World Health Organization (Public Health Papers, 14); 1962.

American Psychiatric Association. Diagnostisches und statistisches Manual psychischer Störungen DSM-5. 2. korrigierte Auflage. Göttingen: Hogrefe; 2018.

Ayres JA, Marr DB. Sensorische Integrations- und Praxisteste. In: Fisher AG, Murray EA, Bundy AC, editors. Sensorische Integrationstherapie. 1. Aufl. Berlin: Springer; 1998. p. 383–407.

Ballesteros S, Reales JM. Intact haptic priming in normal aging and Alzheimer's disease: evidence for dissociable memory systems. Neuropsychologia.

2004;42(8):1063–70. https://doi.org/10.1016/j.neuropsychologia.2003.12.008.
Bär K-J, de La Cruz F, Berger S, Schultz CC, Wagner G. Structural and functional differences in the cingulate cortex relate to disease severity in anorexia nervosa. J Psychiatry Neurosci. 2015;40(4):269–79. https://doi.org/10.1503/jpn.140193.
Baranek GT, Foster LG, Berkson G. Tactile defensiveness and stereotyped behaviors. Am J Occup Ther. 1997;51(2):91–5. https://doi.org/10.5014/ajot.51.2.91.
Bishop DVM. Which neurodevelopmental disorders get researched and why? PLoS One. 2010;5(11):e15112. https://doi.org/10.1371/journal.pone.0015112.
Blakemore S-J, Tavassoli T, Calò S, Thomas RM, Catmur C, Frith U, Haggard P. Tactile sensitivity in Asperger syndrome. Brain Cogn. 2006;61(1):5–13. https://doi.org/10.1016/j.bandc.2005.12.013.
Bleyenheuft Y, Cols C, Arnould C, Thonnard J-L. Age-related changes in tactile spatial resolution from 6 to 16 years old. Somatosens Motor Res. 2006;23(3–4):83–7. https://doi.org/10.1080/08990220600816440.
Bloch MH, Sukhodolsky DG, Dombrowski PA, Panza KE, Craiglow BG, Landeros-Weisenberger A, et al. Poor fine-motor and visuospatial skills predict persistence of pediatric-onset obsessive-compulsive disorder into adulthood. J Child Psychol Psychiatry Allied Discip. 2011;52(9):974–83. https://doi.org/10.1111/j.1469-7610.2010.02366.x.
Boll TJ, Berent S. Tactile-perceptual functioning as a factor in general psychological abilities. Percept Motor Skills. 1977;44(2):535–9. https://doi.org/10.2466/pms.1977.44.2.535.
Boll TJ, Richards H, Berent S. Tactile-perceptual functioning and academic performance in brain-impaired and unimpaired children. Percept Motor Skills. 1978;47(2):491–5. https://doi.org/10.2466/pms.1978.47.2.491.
Bolton CF, Winkelmann RK, Dyck PJ. A quantitative study of Meissner's corpuscles in man. Neurology. 1966;16(1):1–9. https://doi.org/10.1212/wnl.16.1.1.
Bos KJ, Fox N, Zeanah CH, Iii N, Charles A. Effects of early psychosocial deprivation on the development of memory and executive function. Front Behav Neurosci. 2009;3:16. https://doi.org/10.3389/neuro.08.016.2009.
Bos K, Zeanah CH, Fox NA, Drury SS, McLaughlin KA, Nelson CA. Psychiatric outcomes in young children with a history of institutionalization. Harv Rev Psychiatry. 2011;19(1):15–24. https://doi.org/10.3109/10673229.2011.549773.
Bradley RM, Mistretta CM. Fetal sensory receptors. Physiol Rev. 1975;55(3):352–82. https://doi.org/10.1152/physrev.1975.55.3.352.
Bruce MF. The relation of tactile thresholds to histology in the fingers of elderly people. J Neurol Neurosurg Psychiatry. 1980;43(8):730–4. https://doi.org/10.1136/jnnp.43.8.730.
Bystrova K. Novel mechanism of human fetal growth regulation: a potential role of lanugo, vernix caseosa and a second tactile system of unmyelinated low-threshold C-afferents. Med Hypotheses. 2009;72(2):143–6. https://doi.org/10.1016/j.mehy.2008.09.033.
Cameron OG. Interoception: the inside story--a model for psychosomatic processes. Psychosom Med. 2001;63(5):697–710. https://doi.org/10.1097/00006842-200109000-00001.
Capasso M, Manzoli C, Ciccocioppo F, Caulo M, Uncini A. A misleading sensory level. J Neurol. 2009;256(10):1769–70. https://doi.org/10.1007/s00415-009-5199-y.
Cascio CJ. Somatosensory processing in neurodevelopmental disorders. J Neurodev Disord. 2010;2(2):62–9. https://doi.org/10.1007/s11689-010-9046-3.
Cascio C, McGlone F, Folger S, Tannan V, Baranek G, Pelphrey KA, Essick G. Tactile perception in adults with autism: a multidimensional psychophysical study. J Autism Dev Disord. 2008;38(1):127–37. https://doi.org/10.1007/s10803-007-0370-8.
Cascio CJ, Moore D, McGlone F. Social touch and human development. Dev Cogn Neurosci. 2019;35:5–11. https://doi.org/10.1016/j.dcn.2018.04.009.
Cauna N, Mannan G. The structure of human digital pacinian corpuscles (corpus cula lamellosa) and its functional significance. J Anat. 1958;92(1):1–20.
Chapman WP, Jones CM. Variations in cutaneous and visceral pain sensitivity in normal subjects. J Clin Investig. 1944;23(1):81–91. https://doi.org/10.1172/JCI101475.
Chong RK, Horak FB, Frank J, Kaye J. Sensory organization for balance: specific deficits in Alzheimer's but not in Parkinson's disease. J Gerontol A Biol Sci Med Sci. 1999;54(3):122–8. https://doi.org/10.1093/gerona/54.3.m122.
Cole LJ, Farrell MJ, Gibson SJ, Egan GF. Age-related differences in pain sensitivity and regional brain activity evoked by noxious pressure. Neurobiol Aging. 2010;31(3):494–503. https://doi.org/10.1016/j.neurobiolaging.2008.04.012.
Corso JF. Sensory processes and age effects in normal adults. J Gerontol. 1971;26(1):90–105. https://doi.org/10.1093/geronj/26.1.90.
Cosh JA. Studies on the nature of vibration sense. Clin Sci. 1953;12(2):131–51.
Cronin V. Active and passive touch at four age levels. Dev Psychol. 1977;13(3):253–6. https://doi.org/10.1037/0012-1649.13.3.253.
Cury RG, Galhardoni R, Teixeira MJ, Ghilardi DS, Maria G, Silva V, Myczkowski ML, et al. Subthalamic deep brain stimulation modulates conscious perception of sensory function in Parkinson's disease. Pain. 2016;157(12):2758–65. https://doi.org/10.1097/j.pain.0000000000000697.
DeGangi GA, Greenspan SI. The development of sensory functions in infants. Phys Occup Ther Pediatr. 1989;8(4):21–33. https://doi.org/10.1080/J006v08n04_02.
Domschke K, Stevens S, Pfleiderer B, Gerlach AL. Interoceptive sensitivity in anxiety and anxiety disorders: an overview and integration of neurobio-

logical findings. Clin Psychol Rev. 2010;30(1):1–11. https://doi.org/10.1016/j.cpr.2009.08.008.
van Dongen LRG, Goudie EG. Fetal movement patterns in the first trimester of pregnancy. J Obstet Gynaecol. 1980;87(3):191–3. https://doi.org/10.1111/j.1471-0528.1980.tb04516.x.
Dunn W. Sensory profile 2. Test manual. Dt. Fassung. Frankfurt am Main: Pearson; 2017.
Eeles AL, Spittle AJ, Anderson PJ, Brown N, Lee KJ, Boyd RN, Doyle LW. Assessments of sensory processing in infants: a systematic review. Dev Med Child Neurol. 2013;55(4):314–26. https://doi.org/10.1111/j.1469-8749.2012.04434.x.
Eggart M, Lange A, Binser MJ, Queri S, Müller-Oerlinghausen B. Major depressive disorder is associated with impaired interoceptive accuracy: a systematic review. Brain Sci. 2019;9(6):131. https://doi.org/10.3390/brainsci9060131.
Ehlers A, Breuer P. Increased cardiac awareness in panic disorder. J Abnorm Psychol. 1992;101(3):371–82. https://doi.org/10.1037/0021-843X.101.3.371.
Fabrizi L, Slater R, Worley A, Meek J, Boyd S, Olhede S, Fitzgerald M. A shift in sensory processing that enables the developing human brain to discriminate touch from pain. Curr Biol. 2011;21(18):1552–8. https://doi.org/10.1016/j.cub.2011.08.010.
Fagard J, Esseily R, Jacquey L, O'Regan K, Somogyi E. Fetal origin of sensorimotor behavior. Front Neurorobot. 2018;12:23. https://doi.org/10.3389/fnbot.2018.00023.
Fassino S, Pierò A, Gramaglia C, Abbate-Daga G. Clinical, psychopathological and personality correlates of interoceptive awareness in anorexia nervosa, bulimia nervosa and obesity. Psychopathology. 2004;37(4):168–74. https://doi.org/10.1159/000079420.
Ferrell WR, Crighton A, Sturrock RD. Age-dependent changes in position sense in human proximal interphalangeal joints. Neuroreport. 1992;3(3):259–61. https://doi.org/10.1097/00001756-199203000-00011.
Finlayson MAJ, Reitan RM. Tactile-perceptual functioning in relation to intellectual, cognitive and reading skills in younger and older normal children. Dev Med Child Neurol. 1976;18(4):442–6. https://doi.org/10.1111/j.1469-8749.1976.tb03683.x.
Fuentes CT, Mostofsky SH, Bastian AJ. No proprioceptive deficits in autism despite movement-related sensory and execution impairments. J Autism Dev Disord. 2011;41(10):1352–61. https://doi.org/10.1007/s10803-010-1161-1.
Gadsby S. Anorexia nervosa and body representation. Sydney: Macquarie University; 2016.
Gadsby S. Distorted body representations in anorexia nervosa. Conscious Cogn. 2017;51:17–33. https://doi.org/10.1016/j.concog.2017.02.015.
Gambino G, Giglia G, Schiera G, Majo D, Danila, Epifanio MS, La Grutta S, et al. Haptic perception in extreme obesity: qEEG study focused on predictive coding and body schema. Brain Sci. 2020;10(12):908. https://doi.org/10.3390/brainsci10120908.
Gannon L. The role of interoception in learned visceral control. Biofeedback Self Regul. 1977;2(4):337–47.
García-Piqueras J, García-Mesa Y, Cárcaba L, Feito J, Torres-Parejo I, Martín-Biedma B, et al. Ageing of the somatosensory system at the periphery: age-related changes in cutaneous mechanoreceptors. J Anat. 2019;234(6):839–52. https://doi.org/10.1111/joa.12983.
Gescheider GA, Bolanowski SJ, Hall KL, Hoffman KE, Verrillo RT. The effects of aging on information-processing channels in the sense of touch: I. Absolute sensitivity. Somatosens Motor Res. 1994;11(4):345–57. https://doi.org/10.3109/08990229409028878.
Ghanizadeh A. Tactile sensory dysfunction in children with ADHD. Behav Neurol. 2008;20(3):107–12. https://doi.org/10.3233/BEN-2008-0221.
Ghanizadeh A. Sensory processing problems in children with ADHD, a systematic review. Psychiatry Investig. 2011;8(2):89–94. https://doi.org/10.4306/pi.2011.8.2.89.
Ghassemzadeh H, Mojtabai R, Karamghadiri N, Noroozian M, Sharifi V, Ebrahimkhani N. Neuropsychological and neurological deficits in obsessive-compulsive disorder: the role of comorbid depression. Int J Clin Med., 3(03), 200-210. https://doi.org/10.4236/ijcm.2012.33040.
Ghera MM, Marshall PJ, Fox NA, Zeanah CH, Nelson CA, Smyke AT, Guthrie D. The effects of foster care intervention on socially deprived institutionalized children's attention and positive affect: results from the BEIP study. J Child Psychol Psychiatry Allied Discip. 2009;50(3):246–53. https://doi.org/10.1111/j.1469-7610.2008.01954.x.
Gibson SJ, Dostrovsky JO, Carr DB, Koltzenburg M. Proceedings of the 10th world congress on pain. Pain and aging: the pain experience over the adult life span. Seattle: IASP Press; 2003. p. 767–90.
Grant AC, Thiagarajah MC, Sathian K. Tactile perception in blind Braille readers: a psychophysical study of acuity and hyperacuity using gratings and dot patterns. Percept Psychophys. 2000;62(2):301–12. https://doi.org/10.3758/bf03205550.
Gregory SG, Connelly JJ, Towers AJ, Johnson J, Biscocho D, Markunas CA, et al. Genomic and epigenetic evidence for oxytocin receptor deficiency in autism. BMC Med. 2009;7:62. https://doi.org/10.1186/1741-7015-7-62.
Grunwald M. Haptic perception disturbances in eating disorders. In: Grunwald M, editor. Human haptic perception: basics and applications. Basel: Birkhäuser Basel; 2008. p. 335–51.
Grunwald M. Homo hapticus: Warum wir ohne Tastsinn nicht leben können. 1. Auflage. München: Droemer Knaur; 2017.
Grunwald M, Mueller SM. Körperschema und Körperbild. In: Senf W, Broda M, editors. Praxis der Psychotherapie. Ein integratives Lehrbuch. 6., vollständig überarbeitete Auflage. Stuttgart: Georg Thieme; 2020. p. 86–96.

Grunwald M, Weiss T. Inducing sensory stimulation in treatment of anorexia nervosa. QJM. 2005;98(5):379–80. https://doi.org/10.1093/qjmed/hci061.

Grunwald M, Ettrich C, Assmann B, Dahne A, Krause W, Busse F, Gertz HJ. Deficits in haptic perception and right parietal theta power changes in patients with anorexia nervosa before and after weight gain. Int J Eat Disord. 2001a;29(4):417–28.

Grunwald M, Ettrich C, Krause W, Assmann B, Dähne A, Weiss T, Gertz HJ. Haptic perception in anorexia nervosa before and after weight gain. J Clin Exp Neuropsychol. 2001b;23(4):520–9. https://doi.org/10.1076/jcen.23.4.520.1229.

Grunwald M, Busse F, Hensel A, Riedel-Heller S, Kruggel F, Arendt T, et al. Theta-power differences in patients with mild cognitive impairment under rest condition and during haptic tasks. Alzheimer Dis Assoc Disord. 2002a;16(1):40–8. https://doi.org/10.1097/00002093-200201000-00006.

Grunwald M, Ettrich C, Busse F, Assmann B, Dahne A, Gertz H-J. Angle paradigm a new method to measure right parietal dysfunctions in anorexia nervosa. Arch Clin Neuropsychol. 2002b;17(5):485–96. https://doi.org/10.1093/arclin/17.5.485.

Grunwald M, Weiss T, Assmann B, Ettrich C. Stable asymmetric interhemispheric theta power in patients with anorexia nervosa during haptic perception even after weight gain: a longitudinal study. J Clin Exp Neuropsychol. 2004a;26(5):608–20. https://doi.org/10.1080/13803390409609785.

Grunwald M, Weiss T, Assmann B, Ettrich C. Stable asymmetric interhemispheric theta power in patients with anorexia nervosa during haptic perception even after weight gain: a longitudinal study. J Clin Exp Neuropsychol. 2004b;26(5):608–20. https://doi.org/10.1080/13803390490504407.

Guardia D, Conversy L, Jardri R, Lafargue G, Thomas P, Dodin V, et al. Imagining one's own and someone else's body actions: dissociation in anorexia nervosa. PLoS One. 2012;7(8):e43241. https://doi.org/10.1371/journal.pone.0043241.

Güçlü B, Tanidir C, Mukaddes NM, Unal F. Tactile sensitivity of normal and autistic children. Somatosens Motor Res. 2007;24(1-2):21–33. https://doi.org/10.1080/08990220601179418.

Halata Z, Baumann KI. Anatomy of receptors. In: Grunwald M, editor. Human haptic perception: basics and applications. Basel: Birkhäuser; 2008. p. 85–92.

Harlow HF. The nature of love. Am Psychol. 1958;13(12):673–85. https://doi.org/10.1037/h0047884.

Harlow HF. Love in infant monkeys. Sci Am. 1959;200(6):68–74. https://doi.org/10.1038/scientificamerican0659-68.

Hawkes CH, Del Tredici K, Braak H. A timeline for Parkinson's disease. Parkinsonism Relat Disord. 2010;16(2):79–84. https://doi.org/10.1016/j.parkreldis.2009.08.007.

He JL, Wodka E, Tommerdahl M, Edden RAE, Mikkelsen M, Mostofsky SH, Puts NAJ. Disorder-specific alterations of tactile sensitivity in neurodevelopmental disorders. Commun Biol. 2021;4(1):97. https://doi.org/10.1038/s42003-020-01592-y.

Heller, Morton A. (1991): Haptic perception in blind people. In: Morton A. Heller William Schiff: The psychology of touch. New York: Psychology Press, 239–261.

Heller MA, Ballesteros S. Touch and blindness. Psychology and neuroscience. New York: Psychology Press; 2006.

Hepper PG. Haptic perception in the human foetus. In: Grunwald M, editor. Human haptic perception: basics and applications. Basel: Birkhäuser; 2008. p. 149–54.

Herbert BM, Pollatos O. Attenuated interoceptive sensitivity in overweight and obese individuals. Eat Behav. 2014;15(3):445–8. https://doi.org/10.1016/j.eatbeh.2014.06.002.

Hogstel MO. Older widowers: a small group with special needs. Geriatr Nurs. 1985;6(1):24–6. https://doi.org/10.1016/s0197-4572(85)80104-x.

Hooker D. Fetal reflexes and instinctual processes. Psychosomat Med. 1942;4(2):199–205.

Hornix BE, Havekes R, Kas MJH. Multisensory cortical processing and dysfunction across the neuropsychiatric spectrum. Neurosci Biobehav Rev. 2019;97:138–51. https://doi.org/10.1016/j.neubiorev.2018.02.010.

Hsiao S, Yau J. Neural basis of haptic perception. In: Grunwald M, editor. Human haptic perception: basics and applications. Basel: Birkhäuser; 2008. p. 103–12.

Humes LE, Busey TA, Craig JC, Kewley-Port D. The effects of age on sensory thresholds and temporal gap detection in hearing, vision, and touch. Atten Percept Psychophys. 2009;71(4):860–71. https://doi.org/10.3758/APP.71.4.860.

Humphreys KL, Gleason MM, Drury SS, Miron D, Nelson CA III, Fox NA, Zeanah CH. Effects of institutional rearing and foster care on psychopathology at age 12 years in Romania: follow-up of an open, randomised controlled trial. Lancet Psychiatry. 2015;2(7):625–34. https://doi.org/10.1016/S2215-0366(15)00095-4.

Irmak MK, Oztas E, Vural H. Dependence of fetal hairs and sebaceous glands on fetal adrenal cortex and possible control from adrenal medulla. Med Hypotheses. 2004;62(4):486–92. https://doi.org/10.1016/j.mehy.2004.01.001.

James W. What is an emotion? Mind. 1884;9(34):188–205. https://doi.org/10.1093/mind/os-IX.34.188.

Jirikowic TL, Engel JM, Deitz JC. The test of sensory functions in infants: test-retest reliability for infants with developmental delays. Am J Occup Ther. 1997;51(9):733–8. https://doi.org/10.5014/ajot.51.9.733.

Joosten AV, Bundy AC. Sensory processing and stereotypical and repetitive behaviour in children with autism and intellectual disability. Aust Occup Ther J. 2010;57(6):366–72. https://doi.org/10.1111/j.1440-1630.2009.00835.x.

Joosten AV, Bundy AC, Einfeld SL. Intrinsic and extrinsic motivation for stereotypic and repetitive behavior. J Autism Dev Disord. 2009;39(3):521–31. https://doi.org/10.1007/s10803-008-0654-7.

Kaiser MD, Yang DY-J, Voos AC, Bennett RH, Gordon I, Pretzsch C, et al. Brain mechanisms for processing affective (and nonaffective) touch are atypical in autism. Cereb Cortex. 2016;26(6):2705–14. https://doi.org/10.1093/cercor/bhv125.

Kalisch T, Kattenstroth J-C, Kowalewski R, Tegenthoff M, Dinse HR. Age-related changes in the joint position sense of the human hand. Clin Interv Aging. 2012a;7:499–507. https://doi.org/10.2147/CIA.S37573.

Kalisch T, Kattenstroth J-C, Kowalewski R, Tegenthoff M, Dinse HR. Cognitive and tactile factors affecting human haptic performance in later life. PLoS One. 2012b;7(1):e30420. https://doi.org/10.1371/journal.pone.0030420.

Kaplan FS, Nixon JE, Reitz M, Rindfleish L, Tucker J. Age-related changes in proprioception and sensation of joint position. Acta Orthop Scand. 1985;56(1):72–4. https://doi.org/10.3109/17453678508992984.

Karadag F, Tumkaya S, Kırtaş D, Efe M, Alaçam H, Oguzhanoglu N. Neurological soft signs in obsessive compulsive disorder with good and poor insight. Prog Neuropsychopharmacol Biol Psychiatry. 2011;35:1074–9. https://doi.org/10.1016/j.pnpbp.2011.03.003.

Karch D, Freitag H. Sensorische Integrationsstörung und sensorische Integrationstherapie nach Jean Ayres. Stellungnahme der Deutschen Gesellschaft für Sozialpädiatrie und Jugendmedizin. 2017. Online verfügbar unter https://www.dgspj.de/wp-content/uploads/service-stellungnahme-si-2017.pdf, zuletzt geprüft am 12.04.2021.

Keizer A, Smeets MAM, Dijkerman HC, Uzunbajakau SA, van Elburg A, Postma A. Too fat to fit through the door: first evidence for disturbed body-scaled action in anorexia nervosa during locomotion. PLoS One. 2013;8(5):e64602. https://doi.org/10.1371/journal.pone.0064602.

Khan A, Kamran S, Ponirakis G, Akhtar N, Khan R, George P, et al. Peripheral neuropathy in patients with multiple sclerosis. PLoS One. 2018;13(3):e0193270. https://doi.org/10.1371/journal.pone.0193270.

Khazipov R, Sirota A, Leinekugel X, Holmes GL, Ben-Ari Y, Buzsáki G. Early motor activity drives spindle bursts in the developing somatosensory cortex. Nature. 2004;432(7018):758–61. https://doi.org/10.1038/nature03132.

Kinnaird E, Stewart C, Tchanturia K. Interoception in anorexia nervosa: exploring associations with alexithymia and autistic traits. Front Psychiatry. 2020;11:64. https://doi.org/10.3389/fpsyt.2020.00064.

Kleinman JM. Developmental changes in haptic exploration and matching accuracy. Dev Psychol. 1979;15(4):480–1. https://doi.org/10.1037/h0078086.

Kleinman JM, Brodzinsky DM. Haptic exploration in young, middle-aged, and elderly adults. J Gerontol. 1978;33(4):521–7. https://doi.org/10.1093/geronj/33.4.521.

Kokmen E, Bossemeyer RW, Williams WJ. Quantitative evaluation of joint motion sensation in an aging population. J Gerontol. 1978;33(1):62–7. https://doi.org/10.1093/geronj/33.1.62.

Kolb B, Whishaw IQ, Pritzel M. Neuropsychologie. Heidelberg: Spektrum Akad. Verl; 1993.

Konczak J, Krawczewski K, Tuite P, Maschke M. The perception of passive motion in Parkinson's disease. J Neurol. 2007;254(5):655–63. https://doi.org/10.1007/s00415-006-0426-2.

Konczak J, Li K-y, Tuite PJ, Poizner H. Haptic perception of object curvature in Parkinson's disease. PLoS One. 2008;3(7):e2625. https://doi.org/10.1371/journal.pone.0002625.

Konczak J, Corcos DM, Horak F, Poizner H, Shapiro M, Tuite P, et al. Proprioception and motor control in Parkinson's disease. J Motor Behav. 2009;41(6):543–52. https://doi.org/10.3200/35-09-002.

Konczak J, Sciutti A, Avanzino L, Squeri V, Gori M, Masia L, et al. Parkinson's disease accelerates age-related decline in haptic perception by altering somatosensory integration. Brain. 2012;135(Pt 11):3371–9. https://doi.org/10.1093/brain/aws265.

Lautenbacher S. Experimental approaches in the study of pain in the elderly. Pain Med. 2012;13(Suppl 2):S44–50. https://doi.org/10.1111/j.1526-4637.2012.01326.x.

Lautenbacher S, Kunz M, Strate P, Nielsen J, Arendt-Nielsen L. Age effects on pain thresholds, temporal summation and spatial summation of heat and pressure pain. Pain. 2005;115(3):410–8. https://doi.org/10.1016/j.pain.2005.03.025.

Lautenbacher S, Peters JH, Heesen M, Scheel J, Kunz M. Age changes in pain perception: a systematic-review and meta-analysis of age effects on pain and tolerance thresholds. Neurosci Biobehav Rev. 2017;75:104–13. https://doi.org/10.1016/j.neubiorev.2017.01.039.

Lee D, Henriques DY, Snider J, Song D, Poizner H. Reaching to proprioceptively defined targets in Parkinson's disease: effects of deep brain stimulation therapy. Neuroscience. 2013;244:99–112. https://doi.org/10.1016/j.neuroscience.2013.04.009.

Levit-Binnun N, Golland Y. Finding behavioral and network indicators of brain vulnerability. Front Huma Neurosci. 2012:6. https://doi.org/10.3389/fnhum.2012.00010.

Li S-C, Jordanova M, Lindenberger U. From good senses to good sense. A link between tactile information processing and intelligence. Intelligence. 1998;26:99–122.

Li K-y, Pickett K, Nestrasil I, Tuite P, Konczak J. The effect of dopamine replacement therapy on haptic sensitivity in Parkinson's disease. J Neurol. 2010;257(12):1992–8. https://doi.org/10.1007/s00415-010-5646-9.

Libouton X, Barbier O, Plaghki L, Thonnard J-L. Tactile roughness discrimination threshold is unrelated to tactile spatial acuity. Behav Brain Res. 2010;208(2):473–8. https://doi.org/10.1016/j.bbr.2009.12.017.

Mammen MA, Moore GA, Scaramella LV, Reiss D, Ganiban JM, Shaw DS, et al. Infant avoidance during a tactile task predicts autism spectrum behaviors in toddlerhood. Infant Ment Health J. 2015;36(6):575–87. https://doi.org/10.1002/imhj.21539.

Mangeot SD, Miller LJ, McIntosh DN, McGrath-Clarke J, Simon J, Hagerman RJ, Goldson E. Sensory modulation dysfunction in children with attention-deficit-hyperactivity disorder. Dev Med Child Neurol. 2001;43(6):399–406. https://doi.org/10.1111/j.1469-8749.2001.tb00228.x.

Masuhr KF, Neumann M. Duale Reihe Neurologie. 6. Aufl. Stuttgart: Thieme (Das duale Lehrbuch); 2007.

McGoron L, Gleason MM, Smyke AT, Drury SS, Nelson CA III, Gregas MC, et al. Recovering from early deprivation: attachment mediates effects of caregiving on psychopathology. J Am Acad Child Adolesc Psychiatry. 2012;51(7):683–93. https://doi.org/10.1016/j.jaac.2012.05.004.

Metral M, Guardia D, Bauwens I, Guerraz M, Lafargue G, Cottencin O, Luyat M. Painfully thin but locked inside a fatter body: abnormalities in both anticipation and execution of action in anorexia nervosa. BMC Res Notes. 2014;7:707. https://doi.org/10.1186/1756-0500-7-707.

Meyerholz L, Irzinger J, Witthöft M, Gerlach AL, Pohl A. Contingent biofeedback outperforms other methods to enhance the accuracy of cardiac interoception: A comparison of short interventions. J Behav Ther Exp Psychiatry. 2019;63:12–20. https://doi.org/10.1016/j.jbtep.2018.12.002.

Milh M, Kaminska A, Huon C, Lapillonne A, Ben-Ari Y, Khazipov R. Rapid cortical oscillations and early motor activity in premature human neonate. Cereb Cortex. 2007;17(7):1582–94. https://doi.org/10.1093/cercor/bhl069.

Miller NE. Learning of visceral and glandular responses. Science. 1969;163(3866):434–45. https://doi.org/10.1126/science.163.3866.434.

Minshew NJ, Hobson JA. Sensory sensitivities and performance on sensory perceptual tasks in high-functioning individuals with autism. J Autism Dev Disord. 2008;38(8):1485–98. https://doi.org/10.1007/s10803-007-0528-4.

Modahl C, Green LA, Fein D, Morris M, Waterhouse L, Feinstein C, Levin H. Plasma oxytocin levels in autistic children. Biol Psychiatry. 1998;43(4):270–7. https://doi.org/10.1016/S0006-3223(97)00439-3.

Mohr HM, Zimmermann J, Röder C, Lenz C, Overbeck G, Grabhorn R. Separating two components of body image in anorexia nervosa using fMRI. Psychol Med. 2010;40(9):1519–29. https://doi.org/10.1017/S0033291709991826.

Montagu A. Touching. The human significance of the skin. 3rd ed. New York: Harper & Row; 1986.

Moore AR, Clinch D. Underlying mechanisms of impaired visceral pain perception in older people. J Am Geriatr Soc. 2004;52(1):132–6.

Mueller SM. Visuo-haptische Erkennungsleistungen und haptische Schwellenwerte bei neurologischen und psychischen Störungsbildern. Diplomarbeit. Friedrich Schiller Universität Jena; 2011.

Mueller SM, Grunwald M. Haptische Wahrnehmungsleistungen: Effekte bei erfahrenen und unerfahrenen Physiotherapeuten. Manuelle Medizin. 2013;51(6):473–8. https://doi.org/10.1007/s00337-013-1068-y.

Mueller S, Winkelmann C, Grunwald M. Messung und Training der haptischen Wahrnehmung. Vorstellung des Haptik-Schwellen-Tests sowie des Haptik-Figuren-Test und Trainingssets. Online Version. pt - Zeitschrift für Physiotherapeuten. 2014; 66:91–5.

Mueller SM, Stengler K, Jahn I, Grunwald M. Sensory integration capacity is diminished in obsessive compulsive disorder patients with poor insight but not in patients with intact insight. Int Neuropsychiatr Dis J. 2014a;2:141. https://doi.org/10.9734/INDJ/2014/8102.

Mueller SM, Winkelmann C, Krause F, Grunwald M. Occupation-related long-term sensory training enhances roughness discrimination but not tactile acuity. Exp Brain Res. 2014b;232(6):1905–14. https://doi.org/10.1007/s00221-014-3882-4.

Mueller SM, Bernigau D, Muelling C, Grunwald M. Does studying veterinary medicine improve students' haptic perception ability? A pilot study with two age-groups. J Vet Med Educ. 2019;46(3):408–14. https://doi.org/10.3138/jvme.0417-051r.

Müller G, Richter RA, Weisbrod S, Klingberg F. Impaired tactile pattern recognition in the early stage of primary degenerative dementia compared with normal aging. Arch Gerontol Geriatr. 1992;14(3):215–25. https://doi.org/10.1016/0167-4943(92)90022-V.

Nelson CA, Fox NA, Zeanah CH. Romania's abandoned children. Deprivation, brain development, and the struggle for recovery. Cambridge: Harvard University Press; 2014.

Nevalainen P, Lauronen L, Pihko E. Development of human somatosensory cortical functions - what have we learned from magnetoencephalography: a review. Front Hum Neurosci. 2014;8:158. https://doi.org/10.3389/fnhum.2014.00158.

Nico D, Daprati E, Nighoghossian N, Carrier E, Duhamel J-R, Sirigu A. The role of the right parietal lobe in anorexia nervosa. Psychol Med. 2010;40(9):1531–9. https://doi.org/10.1017/S0033291709991851.

Norman JF, Kappers AML, Cheeseman JR, Ronning C, Thomason KE, Baxter MW, et al. Aging and curvature discrimination from static and dynamic touch. PLoS One. 2013;8(7):e68577. https://doi.org/10.1371/journal.pone.0068577.

O'Riordan M, Passetti F. Discrimination in autism within different sensory modalities. J Autism Dev Disord. 2006;36(5):665–75. https://doi.org/10.1007/s10803-006-0106-1.

O'Suilleabhain P, Bullard J, Dewey RB. Proprioception in Parkinson's disease is acutely depressed by dopaminergic medications. J Neurol Neurosurg Psychiatry. 2001;71(5):607–10. https://doi.org/10.1136/jnnp.71.5.607.

Pai YC, Rymer WZ, Chang RW, Sharma L. Effect of age and osteoarthritis on knee proprioception. Arthritis Rheumat. 1997;40(12):2260–5. https://doi.org/10.1002/art.1780401223.

Parush S, Sohmer H, Steinberg A, Kaitz M. Somatosensory functioning in children with attention deficit hyperactivity disorder. Dev Med Child Neurol. 1997;39(7):464–8. https://doi.org/10.1111/j.1469-8749.1997.tb07466.x.

Parush S, Sohmer H, Steinberg A, Kaitz M. Somatosensory function in boys with ADHD and tactile defensiveness. Physiol Behav. 2007;90(4):553–8. https://doi.org/10.1016/j.physbeh.2006.11.004.

Peters UH. Lexikon Psychiatrie, Psychotherapie, medizinische Psychologie. 6. Auflage. München: Elsevier Urban & Fischer; 2007.

Peters RM, Goldreich D. Tactile spatial acuity in childhood: effects of age and fingertip size. PLoS One. 2013;8(12):e84650. https://doi.org/10.1371/journal.pone.0084650.

Peters RM, Hackeman E, Goldreich D. Diminutive digits discern delicate details: fingertip size and the sex difference in tactile spatial acuity. J Neurosci. 2009;29(50):15756–61. https://doi.org/10.1523/JNEUROSCI.3684-09.2009.

Petrella RJ, Lattanzio PJ, Nelson MG. Effect of age and activity on knee joint proprioception. Am J Phys Med Rehabil. 1997;76(3):235–41. https://doi.org/10.1097/00002060-199705000-00015.

Pickard CM, Sullivan PE, Allison GT, Singer KP. Is there a difference in hip joint position sense between young and older groups? J Gerontol A. 2003;58(7):631–5.

Pietrini F, Castellini G, Ricca V, Polito C, Pupi A, Faravelli C. Functional neuroimaging in anorexia nervosa: a clinical approach. Eur Psychiatry. 2011;26(3):176–82. https://doi.org/10.1016/j.eurpsy.2010.07.011.

Pollatos O, Georgiou E. Normal interoceptive accuracy in women with bulimia nervosa. Psychiatry Res. 2016;240:328–32. https://doi.org/10.1016/j.psychres.2016.04.072.

Pollatos O, Traut-Mattausch E, Schroeder H, Schandry R. Interoceptive awareness mediates the relationship between anxiety and the intensity of unpleasant feelings. J Anxiety Disord. 2007;21(7):931–43. https://doi.org/10.1016/j.janxdis.2006.12.004.

Pollatos O, Kurz A-L, Albrecht J, Schreder T, Kleemann AM, Schöpf V, et al. Reduced perception of bodily signals in anorexia nervosa. Eat Behav. 2008;9(4):381–8. https://doi.org/10.1016/j.eatbeh.2008.02.001.

Pollatos O, Traut-Mattausch E, Schandry R. Differential effects of anxiety and depression on interoceptive accuracy. Depress Anxiety. 2009;26(2):167–73. https://doi.org/10.1002/da.20504.

Poncelet AN, Connolly MK. Peripheral neuropathy in scleroderma. Muscle Nerve. 2003;28(3):330–5. https://doi.org/10.1002/mus.10439.

Prätorius B, Kimmeskamp S, Milani TL. The sensitivity of the sole of the foot in patients with Morbus Parkinson. Neurosci Lett. 2003;346(3):173–6. https://doi.org/10.1016/S0304-3940(03)00582-2.

Provost B, Oetter P. The sensory rating scale for infants and young children. Phys Occup Ther Pediatr. 1994;13(4):15–35. https://doi.org/10.1080/J006v13n04_02.

Puéchal X, Said G, Hilliquin P, Coste J, Job-Deslandre C, Lacroix C, Menkès CJ. Peripheral neuropathy with necrotizing vasculitis in rheumatoid arthritis. A clinicopathologic and prognostic study of thirty-two patients. Arthritis Rheumat. 1995;38(11):1618–29. https://doi.org/10.1002/art.1780381114.

Puts NAJ, Harris AD, Mikkelsen M, Tommerdahl M, Edden RAE, Mostofsky SH. Altered tactile sensitivity in children with attention-deficit hyperactivity disorder. J Neurophysiol. 2017;118(5):2568–78. https://doi.org/10.1152/jn.00087.2017.

Ragert P, Schmidt A, Altenmüller E, Dinse HR. Superior tactile performance and learning in professional pianists: evidence for meta-plasticity in musicians. Eur J Neurosci. 2004;19(2):473–8. https://doi.org/10.1111/j.0953-816x.2003.03142.x.

Reissland N, Francis B, Aydin E, Mason J, Schaal B. The development of anticipation in the fetus: a longitudinal account of human fetal mouth movements in reaction to and anticipation of touch. Dev Psychobiol. 2014;56(5):955–63. https://doi.org/10.1002/dev.21172.

Reissland N, Aydin E, Francis B, Exley K. Laterality of foetal self-touch in relation to maternal stress. Laterality. 2015;20(1):82–94. https://doi.org/10.1080/1357650X.2014.920339.

Riancho J, Paz-Fajardo L, de Munaín Adolfo L. Clinical and preclinical evidence of somatosensory involvement in amyotrophic lateral sclerosis. Br J Pharmacol. 2021;178(6):1257–68. https://doi.org/10.1111/bph.15202.

Ribeiro F, Oliveira J. Aging effects on joint proprioception: the role of physical activity in proprioception preservation. Eur Rev Aging Phys Act. 2007;4(2):71–6. https://doi.org/10.1007/s11556-007-0026-x.

Riquelme I, Hatem SM, Montoya P. Abnormal pressure pain, touch sensitivity, proprioception, and manual dexterity in children with autism spectrum disorders. Neural Plast. 2016;2016:1723401. https://doi.org/10.1155/2016/1723401.

Rocchi L, Chiari L, Horak FB. Effects of deep brain stimulation and levodopa on postural sway in Parkinson's disease. J Neurol Neurosurg Psychiatry. 2002;73(3):267–74. https://doi.org/10.1136/jnnp.73.3.267.

Rogers SJ, Hepburn S, Wehner E. Parent reports of sensory symptoms in toddlers with autism and those with other developmental disorders. J Autism Dev Disord. 2003;33(6):631–42. https://doi.org/10.1023/b:jadd.0000006000.38991.a7.

Roley SS, Mailloux Z, Parham LD, Schaaf RC, Lane CJ, Cermak S. Sensory integration and =praxis patterns in children with autism. Am J Occup Ther. 2015;69(1):6901220010. https://doi.org/10.5014/ajot.2015.012476.

van Rosmalen L, van der Horst FCP, van der Veer R. Of monkeys and men: Spitz and Harlow on the consequences of maternal deprivation. Attach Hum Dev. 2012;14(4):425–37. https://doi.org/10.1080/14616734.2012.691658.

Routasalo P, Isola A. The right to touch and be touched. Nurs Ethics. 1996;3(2):165–76. https://doi.org/10.1177/096973309600300209.

Sabourin S, Khazen O, DiMarzio M, Staudt MD, Williams L, Gillogly M, et al. Effect of directional deep brain stimulation on sensory thresholds in Parkinson's disease. Front Hum Neurosci. 2020;14:217. https://doi.org/10.3389/fnhum.2020.00217.

Sathian K, Zangaladze A, Green J, Vitek JL, DeLong MR. Tactile spatial acuity and roughness discrimination: impairments due to aging and Parkinson's disease. Neurology. 1997;49(1):168–77. https://doi.org/10.1212/wnl.49.1.168.

Schaefer M, Egloff B, Witthöft M. Is interoceptive awareness really altered in somatoform disorders? Testing competing theories with two paradigms of heartbeat perception. J Abnorm Psychol. 2012;121(3):719–24. https://doi.org/10.1037/a0028509.

Schaefer M, Egloff B, Gerlach AL, Witthöft M. Improving heartbeat perception in patients with medically unexplained symptoms reduces symptom distress. Biol Psychol. 2014;101:69–76. https://doi.org/10.1016/j.biopsycho.2014.05.012.

Schandry R. Heart beat perception and emotional experience. Psychophysiology. 1981;18(4):483–8. https://doi.org/10.1111/j.1469-8986.1981.tb02486.x.

Schandry R, Weitkunat R. Enhancement of heartbeat-related brain potentials through cardiac awareness training. Int J Neurosci. 1990;53(2-4):243–53. https://doi.org/10.3109/00207459008986611.

Sehlstedt I, Ignell H, Backlund Wasling H, Ackerley R, Olausson H, Croy I. Gentle touch perception across the lifespan. Psychol Aging. 2016;31(2):176–84. https://doi.org/10.1037/pag0000074.

Seilbeck C, Langmeyer A. Ergebnisse der Studie "Generationenübergreifende Zeitverwendung: Großeltern, Eltern, Enkel". München; 2018. Online verfügbar unter https://www.dji.de/fileadmin/user_upload/bibs2018/WEB_DJI_GenerationZeit.pdf, zuletzt geprüft am 12.04.2021.

Shaffer D, Schonfeld I, O'Connor P, Stokman C, Trautman P, Shafer S, Ng S. Neurological soft signs: their relationship to psychiatric disorder and intelligence in childhood and adolescence. Arch Gen Psychiatry. 1985;42:342–51. https://doi.org/10.1001/archpsyc.1985.01790270028003.

Sheffield A, Waller G, Emanuelli F, Murray J, Meyer C. Do schema processes mediate links between parenting and eating pathology? Eur Eat Disord Rev. 2009;17(4):290–300. https://doi.org/10.1002/erv.922.

Shin H-W, Kang SY, Sohn YH. Dopaminergic influence on disturbed spatial discrimination in Parkinson's disease. Mov Disord. 2005;20(12):1640–3. https://doi.org/10.1002/mds.20642.

Siaperas P, Ring HA, McAllister CJ, Henderson S, Barnett A, Watson P, Holland AJ. Atypical movement performance and sensory integration in Asperger's syndrome. J Autism Dev Disord. 2012;42(5):718–25. https://doi.org/10.1007/s10803-011-1301-2.

Smirni D, Smirni P, Carotenuto M, Parisi L, Quatrosi G, Roccella M. Noli Me Tangere: social touch, tactile defensiveness, and communication in neurodevelopmental disorders. Brain Sci. 2019;9(12):368. https://doi.org/10.3390/brainsci9120368.

Smith B, Rogers SL, Blissett J, Ludlow AK. The relationship between sensory sensitivity, food fussiness and food preferences in children with neurodevelopmental disorders. Appetite. 2020;150:104643. https://doi.org/10.1016/j.appet.2020.104643.

Spitz RA. The role of ecological factors in emotional development in infancy. Child Dev. 1949;20:145–56.

Stankov L, Seizova-Cajić T, Roberts RD. Tactile and kinesthetic perceptual processes within the taxonomy of human cognitive abilities. Intelligence. 2001;29(1):1–29. https://doi.org/10.1016/s0160-2896(00)00038-6.

Stevens JC, Choo KK. Spatial acuity of the body surface over the life span. Somatosens Motor Res. 1996;13(2):153–66. https://doi.org/10.3109/08990229609051403.

Stevens JC, Patterson MQ. Dimensions of spatial acuity in the touch sense: changes over the life span. Somatosens Motor Res. 1995;12(1):29–47. https://doi.org/10.3109/08990229509063140.

Suttanon P, Hill KD, Said CM, Logiudice D, Lautenschlager NT, Dodd KJ. Balance and mobility dysfunction and falls risk in older people with mild to moderate Alzheimer disease. Am J Phys Med Rehabil. 2012;91(1):12–23. https://doi.org/10.1097/PHM.0b013e31823caeea.

Symmons MA, Richardson BL, Wuillemin DB. Components of haptic information: skin rivals kinaesthesis. Perception. 2008;37(10):1596–604. https://doi.org/10.1068/p5855.

Tau GZ, Peterson BS. Normal development of brain circuits. Neuropsychopharmacology. 2010;35(1):147–68. https://doi.org/10.1038/npp.2009.115.

Thompson LW, Axelrod S, Cohen LD. Senescence and visual identification of tactual-kinesthetic forms. J Gerontol. 1965;20:244–9. https://doi.org/10.1093/geronj/20.2.244.

Thornbury JM, Mistretta CM. Tactile sensitivity as a function of age. J Gerontol. 1981;36(1):34–9.

Thye MD, Bednarz HM, Herringshaw AJ, Sartin EB, Kana RK. The impact of atypical sensory processing on social impairments in autism spectrum disorder. Dev Cogn Neurosci. 2018;29:151–67. https://doi.org/10.1016/j.dcn.2017.04.010.

Tomchek SD, Dunn W. Sensory processing in children with and without autism: a comparative study using the short sensory profile. Am J Occup Ther. 2007;61(2):190–200. https://doi.org/10.5014/ajot.61.2.190.

Treister R, Eisenberg E, Demeter N, Pud D. Alterations in pain response are partially reversed by methylphenidate (Ritalin) in adults with attention deficit hyperactivity disorder (ADHD). Pain Pract. 2015;15(1):4–11. https://doi.org/10.1111/papr.12129.

Vaugoyeau M, Cignetti F, Eusebio A, Azulay JP. Subthalamic deep brain stimulation modulates proprioceptive integration in Parkinson's disease during a postural task. Neuroscience. 2020;437:207–14. https://doi.org/10.1016/j.neuroscience.2020.04.028.

Vega-Bermudez F, Johnson KO. Fingertip skin conformance accounts, in part, for differences in tactile spatial acuity in young subjects, but not for the decline in spatial acuity with aging. Percept Psychophys. 2004;66(1):60–7. https://doi.org/10.3758/bf03194861.

Verrillo RT. Age related changes in the sensitivity to vibration. J Gerontol. 1980;35(2):185–93. https://doi.org/10.1093/geronj/35.2.185.

de Vries JIP, Visser GHA, Prechtl HFR. The emergence of fetal behaviour. II. Quantitative aspects. Early Hum Dev. 1985;12(2):99–120. https://doi.org/10.1016/0378-3782(85)90174-4.

Weineck F, Messner M, Hauke G, Pollatos O. Improving interoceptive ability through the practice of power posing: a pilot study. PLoS One. 2019;14(2):e0211453. https://doi.org/10.1371/journal.pone.0211453.

Wingert JR, Welder C, Foo P. Age-related hip proprioception declines: effects on postural sway and dynamic balance. Arch Phys Med Rehabil. 2014;95(2):253–61. https://doi.org/10.1016/j.apmr.2013.08.012.

Wolpe N, Zhang J, Nombela C, Ingram JN, Wolpert DM, Rowe JB. Sensory attenuation in Parkinson's disease is related to disease severity and dopamine dose. Sci Rep. 2018;8(1):1–10. https://doi.org/10.1038/s41598-018-33678-3.

Wong M, Peters RM, Goldreich D. A physical constraint on perceptual learning: tactile spatial acuity improves with training to a limit set by finger size. J Neurosci. 2013;33(22):9345–52. https://doi.org/10.1523/JNEUROSCI.0514-13.2013.

Woodward KL. The relationship between skin compliance, age, gender, and tactile discriminative thresholds in humans. Somatosens Motor Res. 1993;10(1):63–7. https://doi.org/10.3109/08990229309028824.

Wright ML, Adamo DE, Brown SH. Age-related declines in the detection of passive wrist movement. Neurosci Lett. 2011;500(2):108–12. https://doi.org/10.1016/j.neulet.2011.06.015.

Yang J, Ogasa T, Ohta Y, Abe K, Wu J. Decline of human tactile angle discrimination in patients with mild cognitive impairment and Alzheimer's disease. J Alzheimers Dis. 2010;22(1):225–34. https://doi.org/10.3233/JAD-2010-100723.

Yang DY-J, Rosenblau G, Keifer C, Pelphrey KA. An integrative neural model of social perception, action observation, and theory of mind. Neurosci Biobehavioral reviews. 2015;51:263–75. https://doi.org/10.1016/j.neubiorev.2015.01.020.

Yaryura-Tobias JA, Neziroglu F, Torres-Gallegos M. Neuroanatomical correlates and somatosensorial disturbances in body dysmorphic disorder. CNS Spectr. 2002;7(6):432–4. https://doi.org/10.1017/s1092852900017934.

Zetler NK, Cermak SA, Engel-Yeger B, Gal E. Somatosensory discrimination in people with autism spectrum disorder: a scoping review. Am J Occup Ther. 2019;73(5):7305205010p1–7305205010p14. https://doi.org/10.5014/ajot.2019.029728.

Zia S, Cody F, O'Boyle D. Joint position sense is impaired by Parkinson's disease. Ann Neurol. 2000;47(2):218–28.

Zoia S, Blason L, D'Ottavio G, Bulgheroni M, Pezzetta E, Scabar A, Castiello U. Evidence of early development of action planning in the human foetus: a kinematic study. Exp Brain Res. 2007;176(2):217–26. https://doi.org/10.1007/s00221-006-0607-3.

Testing, Training, and Rehabilitation

4

Stephanie Margarete Mueller,
Claudia Winkelmann, and Martin Grunwald

Contents

4.1 Training and Rehabilitation

The ability to process haptic, proprioceptive, and tactile stimuli can be trained due to the neural plasticity of the human central nervous system (CNS) (Elbert et al. 1995; Dinse et al. 2008; Mueller et al. 2014a; Weiss 2001). Plasticity, in the neuroscientific sense, describes the ability of the CNS to adapt to changing environmental conditions and requirements. Accordingly, the

S. M. Mueller (✉) · M. Grunwald
Haptic Research Lab, Paul-Flechsig-Institute for Brain Research, Leipzig University, Leipzig, Germany
e-mail: s.mueller@medizin.uni-leipzig.de; mgrun@medizin.uni-leipzig.de

C. Winkelmann
Alice Salomon University of Applied Sciences, Berlin, Berlin, Germany
e-mail: winkelmann@ash-berlin.eu

S. M. Mueller et al., *Human Touch in Healthcare*, https://doi.org/10.1007/978-3-662-67860-2_4

performance of the haptic system can be improved by suitable training measures. Similar to learning complex motor tasks (e.g., riding a bike), an increase in sensory performance requires weeks or months of intensive practice (Krakauer and Shadmehr 2006). Studies have reported a **typical course of sensory training** (Grunwald and Mueller 2017; Gibson 1953; Dinse et al. 2008), which can be divided into two phases:

- A first phase, with rapid and significant improvement in performance
- A second phase, with slower learning progression

The changes in the first phase are likely due to the development of appropriate strategies within the training situation and attentional focus (Ahissar and Hochstein 1993). The second phase is characterized by slower, but usually long-lasting, learning effects, which are associated with changes in cortical processing (neuroplasticity) (Bliss and Lomo 1973).

The **magnitude and speed of training success** are also dependent on several factors:

- Motivation and attention
- Intensity and duration of the training sessions
- The age of the trainees

Depending on the characteristics of these factors, they can either promote or hinder learning success. Furthermore, training success is influenced by feedback. Adequate feedback information, praise, and reinforcement promote performance enhancement; irrelevant feedback and false information hinder positive training effects (Herzog and Fahle 1997). However, feedback or praise is not required to enable training effects. In many training tasks, it is implicitly apparent to the trainee how well or poorly the task was mastered.

In adulthood, two types of neuronal plasticity occur, which are intertwined in the context of rehabilitation processes (Nelles et al. 2018):

1. **Use-dependent plasticity** refers to changes in the CNS due to the intensity of use. In this context, *intensified* everyday use or targeted training lead to increases in synaptic connections in cortical representation areas (Feldman and Brecht 2005). This is usually accompanied by an improvement in performance. In contrast, *reduced* use of a limb leads to degeneration processes and restructuring in the CNS, which can result in motor and sensory impairments (Lissek et al. 2009).
2. **Lesion-induced plasticity** refers to adaptive mechanisms following diseases or injuries to the CNS or limbs (e.g., amputation). These include (a) the reorganization of intact cortical structures for other purposes, and (b) the recruitment of neurons from cortical areas adjacent to a lesion for functional compensation.

▶ **Synopsis** Improvement during sensory training occurs in two phases: the first phase is characterized by rapid and significant improvement in performance, and the second phase is characterized by slower learning progression. Improvements depend on motivation, attention, intensity and duration of the training, and the age of the trainees.

4.1.1 Hands: Training of Manual Perception Thresholds (Healthy Adults to Old Age)

In healthy adults, training of the haptic system can achieve two goals:

- Improvement of the base level
- Counteracting age effects

4.1.1.1 Improvement of the Base Level

Healthy adults of the same age differ greatly in their sensory abilities, and these differences are only partly based on disposition (see Sect. 3.2 Causes of individual differences). Both human and animal studies suggest that sensory sensitivity can be influenced by the intensity and frequency of tactile, haptic, and proprioceptive experiences (Mueller et al. 2014a; Wong et al. 2013; Montagu 1986). This use-dependent effect is retained through adulthood and old age. Therefore, in principle, all perceptual dimensions of the haptic system can be improved with training (Gibson 1953). This includes improvements in the perception of joint positions, weights, pressure stimuli, the discrimination of tactile-spatial stimuli, and solving complex haptic shape, structure, and object recognition tasks. This **perceptual learning (or sensory learning)** refers to the improvement of perceptual ability by repeatedly performing a perceptual task. Usually, only a few practice sessions are required to produce a significant effect. However, most of these effects are highly task-specific. In other words, the sensory learning effects are exclusive to the practiced task, while no changes occur in other tasks. One reason for this lack of generalization is that research settings use primarily tactile tasks. For example, the current predominant settings involve the discrimination of two tactile contact points (two-point threshold) and its improvement through training (Gibson 1953; Gilbert et al. 2001; Harrar et al. 2014).

In contrast, studies on individuals whose daily lives routinely require sensory and fine motor tasks (e.g., physical therapists and pianists) report that it is possible to achieve generalizing effects through training (Mueller et al. 2014a; Ragert et al. 2004). These individuals not only perform exceptionally well in the activities they frequently perform, but they also achieve better average test scores than control persons of the same age when performing haptic tests. Accordingly, physiotherapists with or without additional osteopathic training achieved better mean haptic thresholds than controls (Fig. 4.1) (Mueller et al. 2014a). However, the dispersion (variance) in haptic thresholds was equally high between physical therapists and between control persons. Consequently, the everyday occupational "training" (in the form of palpation for diagnostic and therapeutic purposes) led to a group effect, but interindividual differences persisted. Considering the large differences in sensitivity, even among young professionals (Mueller et al. 2014a; Mueller and Grunwald 2013), appropriate sensory tests and training modules should be established within the framework of physiotherapeutic educational guidelines (Sect. 4.3).

Research suggests that individuals with **poorer baseline performance tend to benefit more from training** than those with high baseline performance (Wong et al. 2013). Individuals with high baseline performance can also improve their sensory abilities through training, but the effects tend to be less pronounced. In general, training effects exhibit **high sta-**

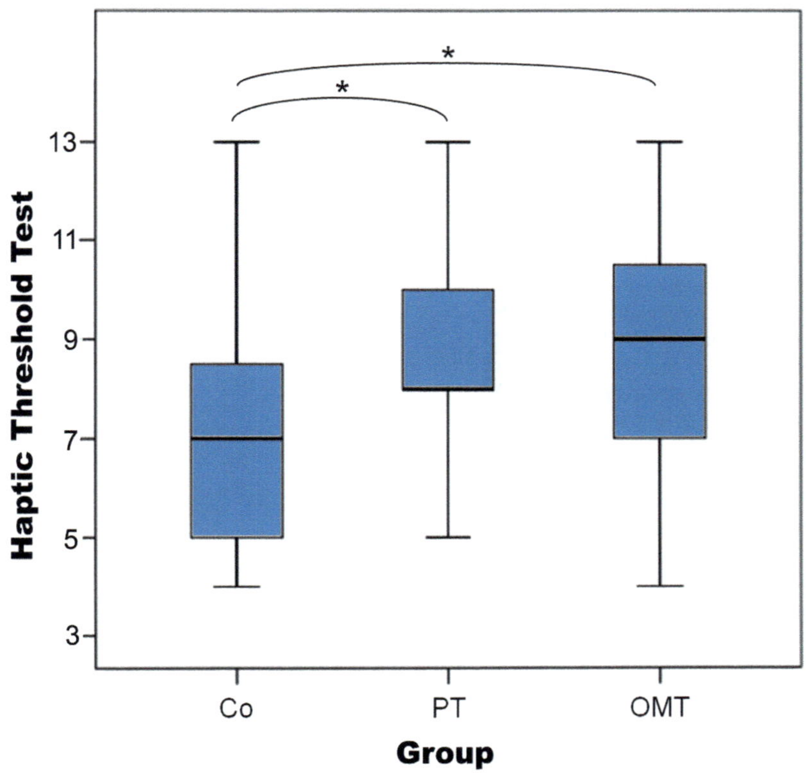

Fig. 4.1 Training effects of demanding sensory and fine motor tasks. Physical therapists (PT) and PT with additional osteopathic training (OMT) achieve better mean haptic thresholds than comparison persons of the same age (Co). Asterisks indicate significant group differences. Variance is similar in all three groups. Higher values in the Haptic-Threshold-Test (Sect. 4.2.3) indicate better perceptual performance. (Fig. from: Mueller et al. 2014a)

bility over time; they persist over long periods without additional training or can be reactivated with little effort (Kaas et al. 2013; Grunwald and Mueller 2017).

4.1.1.2 Counteracting Age Effects

Due to aging processes, sensory abilities progressively decline (Sect. 3.1.4). While it is well known that motor training can maintain mobility and physical strength into old age, the fact that the age-related decline in *sensory* abilities can also be counteracted by exercise and training has only been researched for a few years (Dinse et al. 2006). Research indicates that cortical reorganization after training differs between older and younger adults; learning processes in young people lead to changes in the somatosensory cortex that coincide with perceptual and performance improvements, while in older adults, performance declines despite cortical reorganization processes (Grunwald et al. 2002a; Kalisch et al. 2009). However, training can slow down age-related decline in sensory abilities in older adults substantially. Therefore, it is likely that **age-related decline in CNS functionality** is the primary cause of impaired haptic abilities in older individuals. In contrast, changes in the skin and connective tissue (e.g., decreasing mechanoreceptor density, decreasing nerve conduction velocity) are of secondary importance (Sect. 3.1.4). Therefore, learning new processing strategies can counteract the effects of age-related changes (Dinse et al. 2006).

Various experimental studies provide evidence for the preservation of sensory abilities through continuous training. In these studies, individuals whose everyday life is characterized by high sensory and fine motor demands (e.g., physiotherapists) are compared with a control group without notable haptic demands in everyday life or their occupation. In the control group, a decrease in haptic thresholds was already apparent in the 30–50-year age range. In contrast, no correlation between age and haptic threshold was found in a group of working physiotherapists in the same age range (Fig. 4.2) (Mueller et al. 2014a). Similar effects exist for blind persons who have learned to read Braille. In these persons, tactile discrimination acuity also remains high into old age (Stevens et al. 1996; Legge et al. 2008).

It is currently unknown upto which age consistent haptic sensitivity can be maintained by training. Furthermore, it has yet to be investigated whether increasing training intensity is required to delay the decline in haptic sensitivity with increasing age.

In principle, even manifest age-related deteriorations can be reduced by intense active training or **high-frequency sensory stimulation** (also known as tactile coactivation; see Sect. 4.1.2) (Dinse et al. 2006; Kalisch et al. 2008). Unfortunately, few sys-

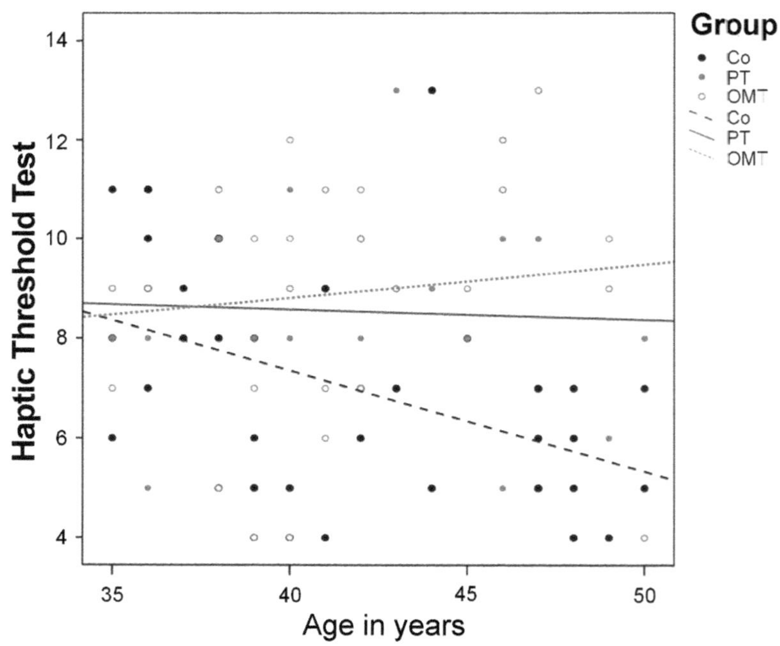

Fig. 4.2 Age effects of haptic perception and training. The graph shows the haptic thresholds of physical therapists (PT), physical therapists with additional osteopathic manual therapy (OMT) training, and healthy controls (Co) between the ages of 35 and 50 years. The three lines indicate the regression lines per group. Higher scores in the Haptic-Threshold-Test (Sect. 4.2.3) indicate better perceptual performance. (Fig. from: Mueller et al. 2014a)

tematic studies have investigated training effects of the upper limb in healthy older age (Dinse et al. 2006; Kalisch et al. 2008; Voelcker-Rehage and Godde 2010). Instead, training of upper limb sensitivity has been investigated mainly in the context of stroke rehabilitation (Sect. 4.1.2). Relatively more studies are dedicated to the improvement of proprioception of the lower limb to maintain stance and gait stability in old age and in the context of diseases (Sect. 4.1.3).

4.1.2 Upper Limbs: Sensory Rehabilitation After Stroke and Other Brain Injuries

Sensorimotor dysfunction and deficits are the most common neurological consequences of CNS injury. Approximately 80% of all individuals who have suffered strokes or other craniocerebral injuries exhibit motor and sensory dysfunction (Nelles et al. 2018). In Western industrialized nations, strokes with hemiparesis are the most common cause of acquired disability in adults (Warlow et al. 2008). Although most patients experience improvement in neurological symptoms in the first few months after the cerebral insult, a large proportion (more than 50%) of stroke patients retain sensory and motor impairments in the long term (Nelles et al. 2018). These namely affect the upper limbs, severely limiting activities of daily living (e.g., eating, dressing, and personal hygiene). Furthermore, **persistent impairment of arm-hand functions** is associated with anxiety, lower perceived quality of life, and reduced well-being. Therefore, improving arm-hand function is one of the central goals of poststroke rehabilitation efforts (Pollock et al. 2014).

Regarding predictors of rehabilitation success, the patient's age and the extent of hemiparesis have the greatest predictive power. The best chances of recovery are expected in patients with only motor deficits, while proprioceptive and cognitive functions are preserved. A recent review reported that patients with neglect have more severe impairments in proprioceptive function than patients without neglect (Fisher et al. 2020). Concomitant neurological deficits (e.g., aphasias, neglect, and deficits in proprioception) are generally considered prognostically unfavorable (Nelles et al. 2018).

▶ **Important** The success of *motor* rehabilitation depends on the extent of sensory (proprioceptive/haptic) impairment. Severe sensory impairment is a poor prognostic factor for motor rehabilitation.

Sensory deficits after stroke often affect both proprioception and skin sensitivity. As described in Chaps. 1 and 2, information from mechanoreceptors of the skin, connective tissue, joints, and muscles forms the basis for goal-directed movements. Consequently, disturbances in any of these perceptual dimensions can interfere with motor abilities, even with intact motor brain regions. This affects posture, balance, gait stability, and the fine motor processes required for activities of daily living. Therefore, functional disorders of a limb can be caused by motor or sensory impairments due to the close **interactions between motor and sensory systems.** With this in mind, it is not surprising that the success of motor rehabilitation depends on the extent of proprioceptive and haptic impairment (Tyson et al. 2008; Meyer et al. 2014; Krewer 2019).

▶ **Important** Disturbances in sensory abilities, even with intact motor brain regions, lead to impairment of motor skills.

Current standard poststroke therapy focuses on rehabilitating motor function. Despite the frequency of concomitant sensory disorders after stroke, approaches to their specific treatment are not part of the standard clinical therapy.

The reason for this likely lies in the inconclusive and confusing nature of research on the effectiveness of sensory training approaches. Although many promising techniques exist, few high-quality studies have examined their effectiveness (Doyle et al. 2010). Consequently, only a few evidence-based **therapeutic methods** exist **to improve sensory deficits after stroke** (Findlater and Dukelow 2017), which will be introduced below.

▶ **Important** To achieve motor rehabilitation in the presence of sensory impairments, sensory skills must first be trained.

Sensory improvements can be achieved through repeated performance of discrimination tasks. It is thereby possible to achieve poststroke haptic and proprioceptive discrimination ability similar to the unimpaired half of the body (Carey et al. 1993). However, changes in sensitivity that are achieved in this way are often extremely task-specific (Carey et al. 1993); the training effects from discrimination tasks have little effect on sensitivity in other tasks and do not have positive effects on motor function (Mehrholz 2019). Therefore, sensory training that achieves cross-task effects is required. In recent years, randomized controlled studies have reported promising results. **Sensory training that achieves cross-task effects** can be divided into three groups:

- Proprioception training through goal-directed movement and grasping with adaptive haptic support
- Proprioception training through joint movement with amplification of sensory perception using vibration
- Electrical and repetitive sensory stimulation

4.1.2.1 Proprioception Training Through Goal-Directed Movement and Grasping with Adaptive Haptic Support

The term "proprioception training" does not denote a specific exercise; instead, proprioceptive performance can be trained through various exercises. **Proprioception training** usually refers to exercises of a specific joint to improve the ability to perceive joint position. In contrast, in neurorehabilitation, **sensorimotor training (SMT)**, balance training, and exercise therapy usually place simultaneous demands on multiple muscle groups and cognitive resources. This increases the difficulty of the training, as strength, balance, and joint position information from multiple body parts must be processed simultaneously. Consequently, intact sensory processing is required for active execution of these exercises. Therefore, improvements in sensory control, especially of the upper limbs, needs to be achieved by antecedent proprioception training of individual joints (Aman et al. 2014).

▶ **Important** Sensorimotor and balance training requires a minimum level of sensory/proprioceptive abilities. In the case of sensory impairments and paresis, sensory/proprioceptive abilities must be trained first.

The decision to initiate proprioception training should be based on the patient's abilities and limitations. For example, SMT also improves proprioception and balance in patients after stroke (Nelles et al. 2018; Lim 2019); however, the primary goal of SMT is to restore and maintain motor abilities, strength, and movement coordination. Without a rudimentary level of proprioception, complex sensorimotor and balance exercises like SMT cannot be performed.

▶ **Definition: Proprioception Training** To date, there is no comprehensive definition for proprioception training. In the context of this book, proprioception training is defined as exercises performed on specific joints that improve the ability to perceive joint position without placing additional demands on balance, muscle strength, or cognitive resources.

Unfortunately, sources differ in their use of the terms proprioception training, SMT, and balance training, and the terms are sometimes used synonymously.

Purposeful movements and grasping are the basis for executing all activities of daily living. Accordingly, a core element of stroke rehabilitation is active, repetitive motor training of action sequences and movements in addition to occupational therapy to improve activities of daily living. Active exercise of the paretic half of the body at the individual performance limit can also be trained by constraint-induced movement therapy (Taub's training) (Nelles et al. 2018). These techniques, which are already well established in the rehabilitation of sensorimotor disorders, require a minimum level of movement ability and control; therefore, their use is only possible in patients with mild-to-moderate impairments. In contrast, patients with high-grade paresis must relearn the voluntary activation of individual muscle groups and practice processing sensory stimuli. For this purpose, individualized impairment-oriented training, such as the **Arm Basis Training** developed by Eickhof (2001), has proven to be more effective than Bobath therapy (Nelles et al. 2018; Eickhof 2001; Platz et al. 2005). In addition, device-assisted (e.g., computer-assisted) methods can be used for patients with severe arm paralysis. **Computer-assisted training with minimal haptic support** is currently considered an effective method (Aman et al. 2014; Casadio et al. 2009). Such systems allow repetitive, interactive, and highly intensive training of the paretic hand or arm, adapted to individual needs (Veerbeek et al. 2014). In addition, an advantage of computer-assisted methods is that movement accuracy and training effects can be measured accurately. The improvements achieved in this way can be used as feedback to motivate the patient and document their successes.

An advantage of computer-assisted procedures is that the support functions are adaptive; they can be adapted to the patient's changing functional range. As the functional range increases, haptic feedback and computer-controlled cues can be gradually reduced (de Santis et al. 2014). In general, actively executed training movements produce larger positive effects than passive movements (Kaelin-Lang et al. 2005; Wong et al. 2011; Beets et al. 2012). Correspondingly, computer-controlled haptic support ranges from passive-guided movement to minimal cues during active movement.

▶ **Important** Active movements lead to larger training effects of proprioception than passively guided movements. Therefore, assisted (e.g., computer-assisted) support should be adaptively reduced.

Patients with chronic stroke (disease duration 12–76 months) showed substantial improvements in motor performance after 10× 1-h computer-assisted training sessions (one session per week). This improvement was observed both in patients **with moderate and severe impairments.** On average, the number of nontargeted movements declined, and the deviation from the movement target decreased significantly (from 4.3 to 0.8 cm with eyes open and from 5.9 to 1.1 cm with eyes closed) (Casadio et al. 2009). Even in patients with a disease duration of up to 15 years and pronounced arm paresis, successive improvements were achieved after several training sessions (de Santis et al. 2014; Lo et al. 2010). Moreover, these improvements persisted 6 months after completion of the training.

Interestingly, comparing computer-assisted therapy with conventional therapy without technical support (at the same intensity and duration of exercises) produced equivalent positive effects in patients (Lo et al. 2010). Consequently, the frequently reported improved outcome of computer-assisted training methods compared with standard therapy is mainly attributable to higher training intensity.

Note

Computer-assisted training, which provides minimal haptic support, produces positive effects, even in patients with chronic stroke and severe paresis. The higher intensity of computer-assisted training methods explains the better outcomes of computer-assisted training compared with standard therapy.

4.1.2.2 Proprioception Training by Joint Movement with Amplification of Sensory Perception Using Vibration

Another method to train proprioceptive processes involves using vibratory stimuli. For this purpose, two vibrating elements are attached to the joint: one above the tendon of the flexor muscle and one above the tendon of the extensor muscle. When the patient performs a movement, a vibratory impulse stimulates the stretched tendon. Usually, the vibration is computer controlled and is linked to a flexor-extensor movement system. The patient is instructed to follow the stretching impulses and perform the movement together with the device. With each change of direction of the movement, the vibration changes between the flexor and the extensor tendon. Vibration stimulation is always applied to the respective antagonistic (i.e., stretched) muscle and should be between 30 and 100 Hz (Aman et al. 2014; Conrad et al. 2011; Marconi et al. 2011).

Exemplary for the possible effects of **amplification of sensory perception by vibration** is a longitudinal study on chronic stroke patients (disease duration 1–10 years) who had very low muscle strength (on average 10–25% of the hand strength of healthy comparison persons) and severe muscular cocontraction. They trained independently at home and performed 30 min of exercise training with vibration amplification (60 Hz) daily for 6 months. At the end of the 6-month period, muscular cocontraction had significantly decreased, extension and flexion strength had increased by at least 10%, and the ability to determine joint position had improved by 73% (arm) and 109% (leg) (Cordo et al. 2009).

In addition, there were significant positive effects on activities of daily living, step size, and step speed that persisted 6 months after the completion of training and even continued to increase on average.

With this vibration stimulation of the affected muscle group, the sensory perception of muscle stretch is enhanced. This type of **vibration synchronized with movement** is very different from the application of **vibrotactile feedback**. Vibrotactile feedback is used as cue stimuli, for example, to indicate errors or announce direction changes. These signals can be triggered at body locations that are far away from the trained muscle group (Cuppone et al. 2016).

> **Important** For proprioception training with amplification of sensory perception by vibration, vibration is applied to the antagonistic muscle tendon during movements. This synchronized vibration enhances stretch perception, which improves proprioception and reduces muscle cocontraction.

4.1.2.3 Electrical and Repetitive Sensory Stimulation

Electrical stimulation procedures are not primarily aimed at improving proprioception. Instead, electrical stimulation can have positive effects on both motor and sensory abilities. The electrical procedures differ primarily in the intensity of the applied stimulation. The intensity can range from involuntary muscle contractions (neuromuscular electrical stimulation [NMES]) to mild tingling sensations (peripheral nerve stimulation [PNS] and repetitive sensory stimulation [RSS]) to stimulation below the sensory perception threshold (transcutaneous electrical nerve stimulation; sensory noise method) (Pollock et al. 2014; Yang et al. 2019).

Many rehabilitation facilities offer **neuromuscular electrical stimulation (NMES)** and **electromyography-triggered neuromuscular electrical stimulation (EMG-NMES)**. In NMES, adhesive electrodes are attached to the patient's forearm, and electrical stimuli are used to stimulate the extensors and flexors of the hand/finger to trigger visible **muscle contractions**. In coupled EMG-NMES, NMES is activated only when the patient shows active muscle activity which is measured by EMG. This allows muscle movements and sensory feedback to be simultaneously and specifically reinforced. Both techniques have significant positive effects on the functional range of the upper limb, especially muscle strength (Pollock et al. 2014; Veerbeek et al. 2014).

Less intense electrical stimulation is used for PNS and RSS training than for NMES. The two forms of stimulation are used for different areas of application (forearm vs. finger), resulting in different effects.

For **peripheral nerve stimulation (PNS)**, electrodes are attached above the ulnar and median nerves of the paretic forearm. Pulses with a duration of 1 ms and a frequency of 10 Hz are applied. Activation of the electrodes is simultaneous. The stimulus intensity triggers a **slight tingling sensation,** but no visible muscle movement. Large positive effects on the motor function of the upper limb have been achieved when PNS was applied simultaneously with exercise training at the performance limit (Celnik et al. 2007; Ikuno et al. 2012). In this case, the PNS acts as an amplifier for the nerve signals triggered by the movement, producing faster and long-lasting cortical reorganization.

By using PNS daily for 1 h in combination with task-oriented training, permanent motor improvements can be achieved as early as after 1 week (measured with the Wolf Motor Function test [WMFT]; Ikuno et al. 2012). More intensive and prolonged training result in sustained improvements in the Fugl-Meyer Assessment (FMA) and the Action Research Arm Test (ARAT) (Carrico et al. 2018; Conforto et al. 2018).

In addition, PNS is suitable for **patients with chronic stroke, severe motor impairments, and severe hemiparesis.** Significant improvements in motor skills can be achieved after only 10 days of intensive training, and these improvements are maintained for at least 1 month after the completion of training (Carrico et al. 2016). Accordingly, PNS combined with intensive task-oriented training produced significantly stronger positive effects than task-oriented training alone: An increase in FMA score, reduction in WMFT score, and improvement in ARAT were reported.

> **Important** In NMES and PNS, electrodes are used to apply electrical stimuli to the patient's forearm. Simultaneously, the patient performs simple movements. In this way, motor skills can be improved, even in patients with chronic stroke and severe sensory and motor impairments.

In contrast with PNS, **repetitive sensory stimulation (RSS)** is usually performed directly on the fingers to affect sensory abilities. To perform the training, self-adhesive electrodes are attached to each distal phalanx. The application can be simplified by using a glove in which the electrodes are firmly integrated (TipStim® BOSANA Medizintechnik GmbH) (Kattenstroth et al. 2018). The electrodes stimulate the finger for 1 s at a frequency of 20 Hz, followed by a 5 s pause.

Studies on healthy persons of different ages report that RSS can achieve substantial **improvements in tactile, haptic, and proprioceptive perception**, which are associated with cortical reorganization (Höffken et al. 2007). The simultaneous stimulation of *several* mechanoreceptors in one area (e.g., an entire fingertip) is crucial for the stimulation training to be effective. For this reason, the technique is also called **tactile coactivation.** Comparative studies show that repeated stimulation of a single receptor does not induce sensory changes or cortical reorganization (Pleger et al. 2003).

Results from feasibility studies examining the effects of RSS in stroke patients are promising (Smith et al. 2009; Kattenstroth et al. 2018). When used for 45 min per day for 10 out of 14 days, significant effects on both sensory and motor measures were achieved in a randomized controlled trial (Kattenstroth et al. 2018). Both groups (RSS and control) received standard rehabilitation, occupational, and physical therapy according to the Bobath, Affolter, or Perfetti concept, training in activities of daily living, and mental activation training during the study. At the end of the 2-week intervention, only participants in the group that had received RSS showed significant changes compared with pretest levels. Improvements in tactile sensitivity were measured using von Frey monofilaments (Sect. 1.1.1) and the Grating Orientation Test (Sect. 4.2.4). Proprioceptive and motor improvements were assessed using the Jebsen–Taylor Hand Function Test, the Nine-Hole Peg Test, and by the ability to determine joint position (Kattenstroth et al. 2018). In a feasibility study without a control group, the effects were maintained 4 weeks after the completion of training (Smith et al. 2009). The uniqueness of this method is the **complete passivity of the treated person** during the application. To date, mainly patients in the subacute stage of recovery after stroke have been studied. Future studies are needed to investiagte what effects can be achieved in chronic stroke patients with severe motor and sensory impairments. Analogous to PNS, future studies should also investigate whether RSS with concurrent exercise training can achieve additional functional progress.

> **Important** In RSS, electrical impulses are applied directly to the fingers. The uniqueness of this method is the complete passivity of the treated person during the application. Substantial improvements in tactile, haptic, and proprioceptive performance can be achieved through RSS.

4.1.3 Lower Limbs: Balance and Proprioception Training in Different Diseases and Old Age

Sports activity, sensory-motor training, and reactive balance training of the lower limb can help improve proprioception and strengthen the musculature. The primary field of application is fall prevention (see list of applications). In addition, these procedures aim to strengthen motor control and improve stance and gait stability, which can increase mobility, strength, and range of motion and reduce pain.

Selected applications for balance training include:

- Gait instability in old age and after ankle or knee injuries
- Exercise therapy for physical fitness in old age
- Infantile cerebral palsy
- Multiple sclerosis
- Peripheral neuropathy (PNP)
- Rehabilitation after surgery (e.g., hip or knee surgery)
- Osteoporosis
- Diseases or damage of the vestibular organ/vertigo
- Rehabilitation after stroke

Age-related decline in postural control and balance occurs as early as 40 years of age and accelerates after the age of 60 years (Nicholson et al. 2015). While limitations in balance correlate strongly with age, the underlying processes are not exclusively age-related degeneration processes. Instead, **lack of exercise and predominantly sedentary activities** strongly contribute to declines in stance and gait stability. Diseases and injuries that additionally limit the extent of physical activity accelerate the degeneration process. In addition, **inflammatory or degenerative disorders** can lead to declining sensory and motor functions. For example, individuals with chemotherapy-induced polyneuropathy (mean age of study participants = 55 years) are similarly impaired in stance and gait stability as individuals 15 years older without cancer (Schmitt et al. 2017).

An increasing number of studies report that postural control and balance can be improved through physical activity and specific exercises at any age and in the context of many diseases.

The various exercises that can be used to improve balance and motor control differ in the degree to which they **affect motor, strength, or sensory functions**. For example, some exercises specifically affect single aspects (e.g., joint position training mainly affects proprioception), while others are more complex and extensive (e.g., partner dance). In addition, different tasks differ in the required activity level (Tai chi vs. focal muscle vibration). Techniques in which the person is treated passively, as in focal muscle vibration, are suitable, for example, as a supplemental therapy method (e.g., for persons with Parkinson's disease) or for persons who are easily exhausted.

4.1.3.1 Static and Dynamic Balance Training to Treat Peripheral Neuropathies

Both static and reactive balance exercises are commonly used to train balance. The main difference between exercises is the trigger of the instability. Instability can be achieved either through moving surfaces or by applying forces to the body. Depending on the biomechanical property that causes the instability, different motor strategies are required to stabilize the body. For example, **static (sensorimotor) balance training** on soft or wobbly surfaces causes strong torque forces at the ankles (Freyler et al. 2016). In contrast, during **reactive balance tasks** on horizontally moving plates, the forces act on multiple joints (ankles, knees, and hips). Consequently, the training effects vary depending on the type of balance task and the center of mass of the training person. In other words, different balance workouts result in different functional and neuromuscular effects (Freyler et al. 2016). This is relevant for evaluating the achieved changes and selecting the appropriate tasks for each indication. Furthermore, it is helpful to question what causes balance problems in a person and which exercises—depending on the indication—promise the highest benefit. To measure the effects achieved after a training session, it is important to conduct tests that are sensitive to the same dimensions as the training performed.

▶ **Important** Different balance tasks place different demands on the neuromuscular system, which can produce different effects, that is, exercises vary in the extent they influence motor, strength, or sensory abilities.

A relatively new area of application for balance training is **peripheral neuropathies (PNP)** of various etiologies. Recent research suggests that physical activity, namely balance training, can have positive effects on motor and sensory symptoms in all types of PNP (Kluding et al. 2017; Streckmann et al. 2014).

PNP comprises a group of disorders that can lead to the impairment of motor, sensory, and autonomic nerve fibers. Typical symptoms include neuropathic pain, paresthesia (e.g., tingling, burning, and numbness), hypersensitivity to touch stimuli (hyperesthesias), reduced touch sensitivity (hypesthesias), reduced proprioception, muscle weakness, reduced balance, and gait unsteadiness (Streckmann et al. 2014). These symptoms usually start in fingers or toes and spread in a distal-to-proximal direction. As the intensity of the symptoms increases, activities of daily living become more difficult, and the risk of falls increases, severely affecting the patient's quality of life. Diabetes mellitus is the causative factor in approximately one-third of patients with PNP. Other common causes are side effects of drugs (e.g., chemotherapy), autoimmune diseases, metabolic disorders, vitamin deficiencies, and unknown causes (idiopathic neuropathy).

Note
Physical activity, especially balance training, has a positive effect on motor and sensory symptoms in all types of PNPs.

Strength, balance, and endurance training can help prevent **diabetic polyneuropathy (DPN)** and diabetic foot syndrome (Streckmann et al. 2014). However, special care is required to prevent injuries and treat them appropriately. If symptoms of diabetic foot syndrome are already present (Table 4.1), activities that are as gentle on the foot as possible (e.g., ergometers) should be preferred (Kluding et al. 2017).

Table 4.1 Risk factors for diabetic foot syndrome in DPN

Functional system	Risk factor
Skin	Diabetic foot ulcer
	Callus formation, blisters, redness
	Dry, cracked skin/peripheral hair loss
	Ingrown toenails
Nervous system	Absence of Achilles tendon reflex
	Absence of vibration perception
Musculoskeletal system	Foot deformations
	Inappropriate shoes (wrong size, insufficient protection of the foot)
Vascular system	Disturbed blood flow/no measurable distal pulse

Adapted from Kluding et al. (2017)

In recent years, increased research efforts have been directed at reducing the symptoms of **chemotherapy-induced polyneuropathy (CIPN)** through physical activity (Streckmann et al. 2014; Hilkens and ven den Bent 1997). CIPN is the most common neurological side effect of chemotherapeutic interventions (Quasthoff and Hartung 2002). Its occurrence is clinically relevant in two ways:

- First, the physical limitations caused by CIPN can trigger a vicious cycle of physical inactivity and avoidance that ultimately leads to patients being unable to independently perform activities of daily living (Duregon et al. 2018).
- Secondly, the occurrence of neuropathy requires a reduction in the treatment dose or even a pause or termination of chemotherapy, which may have adverse effects on the course of therapy and possibly on survival (Streckmann et al. 2014; Stubblefield et al. 2009).

Previous treatment approaches for CIPN have been limited to the medicinal treatment of neuropathic pain; however, these interventions have no effects on motor or sensory symptoms. Instead, drug treatment is often associated with additional side effects (Streckmann et al. 2014).

To date, few clinical trials have systematically examined which exercise activities are best suited to counteract CIPN symptoms. However, the existing studies provide robust evidence that improvements in functional limitations and fatigue can be achieved through sports, occupational, and physical therapy. Initial meta-analyses provide evidence that **sensorimotor and balance training is particularly useful in reducing CIPN symptoms**, improving balance and postural control, and enhancing quality of life and physical performance (Streckmann et al. 2014; Duregon et al. 2018). Studies in which only strength or endurance were trained produced smaller effect sizes (Streckmann et al. 2014). Therefore, sports and exercise programs that include endurance and strength and sensorimotor/balance training sessions are likely to produce the most comprehensive positive effects (Duregon et al. 2018). No undesirable side effects are reported when practitioners adhere to the usual contraindications (see Table 4.2). To achieve positive effects on CIPN symptoms, training programs should be conducted two or three times a week for at least 10 weeks (Mizrahi et al. 2015). Depending on the type of exercise, after at least 15 training sessions, patients reported a decrease in pain and tingling symptoms and improvements in pressure and vibration perception of the lower limbs (Hilkens and ven den Bent 1997).

> **Important** Sensorimotor and balance training is superior to strength and endurance training in reducing the symptoms of CIPN, improving balance and postural control, and enhancing quality of life and physical performance in oncology patients.

Table 4.2 Contraindications and precautions for sporting activity in cancer

Variable	Contraindication
Treatment factors	Days on which intravenous chemotherapy is administered
Blood count changes	Low platelet/neutrophil count
	Low hematocrit value
	Low hemoglobin level
Musculoskeletal disorders	Severe muscle weakness
	Severe weakness (fatigue)
	Pronounced cachexia (>35% weight loss since onset of disease)
Gastrointestinal disorders	Severe nausea, vomiting, or diarrhea in the last 36 h
	Dehydration
	Malnutrition (inadequate fluid/nutrition intake)
Cardiovascular disorders	Chest pain
	Increased resting pulse/irregular heartbeat
	Swollen ankles/lymphedema (wear compression stockings)
Pulmonary disorders	Respiratory disorders/shortness of breath
	Cough/chest pain
Neurological symptoms	Strongly declining cognitive abilities
	Dizziness/disorientation/ataxia
	Blurred vision
	Increased postural instability
Systemic factors	Acute infection
	Fever
	Surgical intervention within 8 weeks

Table from Stefani et al. (2017)

4.1.3.2 Exergames

In recent years, an increasing number of studies have examined whether interactive computer game technology (e.g., Nintendo Wii or Microsoft Kinect) can be used to promote mobility and balance. In these so-called "exergames," figures (avatars) or objects on a screen are controlled using body movements. Large body movements are registered by a camera or motion sensor and replace the joystick, keyboard, and controller. For example, upper body movements and shifts in balance can be used to move a figure into a ski slalom, or corresponding arm movements can be used to play tennis, golf, or bowling.

It has long been understood that physical activity positively affects the maintenance and regeneration of motor skills and balance and that individuals who are more physically active (e.g., through dance or Tai chi) experience fewer age-related changes. By using interactive game-based training methods, both motivation and enjoyment of physical activity can be increased. In addition, the activities can be performed independently at home, alone, or in small groups, which may make them more attractive to some individuals than playing sports together with strangers in sports facilities (Yardley et al. 2006). Commercial fitness and balance games are usually used in studies. Study results are promising and suggest that balance exergames can achieve similar preventive effects to conventional balance training programs (Nicholson et al. 2015; Jeon et al. 2020; Toulotte et al. 2012). Both **seniors and younger adults benefit** from this training (Gioftsidou et al. 2013; Nitz et al. 2010). Younger (20–22-year-old) and middle-aged (30–60-year-old) adults showed significant improvements in single-leg balance (eyes open) and leg muscle strength after 8 weeks of training.

Further potential applications exist for various diseases and surgical rehabilitation. For example, improvement in leg proprioception and reductions in postural instability were achieved in individuals aged between 60 and 70 years with **diabetes mellitus type 2** after 12 weeks of training (3 times per week for 40 min each time) (Morrison et al. 2018). Specifically, the group that performed balance exergames (without supervision) experienced effects similar to those of participants who completed supervised conventional balance training.

Studies have reported that exergames are also suitable after **cruciate ligament surgery** (mean age of patients: 29 years). Twelve weeks of training with Wii balance exercises resulted in the same positive effects as a conventional rehabilitation program and improved muscle strength, dynamic balance, and range of motion (Baltaci et al. 2013).

Patients with **Parkinson's disease** also benefit from exergames (two or three times per week) at least as much as from analogous balance training. Some studies even suggest larger positive effects from exergames than from traditional training methods (Garcia-Agundez et al. 2019). After 8 weeks of training, patients with Parkinson's disease showed significant improvements on the Berg Balance Scale, the Timed Up and Go Test (Shih et al. 2016), one-leg stand with eyes closed, cognitive skills, and activities of daily living (Garcia-Agundez et al. 2019; Esculier et al. 2012; Pompeu et al. 2012). Depending on disease status, exercises can be performed at home or with supervision. The current commercially available exergames are not specifically designed for seniors or individuals with disabilities. For individuals without computer game experience or with mild cognitive impairments, it is recommended that at least one supervised introductory training session be conducted to assess suitability and prevent frustration. Games tailored to seniors with more severe physical (and cognitive) limitations are currently under development (Brox et al. 2016).

4.1.3.3 Vibration Training (Vibrating Plates)

This section refers to vibration training using vibrating platforms.

A large body of early research on the effectiveness of vibration plates comes from the sports science community. Athletes use vibration training to supplement strength and cardio workouts. For this purpose, they perform various static and dynamic exercises, such as squats, forearm planks, or push-ups, on the vibrating platform. Studies indicate that training on a vibrating platform (alternative names: **stochastic resonance training (SRT)**, whole-body vibration, and biomechanical stimulation) can increase muscle strength, mobility, and balance (Jones 2014; Jones et al. 2011; Bush et al. 2015).

▶ **Important** ***Note!*** The term "stochastic resonance training" should not be confused with the application of local vibration stimuli below the perceptual threshold, which is sometimes also referred to as "stochastic resonance" see below in this chapter.

The unique feature of vibration training is that the required training time is very short (a few minutes), and the intensity can be varied by adjusting the vibration speed and adding dynamic exercises. In addition, less muscle soreness and muscle stiffness occur after this type of training than after conventional aerobic exercises (Aminian-Far et al. 2011). Because of these characteristics, whole-body vibration is also suitable for untrained individuals or individuals with limitations, and the number of studies investigating the effects of vibration training in various patient groups is rapidly increasing. The results of these studies indicate the **versatile effects and wide-ranging applications** of vibration training.

The key effects of vibration training include:

- Improvement of proprioception (especially in the lower extremity)
- Increased balance and postural control
- Increased muscle strength
- Preservation/increase of bone density (e.g., postmenopausal or in rheumatoid arthritis)
- Improvement of motor control and mobility (e.g., Parkinson's syndrome, after stroke, after surgery of the anterior cruciate ligament)
- Pain reduction (e.g., lower back, musculoskeletal pain, and fibromyalgia)
- Reduction of fatigue and improvement of general well-being (e.g., fibromyalgia, rheumatoid arthritis)
- Reduction of tremor and rigidity (Parkinson's syndrome)

► **Important** *Note!* Vibration plates used for whole-body vibration training are available in assorted designs with different vibration characteristics. Devices that generate stochastic vibration patterns are preferable due to the more joint-friendly and versatile movement.

The intensity of vibration training can be adjusted according to the initial level of athletic fitness, age, and pre-existing conditions. Accordingly, training sessions with low vibration frequency and amplitude, in which the person merely stands on the platform with both or one leg, are possible. Handles are available for additional support and as a safety aspect. During a training program lasting several weeks, the intensity can be increased by increasing the vibration frequency, duration, and number of weekly training sessions or by adding static or dynamic exercises. For example, in individuals **after cruciate ligament surgery**, significantly greater improvements in postural control and proprioception of the operated and healthy knee were achieved by 4 weeks of vibration training than by standard rehabilitation exercise (strength training, stretching, and proprioception training on a wobble board) (Moezy et al. 2008). Vibration training occurred three times per week and was slowly increased from 30 to 50 Hz, from 2.5 to 5 mm amplitude, and from 4 to 16 min total training duration.

In a long-term study over 12 months, **healthy individuals aged 60–80 years** were randomly assigned to 1 of 3 exercise groups: vibration training, fitness training, and a control group with no training. The two training groups trained three times per week. In the fitness group, this training included 1.5 h of endurance and weight training in addition to balance and stretching exercises. The vibration training group completed a total of 4–15 min of exercises on a vibration plate per training session. Duration of the training sessions increased in slow progression. The individual exercises lasted between 30 and 60 s, each followed by 15–60 s of recovery. Compliance was very high; 87% of participants completed the entire study period and participated in at least 80% of the training sessions. Fitness training and vibration training achieved comparable positive effects on the likelihood to fall during a balance test with eyes closed (Bogaerts et al. 2007) despite the **different time intensities of the training programs**. Meta-analytic evaluations suggest that less fit seniors may benefit more from vibration training than more fit seniors (Lam et al. 2012).

Experimental comparisons of vibration training and balance training on a wobble board showed similar positive effects in **patients with Parkinson's syndrome** and preexisting balance impairment. After 3 weeks of training, both training programs produced comparable improvements that were maintained 4 weeks after the completion of training (Sharififar et al. 2014; Ebersbach et al. 2008). In patients with Parkinson's syndrome, vibration training can also produce immediate short-term effects on tremors, rigidity, and the motor score of the United Parkinson Disease Rating Scale (UPDRS) (Kaut et al. 2011; Haas et al. 2006).

Patients after stroke showed comparable improvements in balance and movement measures after either 6-week vibration training or movement therapy to music. These effects persisted for at least 6 weeks after the completion of the training (van Nes et al. 2006). All patients also participated in a regular rehabilitation program.

▶ **Important** Vibration training can produce positive effects that are comparable to comprehensive training programs (e.g., sports rehabilitation) but with a much shorter time requirement.

In addition, there is evidence that vibration training has a positive effect on fracture healing and bone density (Edwards and Reilly 2015). Positive effects have been shown in women with **postmenopausal osteoporosis** and **patients with rheumatoid arthritis** (Stolzenberg et al. 2013; Verschueren et al. 2004; Prioreschi et al. 2016). In healthy persons, vibration training has been shown to positively affect tryptophan-kynurenine metabolism (Kepplinger et al. 2011). Tryptophan-kynurenine metabolism is suspected to be impaired in patients with chronic inflammatory, degenerative, and neuropsychiatric diseases. Therefore, reducing kynurenic acid in the body through vibration training could contribute to symptom improvement in various diseases (e.g., Alzheimer's dementia, schizophrenia, and depression). However, further studies are needed to confirm these effects.

Contrary to expectations, vibration training has **not yet shown any effects in patients with multiple sclerosis** (Sitjà Rabert et al. 2012; Kang et al. 2016). Studies analyzed muscular and functional abilities after 10 and 20 weeks of vibration training. However, compared to the control group, no improvements were observed in the Timed Up and Go Test, the Berg Balance Scale, or the 2-Min Walk Test.

▶ **Important** Due to the novelty of the application, there are few studies on the adverse effects of vibration training. Therefore, **contraindications** must be derived from prior knowledge of sports and rehabilitation medicine.

4.1.3.4 Focal Muscle Vibration

Focal muscle vibration is a passive method by which vibrations with low amplitude (300–500 μm) and high frequency (at least 100 Hz) are applied to narrowly defined body areas. **Punctual vibration** is applied directly to the muscle. Through this passive stimulation, positive effects on strength and endurance can be achieved. In addition, muscle pain after intensive training can be prevented.

While athletes have used this method since the 1970s, its use for rehabilitation after surgery and for the prevention of falls is still relatively new. The unique feature of this method is that very short interventions can achieve positive effects. For example, as little as 30 min of stimulation (3 times 10 min with a 1-min break) over 3 consecutive days improved muscle strength, movement control, and stability in single-leg stance by 20–65% (Brunetti et al. 2006; Filippi et al. 2009). The effects persisted for at least 90 days after the intervention and even increased further without additional training. Therefore, focal muscle vibration is also **suitable for untrained individuals** and can be the groundwork for subsequent training.

For relevant effects, the muscle must be slightly contracted during treatment (Filippi et al. 2009). Lower vibration frequencies, shorter application times, and relaxed muscles lead to significantly lower effects.

Because improvements are measurable immediately after the completion of a 3-day intervention, it is unlikely that the effects are due to an increase in muscle mass. Instead, the intense stimulation likely activates muscle spindles, tendon organs, and other mechanoreceptors, which causes **long-term potentiation and restructuring in the spinal cord and cortex.** Therefore, focal muscle vibration leads to reorganization processes in the CNS that are triggered by the strong and relatively long-lasting increase in afferent impulses.

Therapeutic applications of focal muscle vibration include fall prevention and the reduction of skeletal muscle hypertonia in patients with multiple sclerosis (Camerota et al. 2017) and after stroke (upper and lower extremity)

(Paoloni et al. 2010; Costantino et al. 2017) or spinal cord injury (Ahn and Song 2016; Murillo et al. 2011). In addition, in patients with Parkinson's disease, positive effects were observed on gait speed and step size (Camerota et al. 2016) and on the duration of freezing of gait (Pereira et al. 2016). Vibration stimuli may also cause a short-term reduction in tremors and rigidity in patients with Parkinson's disease (Jöbges et al. 2002). However, the effects on tremor and rigidity are not trainable and last only for the duration of vibration stimulation. Based on this finding, wearable applications ("wearables") are currently under development. In the future, they are intended to reduce hand tremors in patients with Parkinson's disease and may thereby facilitate everyday activities (e.g., writing, eating, and personal hygiene).

▶ **Important** Focal muscle vibration is the passive, punctual stimulation of a muscle. This method can achieve relatively large improvements in muscle strength, movement control, and balance, even with very brief interventions. In addition, abnormally increased muscle tone can be reduced.

4.1.3.5 Subliminal Vibration (Vibro-Tactile Noise)

The effects of subliminal vibration are also referred to as stochastic resonance. The term "stochastic resonance" originated in physics; it refers to the phenomenon that periodic signals can be detected best when minor signal noise is additionally present instead of being completely free of noise. This mechanism has been described for both technical systems and human sensory perception. The sensory perception of weak stimuli can be improved by adding noise. Evidence exists for acoustic, visual, and touch stimuli (Itzcovich et al. 2017; Moss et al. 2004). **Vibratory stimuli below the perception threshold** are used to improve perception in the haptic system (Severini and Delahunt 2018). By applying such vibro-tactile noise to the skin, immediate improvements in sensory functions can be achieved (Collins et al. 1996). However, the effects persist only for the duration of the stimulation.

▶ **Important** ***Note!*** The effects of stochastic resonance should not be confused with "stochastic resonance training (SRT)." SRT is an alternative name for vibration training, where a person performs static or dynamic exercises on a vibration platform (see "Vibration Training" in Sect. 4.1.3.3.). Unfortunately, these similar names are misleading because the interventions use distinct types of stimuli. SRT uses low-frequency, high-amplitude vibrations that cause the entire body to move visibly, depending on body tension. The effects of SRT are based on muscular training, which results from the force the person uses to oppose the vibration.

In contrast, stochastic resonance refers to subliminal vibro-tactile noise that causes temporary improvements in sensory functions.

No training effects can be achieved using vibro-tactile noise; instead, only temporary changes occur for the duration of the noise. Nevertheless, vibro-tactile noise produces interesting effects.

For example, the tactile perception threshold at the tip of the index finger is lower when the finger is simultaneously stimulated with vibro-tactile noise. This is true for poststroke patients, patients with diabetic neuropathy, and healthy elderly persons (Liu et al. 2002; Seo et al. 2014). Similarly, applying vibro-tactile noise to the foot improved tactile sensitivity in younger and older healthy individuals (Wells et al. 2005) and in persons with diabetic neuropathy (Liu et al. 2002). Other studies reported that this effect can **reduce body sway and improve gait stability**. The positive effects of vibro-tactile noise on stance and gait stability have been demonstrated in patients after stroke, patients with diabetes type 2, children with cerebral palsy, and healthy older adults (Priplata et al. 2003, 2006; Zarkou et al. 2018; Aboutorabi et al. 2018).

In recent years, wearable applications (e.g., insoles) have been developed that utilize vibrotactile noise to improve stance and gait stability. Studies on vibrating insoles suggest promising effects in patients with Parkinson's disease (Novak and Novak 2006), polyneuropathy (Priplata et al. 2006; Hijmans et al. 2007), and in elderly persons with a tendency to fall (Priplata et al. 2003). The first products are already available commercially.

4.2 Neuropsychological Tests and Training

Neuropsychological tests and training systems for education and clinical use must meet specific requirements that also apply to scientific purposes. First, they must be able to measure a specific characteristic or ability with a high degree of dependability (**reliability**), even with repeated measurement (**validity**), regardless of who administers or evaluates the test (**objectivity**). Second, the measurement results must be readily interpretable. Interpretation of test results is only possible if the tests have been standardized on large samples so that normative values are available. Individual test results can subsequently be compared to the **norm data**.

Except for intelligence tests, most neuropsychological tests are used to identify deficits. This is also true for extero-, intero-, and proprioception tests. Most tactile-haptic or proprioceptive tests are used to diagnose psychomotor developmental disorders and neurological diseases. Because they were developed to detect deficits, they are often simple or not validated for a higher performance range; consequently, they are not suitable for aptitude or performance testing. Internationally, few tactile and haptic examination procedures exist beyond testing neurological dysfunction. However, in recent years, the first test and training systems for **tactile-haptic or proprioceptive dimensions of healthy adults** have been developed (Sects. 4.2.2, 4.2.3 and 4.2.4).

4.2.1 Clinical Diagnostic Test Batteries for Children and Adults

4.2.1.1 Sensory Integration Test (SIT) and Göttingen Developmental Test of Tactile-Kinaesthetic Perception (TAKIWA)

The **TAKIWA** is normed for children 3–6 years of age and consists of seven predominantly tactile subtests: two-point discrimination, touch localization on the forearm and hands, pressure sensitivity, and graphesthesia (Kiese-Himmel 2003). In the graphesthesia subtest, the test administrator draws a geometric figure in the child's palm with a cotton swab. The child must then select the figure out of six possible images. In addition to the tactile tests, the battery includes two haptic subtests: a haptic stereognosis test (haptic recognition of everyday objects) and a test for distinguishing object properties (e.g., hard/soft, long/short). The theoretical foundation and conception of the TAKIWA are based on the Sensory Integration Theory and the **Sensory Integration and Praxis Test (SIPT)** developed by Jean Ayres (1972). The sensory integration theory (Sect. 1.1.3) assumes that development and learning can only occur if sensory integration processes are intact, that is, only if information from different sensory channels is appropriately merged in the brain. The SIT is a comprehensive test system for children that measures visual, tactile, and proprioceptive perception, motor skills, and integration ability using 17 subtests.

There are no objective test procedures for children younger than 3 years of age or infants, as their ability to follow instructions is limited. Therefore, assessments in this population are always made subjectively by caregivers or medical staff (cf. Sect. 3.4.2).

4.2.1.2 Luria-Nebraska Neuropsychological Battery (LNNB)

The **LNNB** has a version for children aged 8–12 years and an adult version for persons aged 15 years and older. It is used to distinguish psychiatric, pseudoneurological, and neurological disorders (Golden et al. 1978, 1985). The LNNB measures motor skills, tactile perceptual abilities, language, visuospatial, auditory, and cognitive functions. The tactile portion of the LNNB is composed of tasks for the localization of touch on the arm and hand, pressure and movement thresholds, and tasks for the haptic recognition of everyday objects (stereognosis). Motor skills are evaluated using simple movement and imitation tasks.

4.2.1.3 Halstead–Reitan Test Battery

The Halstead–Reitan test battery is one of the few sets that offer more complex haptic diagnostic instruments for adults. The Tactual Performance Test (TPT) and the Tactile Form Recognition (TFR) subtests require active, haptic exploration of various stimuli (Reitan and Davison 1974; Reitan and Wolfson 1993). When used as instructed, these tests effectively distinguish healthy individuals from those with brain lesions.

The TPT consists of ten wooden figures and a board with cut-out shapes into which the figures must be fitted (Fig. 4.3). During testing, the figures, board, and exploring hands are covered by a box. The test is performed three times, with the dominant hand, nondominant hand, and both hands. Subsequently, the test participants must draw the board with the figures in the correct positions from memory.

The TFR subtest of the Halstead–Reitan test battery requires that four flat shapes (circle, cross, triangle, and square) made of plastic must be explored in succession and recognized as quickly as possible on a picture (Reitan and Wolfson 2002). During exploration, the hands are covered. The test is performed once with each hand.

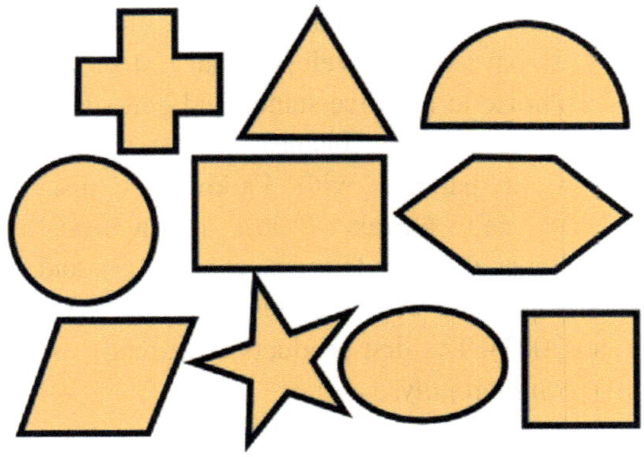

Fig. 4.3 Tactual Performance Test (TPT). The task involves haptic exploration of the test board and figures and placing the 10 three-dimensional figures into the corresponding omission of the TPT test board without visual information. (Fig. from: van Dijk et al. 2013)

4.2.2 Tactile Threshold Tests

Widely used and often part of standard neurological examinations are tactile threshold tests in the form of **two-point discrimination** (Sect. 1.1.1), point localization, and **Grating Domes** to measure tactile spatial resolution, **von-Frey monofilaments** (Sect. 1.1.1) to determine skin sensitivity, and the **tuning fork test** (Sect. 1.1.2) to assess peripheral nerves (vibration threshold). These tests can be used as diagnostic tools in patients and to determine interindividual differences in healthy individuals. The Grating Orientation Task (Grating Domes, Fig. 4.4) (van Boven and Johnson 1994; Johnson and Phillips 1981) is an advancement of two-point discrimination, with more objective implementation. For this test, norm data are available for healthy individuals up to old age (Tremblay et al. 2000).

4.2.3 Haptic Threshold and Perception Tests

For research, haptic thresholds are determined using various settings. The disadvantage of these examination settings is that they are only feasible under laboratory conditions because they require a high degree of structural and technical effort and a large amount of time. In addition, these examination conditions require covering the eyes or hands or closing the eyes during testing, which is different from everyday practice. Research shows that the haptic recognition abilities of individuals who can see their hands during exploration and individuals whose hands are covered differ significantly in their performances (Mueller et al. 2013). Visibility of one's own exploration

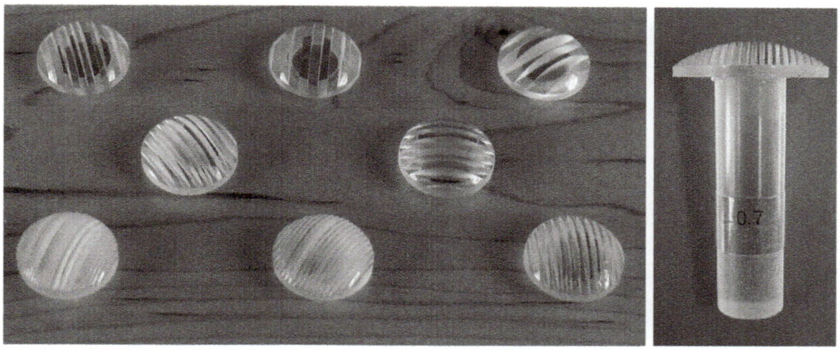

Fig. 4.4 Grating Domes (Grating Orientation Test; Stoelting Co., Wood Dale, IL) consist of plastic stamps with groove reliefs of varying spacing (0.35, 0.5, 0.75, 1.0, 1.2, 1.5, 2.0, and 3.0 mm). Each of the stamps is lightly pressed on the fingertip of the index finger a total of 20 times for 1 s each. During this process, the orientation of the relief lines is randomly alternated between vertical and horizontal. The perception threshold corresponds to the groove spacing that is still correctly recognized in at least 75% of the trials. (Fig. from: Haptic Research Lab, University of Leipzig)

movements results in significantly poorer haptic perception; therefore, the visibility of one's own hands increases the difficulty of perception in haptic exploration.

The following haptic tests are designed to be portable and allow exploration while the eyes remain open.

4.2.3.1 The Haptic Threshold Test

The Haptic Threshold Test (HTT; Haptik-Forschungszentrum, Germany) is currently the only internationally available portable test system that measures a person's haptic threshold during active haptic exploration in the range of micrometers (Mueller et al. 2014a; Mueller and Grunwald 2013; Grunwald and Mueller 2017). Furthermore, the eyes of the test person can remain open during the test, and free exploration is possible with both hands. Therefore, the HTT ensures relatively naturalistic conditions and is suitable for testing healthy adults.

The HTT consists of 13 stimuli (haptic pads) with raised, parallel relief lines covered by a separation film. This separation layer is 252-μm thick and opaque, so the underlying relief lines can be palpated but not visually perceived. With each stimulus, the distance between the relief lines decreases by 200 μm. The line distance of each haptic pad and the technical deformation measures of the separation film are shown in Table 4.3. These measurement values represent mean values of the palpable deformation at medium pressure levels.

Table 4.3 Threshold values of the Haptic Threshold Test

Haptic pad number	Line distance (mm)	Deformation-values (μm)[a]
1	3.0	54.71
2	2.8	45.62
3	2.6	39.40
4	2.4	26.11
5	2.2	25.57
6	2.0	23.42
7	1.8	15.23
8	1.6	12.22
9	1.4	10.69
10	1.2	8.25
11	1.0	7.14
12	0.8	6.48
13	0.6	2.16

[a] Mean deformation values of the PVC layer of each haptic pad of the Haptic Threshold Test, measured with an applied force of 150 mN of a vertical indenter tip

The participant's task is to align the round haptic pads so that the relief lines are oriented horizontally to the test board (Fig. 4.5). Participants complete two full iterations of all 13 haptic pads, starting with the easiest, and an additional validation measurement of those haptic pads with ambiguous results. The haptic threshold is the haptic pad with the smallest line spacing that was correctly aligned in at least two of three iterations.

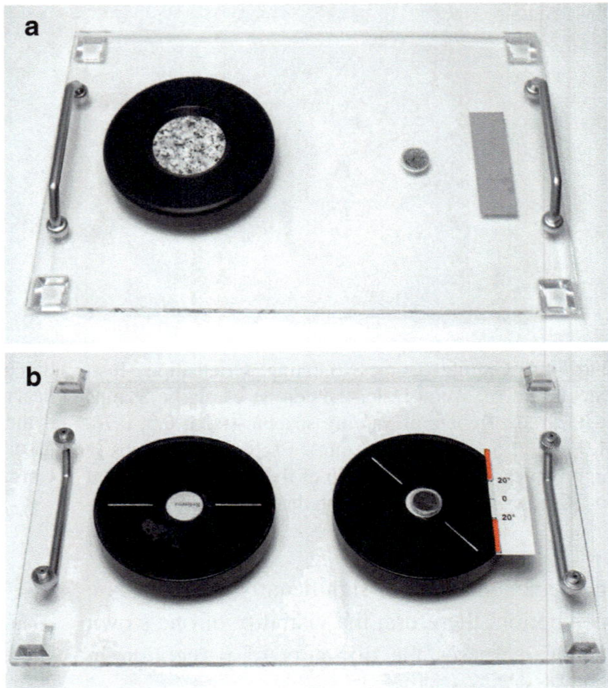

Fig. 4.5 Haptic Threshold Test. (**a**) Front side of the test board with a reference pad (7 mm line spacing) fixed in horizontal orientation. (**b**) Back side of the test board with the horizontal reference (left) and a threshold pad aligned outside the 20° mark (right). (Source: Haptic Research Lab, University of Leipzig)

For validation, the back of each haptic pad is marked with a horizontal line, and a degree scale is fixed on the back of the transparent test board. This allows the investigator to determine whether each haptic pad has been set within the range of ±20°. Haptic pad settings that exceed the range are considered false detections (i.e., not detected).

▶ **Important** Video instruction can be found on YouTube under the keyword "Haptic Threshold Test." https://www.youtube.com/watch?v=sw2XMMY7krg.

The average haptic threshold of $N = 285$ healthy participants (age 18–60 years) is $M = 8.72$ (SD = 2.30) (Grunwald and Mueller 2017). Haptic pad No. 8, with an average deformation measure of 12.22 µm, is reliably recognized by healthy participants. The re-test reliability of the HTT after at least 6 months is high ($r = 0.845$, $p < 0.0001$) (Mueller et al. 2014a).

4.2.3.2 Haptic Figures Test

The Haptic Figures Test (HFT, Haptik-Forschungszentrum, Germany) measures general haptic perceptual ability (Mueller et al. 2013, 2014a; Grunwald 2010) and visual-haptic integration ability (Mueller et al. 2014b). Due to the complexity of the test requirements, the HFT is well-suited for examining a broad age spectrum. In principle, the test is applicable from the age of 6 years; however, the primary target group is adults from adolescence to old age.

The test consists of 16 different raised relief stimuli (Fig. 4.6a). Each stimulus is enclosed in a rectangular frame and covered by an opaque separating layer (Fig. 4.6b). The structure of the HFT is like that of the HTT. By applying light exploratory pressure to the separating layer, the relief shapes underneath can be felt but not seen. The participant is instructed to recognize the explored shape on a visual display. The required exploration time and the number of errors are recorded. If the exploration time exceeds 3 min, the stimulus is marked as "not recognized."

In an alternative version of the test, with increased difficulty, the stimuli are presented without a visual display, and the recognized shapes must be drawn after exploration (cf. Sect. 4.2.5 Training Set). A gamification approach is also available as a memory game-type version.

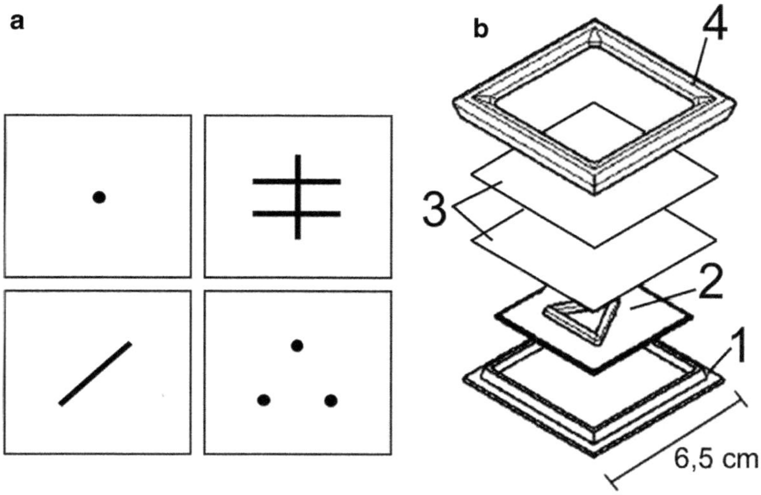

Fig. 4.6 Haptic Figures Test. (**a**) Schematic representation of four two-dimensional relief stimuli. (**b**) Exploded diagram of a stimulus: 1, base plate; 2, two-dimensional geometric shape as raised relief; 3, opaque separating layers; 4, holding frame. (Fig. from: Grunwald 2010)

4.2.4 Proprioception Tests

Proprioceptive abilities are commonly tested as part of neurological examinations to determine disorders of motor function, depth perception, or coordination. Standard tests include the knee-heel test, finger-finger test, finger-nose test, and reproducing joint positions. Test results are evaluated by visual estimate and are difficult or impossible to interpret objectively. Accurate and reliable measurements of force, position, and movement are only possible with elaborate computer-aided technology and are usually only performed for research purposes under laboratory conditions (Han et al. 2016).

Another challenge of measuring proprioceptive abilities is their versatility. There is currently no method that simultaneously measures all three proprioceptive dimensions (motion, position, and force). In addition, it is unclear to what extent proprioceptive dimensions are mutually dependent; for example, to what extent motion and force information contribute to position perception (Han et al. 2016). Furthermore, injuries and diseases can disturb the proprioception of individual joints (e.g., osteoarthritis; For disorders of the haptic system, see Sect. 3.3). Therefore, results from disordered joints cannot be used to conclude the proprioceptive ability of other body parts.

Currently, to our knowledge, there is only one portable method (Haptimeter; Grunwald et al. 2002b) that has the potential to measure the accuracy of movement and position stimuli. However, this method is currently in the evaluation and norming phase.

4.2.4.1 Haptimeter

The test setup of the Haptimeter (Haptik-Forschungszentrum, Germany) consists of two movable angle legs (Fig. 4.7). The test person must bring one of these angle legs into a predetermined position. The person's eyes are covered during the entire test procedure. A distinction is made between the two task types, with the orientation of the two angle legs being either parallel or mirrored. One angle leg is fixed in a predetermined angular position according to the protocol, and the other angle leg is brought into a vertical starting position. The task is to recognize the fixed angular position and align the other angular leg at the same inclination, either parallel or mirrored. Each task type is performed both with the left hand and with the right hand. Accordingly, a

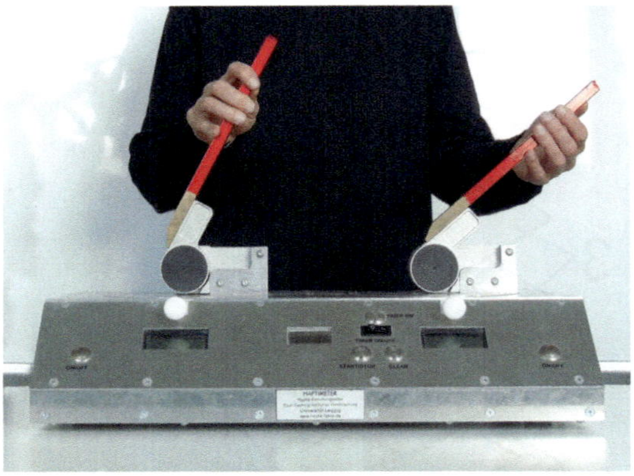

Fig. 4.7 Haptimeter. Execution of a parallel task. One angle is preset, and the other angle is brought into a parallel position with the same angular inclination by the test person. The eyes are covered during testing. (Fig. from: Grunwald and Mueller 2017)

total of four tasks are performed: right-parallel, left-parallel, right-mirrored, and left-mirrored. Each task is performed five times with different inclinations. The deviation from the target angle is measured in degrees (Grunwald and Weiss 2005; Grunwald et al. 2002b; Grunwald and Gertz 2001).

4.2.5 Training Set for Healthy Adults

Repeated performance of specific tasks, actions, and motor sequences usually leads to a shorter duration of performance and fewer errors. Therefore, haptic training can be used for both rehabilitation (Sect. 4.1.2) and **skills training**. Trainings are usually tailored to a situation; for example, grasping movements can be relearned after a stroke, or highly specialized skills, such as performing a lumbar puncture, can be practiced with the help of a simulator (Patton et al. 2006; Gorman et al. 2000; Sutherland et al. 2013). However, the effects that can be achieved by such training are usually selectively limited to the action practiced or aimed at reducing disease-related limitations.

One extraordinary characteristic of the sense of touch in contrast with other sensory systems is that an improvement in sensitivity can be achieved even in healthy individuals through suitable sensory training. Furthermore, age-related deterioration in sensitivity can be counteracted (Sect. 4.1.1). Haptic perceptions require the complex interaction of peripheral sensors and cognitive processing, including working memory, sensory integration, and spatial ability. Therefore, haptic training that requires the palpation of complex shapes without visual feedback can improve individual haptic thresholds.

Despite this potential, only one validated training procedure exists to date, which is designed to improve haptic perception ability and sensory threshold in healthy adults. All other commercially available procedures are used to promote development in children (Sect. 3.4.2 and 4.2.1) or for rehabilitation after severe illness (Sect. 4.1).

4.2.5.1 Leipzig Haptic Training Set

The Haptic Training Set (Haptik Research Center, Leipzig) aims to improve the haptic perception of **healthy individuals in the age range of 18–60 years** (Grunwald and Mueller 2017). Target groups are manual therapists and students of physiotherapy, osteopathy, or manual medicine. However, the training is feasible for all professional groups whose work involves palpatory tasks, including gynecologists, general practitioners, midwives, dentists, and speech therapists.

Prerequisites The prerequisites for participation in the training are that the person shows diminished haptic perception, as determined by the HTT and HFT (for both tests, see Sect. 4.2.3). Haptic thresholds of HTT < 8 or an increased error rate on the HFT without visual stimulus presentation (number of errors ≥ 5) suggest that training should be performed (Mueller et al. 2014a). In persons with such low values, it can be safely assumed that haptic perception is not sufficiently developed for the occupational applications of the target groups mentioned above. For successful participation, training should be self-motivated, voluntary, and without external pressure for results.

Procedure During the training sessions, the trainer presents the haptic figure pads from the training series in random order and orientation (Fig. 4.8; Grunwald and Mueller 2017). The trainee explores the structure of each haptic figure pad through haptic exploration. Visual or other information is not present to the trainee during exploration. The trainee may use any finger for exploration, and they may verbally report on their exploration experiences, if helpful. The pad can be placed on a table or held in hand, and there is no time limit. However, care must be taken to ensure that the trainee does not perform the exploration with the fingernail and that the temperature of the exploring hands is not lower than 23 °C.

After exploration, the haptic pad is put away and the trainee is asked to reproduce the recognized structure or parts of it on paper. Later, the trainer uses the reproductions to show which aspects of the stimulus still need to be correctly recognized and asks the trainee to explore the same haptic pad again. In this way, the trainee should successively develop adequate haptic-visual imagery of the exploration process.

The same procedure is followed with each haptic pad in the series. The stimuli of the training series are presented to the trainee as often as necessary until no further errors occur.

Usually, four or more training sessions are required (Fig. 4.9). The number of sessions cannot be determined in advance because learning progresses individually. To limit the visual information transfer to the trainee and for documentation purposes, the drawings/reproductions should remain with the trainer after the training sessions. If all stimuli of the series are recognized by the trainee without errors, the training can be terminated.

During the training, the trainer must consider the individual learning processes. Impatience and degrading feedback from the trainer do not promote learning performance. After completing all training sessions, the haptic threshold is re-tested using the HTT, and the haptic integration ability is assessed using the HFT. In this way, the training effects can be evaluated objectively. The training sessions should take place once a week. Per single session, 1–1.5 h should not be exceeded because attention and concentration may decrease.

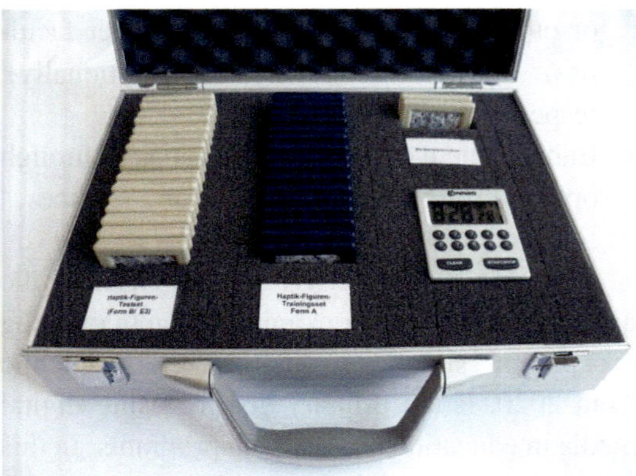

Fig. 4.8 Haptic Training Set. The set consists of a Haptic Figures Test (beige) for status assessment before and after training and a Haptic Training Set (dark blue) for conducting the practice sessions. (Source: Haptic Research Lab, University of Leipzig)

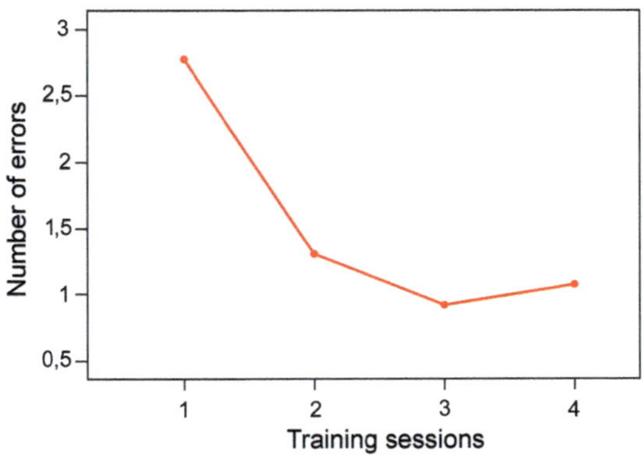

Fig. 4.9 Training effects after four training sessions. Active training with the Haptic Training Set. (Fig. from: Grunwald 2010)

4.3 Propaedeutic Course on Active Tactile Performance (PakT) in the Framework of Education and Training

4.3.1 Didactic Preliminary Considerations

4.3.1.1 Design of Learning Processes in Blended Learning Format

The scientific testing of tactile performance shows strongly fluctuating interindividual differences. In this respect, it is urgently required within the framework of training guidelines to establish corresponding sensory tests and training modules at least accompanying training (Mueller and Grunwald 2013). To ensure the quality of health care, appropriate training and tests should be an integral part of the curricula in the training and continuing education programs of the health care professions (see also Sects. 4.1.1. and 4.2.5). In particular, this applies to activities that include active exploration with the fingers as part of clinical examinations and therapy (e.g., manual therapy) as a core.

In order to be able to offer learners the testing of the haptic threshold and related training units on an interim basis under the current conditions in education and training programs, a propaedeutic course on active tactile performance (PakT) was developed. This is an online module designed as a blended learning format. The proportion of face-to-face lectures as well as the binding of teaching staff are reduced to a minimum. The proportion of guided self-learning is accordingly high. This requires good preparation, a high level of intrinsic motivation and and learning stops for the learners to check their progress.

The use of digital media in the educational landscape in the health professions initially incurs high costs, e.g., for technical equipment, media didactic qualification, expansion of the support structure of the IT facility, which are only amortized through repetition of the course. This does not apply exclusively to online teaching, but is generally true for every first-time activity and therefore also for every first-time course offered. Due to the pandemic, online teaching in Germany experienced a boost in 2020. Due to the closure of training and continuing education institutions, instructors had to make an ad hoc switch from face-to-face to online teaching. Likewise, institutions were challenged to implement technical equipment, e.g., for mobile work. Workplaces were temporarily set up in the home, as educational institutions were not allowed to be entered. Thus, for PakT, there is a conducive infrastructure that teachers in education and training programs, as well as learners as trainees, students, or professionals undergoing further training, can access.

The advantages of digital media in teaching and learning processes are:

- Improving the quality of teaching
- Improving the learning processes of learners, regardless of educational level
- Create new application and training opportunities, e.g., participation through selection options
- Higher learning success, respectively, motivation of the learners
- Reaching different target groups, e.g., single parents, working people
- Stronger opportunities for cooperation with other institutions (e.g., institutions of the same or other educational levels, with other faculties, locally, regionally, internationally), respectively, benchmarking
- Enhancement of face-to-face teaching through optional offerings, information and service

Reaching new target groups and ensuring the quality of teaching, for example, even in ongoing exceptional situations, such as the pandemic from 2020, is the primary goal of using digital media in education and training programs. In this context, the use of digital media merely represents an expansion of the teaching material that can be used. Instead of blackboard and chalk or flipchart and marker, smart device-based digital media (e.g., mixed reality) are also available.

Without an appropriate didactic concept, the analog and digital tools are worthless.

> **Important** The basic principle in the preparation of courses is: Didactic conception before media conception.

First of all, teachers must therefore clarify what they can use digital media, including smart device-based digital media, for in order to plan and implement them in a meaningful way. Digital media can improve the learning processes of the participants, for example, through supplementary visualizations, to highlight processes and to underline important points, which the learners can also call up frequently and at their own learning pace after the classroom event. The effect is least pronounced with individual still images, such as those found in textbooks. The advantage of digital media is more apparent with visualized processes in which learners have to intervene creatively. Interactive visualization can be suitable for demonstrating different approaches to knowledge and learning paths, transferring content in speech, writing, images, sound, etc., and preparing it in different ways and using multimedia. In this way, individual knowledge growth and its sustainable implementation in terms of competence and performance can be positively influenced. can be positively influenced. For example, it is more conducive to learning to use auditory information in combination with visualization instead of text. Pictures should always be presented in addition to text, e.g., directly on a slide. The **retention effects of texts read on screen are lower** than those of texts read offline (Tulodziecki and Herzig 2004). It has proven useful to present the courses prepared in this way online on teaching-learning platforms (e.g., Moodle) to learners with appropriate access rights. These teaching-learning platforms have been well tested in the meantime and fulfill several functions. For example, learners can exchange information in forums, set up their own virtual course rooms for small group work, or present their work results to monitor learning progress.

Conclusion

In the preparation, answers to the following questions become relevant: For whom and for what do I teach, what content with what media, when, how long, and how often.

4.3.1.2 Blended Learning Format as Best Practice

In terms of didactic design, the question arises as to how online teaching should be integrated into the course. Here, it is not trivial whether the course is an optional lecture at a state university without tuition fees or a compulsory course as part of a continuing education program financed by the participants themselves and completed in their free time. Learners can use content in advance to prepare for the course, then to follow-up on the course, alone or with other participants, mandatory or optional as a supplement. In principle, it must be clarified how online teaching is to be embedded in the overall course or which scenarios lend themselves particularly well. In view of the effort involved in creating videos or podcasts, for example, it should be considered whether the offering can also be utilized in other educational programs. Here, the interlacing of education and training offers or the cooperation of institutions in the form of study lines or tracks are possible.

> **Important** In the blended learning format, parts of classroom teaching are combined with online teaching in a meaningful way.

Blended learning is often preferred to exclusively online teaching and at the same time offers itself to **compensate for the weaknesses of face-to-face teaching** (Meyerhoff and Brühl 2015). These can lie in a high number of participants with the consequence of anonymity. Also, knowledge transfer with enrichment of visualization and interactive elements does not necessarily require the personal presence of learners and teachers. Tandem teaching, which requires and ties up correspondingly high personnel resources, especially for courses in which group preparation, preparation and post-processing of the content is purposeful, can be implemented through blended learning with lower personnel requirements. Blended learning is **considered best practice** when face-to-face events, exercises, meetings, and individual needs for competence development are to be combined efficiently. Blended learning also has the advantage that learning can take place asynchronously during the online phases. This practically eliminates time bottlenecks or time pressure on the part of the learners. Prerequisites for the blended learning format are, in addition to motivation on both sides, the available equipment and media competence. In terms of equal treatment, teachers must be able to offer alternatives or support structures if learners have unfavorable conditions in this regard.

4.3.1.3 Intrinsic and Extrinsic Motivation in the Context of Learning Outcome Assessments

Feedback for learners on their learning progress can be provided in various ways. It is common to provide a sample solution, which enables the learner to repeat the test if necessary, e.g., in the case of online self-tests. Such tests are particularly useful for reproducing knowledge about an area (e.g., functional anatomy and biomechanics). Therefore, they can also be used by learners in preparation for courses (e.g., from German Qualifications Framework DQR level 6) that do not teach this knowledge but build on it (DQR 2017). Moreover, this variant is the means of choice to introduce newcomers or re-entrants to the educational level and to studying in general. Self-tests can be used to develop motivation to close knowledge gaps, and evidence-based knowledge (e.g., functional anatomy) should be available at a low threshold to channel motivation accordingly. The risk of recognizing the correct solution by mere trial and error can be reduced if the evaluation is performed with a time delay, e.g., at the end of the entire test.

▶ **Important** The challenge for teachers is to create self-motivating incentives in learners through tests that take into account educational level, i.e., neither under- nor over-challenge, and in any case overcome the trial-and-error phase.

In order to support the learners' reflection processes, it can be useful to simply point out the success rate to the learners by the system before issuing the assessment or solution and to offer to revise the answers without already specifically naming the wrong solutions in this step.

Cloze texts, math tasks, assignment tasks, single- and multiple-choice tests, quizzes, crossword puzzles, text tasks with and without pictures, video and audio have proven successful as online test formats. In the context of healthcare, tests in which learners view videos and images or listen to audio recordings in order to subsequently answer questions, e.g., about findings, conversational situations, or grip techniques, are also suitable.

Teaching-learning platforms, such as Moodle, offer teachers a variety of tools to prepare tests in a didactically meaningful way. The more complex the case to be solved, the more individual feedback and accompanying tutorials are necessary, which tie up corresponding personnel resources. Motivation for self-reflection is promoted by learning success checks in which corrective action is only taken after efforts have already been made to solve the task. In this case, either appropriate criteria must be defined in advance for which the teachers actively intervene, or the learners themselves must demand support. The assurance of results can be increased if the learners compare their solution (also results as a team effort) with the best-practice solution (in the sense of benchmarking) and revise their solution with their own words and, if necessary, illustrations based on this.

Test, exercise, and application options, which can be used without obligation and independently of teachers or course participants, for example, support the individual assessment of one's own level of knowledge. They can be used anywhere and often at any time and can be repeated several times. They can be used before and after the course as well as during the learning process as intermediate tests for self-assessment. More complex cases can also be solved in groups, in which case experts can give advice on how to solve them.

Example

Self-tests are particularly suitable for highly structurable content. Complex tasks that require additional professions or a group solution, especially in healthcare, should be completed, for example, with tutorials and evaluation discussions based on the logbook. ◀

4.3.1.4 Structure Learning Processes Through Online and Classroom Phases

Testing, practice, and application options are provided by instructors on an optional basis (**enrichment approach**) or can be an integral part of the entire module (**integration approach**). In this context, the test format also fulfills the goal of structuring the learning process in terms of time and content. At the same time, the motivation of the learners should be maintained to develop their competencies independently and continuously with regard to the learning objectives of the course (Kerres and Jechle 2000). Thus, exam learning, so-called bulimic learning, can be avoided. The possibility of receiving qualified feedback on the status quo along the learning process provides orientation for learners, especially in the case of new teaching-learning content (e.g., basic or foundation courses), new qualification levels (e.g., freshmen), or re-entry (e.g., extra-occupational training). Teachers can develop a choreography in which certain test formats encourage students to deepen their knowledge of the content during the online phases, and the content and methodology of the classroom phases are based on this. This approach in the sense of **problem-based learning or research-based learning** also optimizes the self-management skills of learners and contributes to the realization of lifelong learning in dynamic change processes (e.g., through digitalization).) in health and social care as well. In choreographing, teachers must take as a basis the total number of hours available for the module. Tests, exercises, and assignments should be feasible in the online phase. This refers to the learners as well as to the teachers who, for example, have to evaluate the results and give feedback to the learners before the next phase (e.g., next self-learning phase or next presence phase). In the presence phase, the results of the online phase must be addressed indirectly or directly, in which the learners can also be guided by several tests over a longer period of time.

The exclusive online teaching (virtualization approach) must be critically questioned (Bremer 2005b; Bachmann et al. 2001). Particularly in the case of participants who are qualified for healthcare, i.e., interaction with patients and relatives as well as teamwork and cooperation, the lack of social relationships (see also Sect. 5.5) with other course participants and with the instructor can lead to high dropout rates or to an extension of the training period.

▶ **Important** The choreography of online and face-to-face phases—also of different durations—takes into account learning objectives, scope, test and exercise options, and structures the learning process. In online phases, material can be provided compulsorily (integration approach) and/or optionally (enrichment approach). Exclusively online teaching (virtualization approach) must be questioned didactically.

In addition to time resources for the preparation of qualified feedback by the teachers, support efforts for possible comprehension questions, conflicts or uncertainties must be planned in the online phase. Teachers determine how this support for learning progress is to be provided and at what intervals, and may also make exceptions for urgent matters. The most common forms are chats and forums via the teaching-learning platform (e.g., Moodle), video conferences via the teaching-learning platform or special conference software, telephone or email contact. The advantage of offering mentoring on a rotational (e.g., weekly) basis is that resources can be planned. The regularity helps structure the learning process. In addition, this offer can positively influence the group dynamics. It is not uncommon for these offers to require a start-up phase, especially in newly formed groups. The team-building phases are therefore to be included by the teachers as well as the typical patterns of extro- and introverted participants. Contact in the form of email or phone call also seems to provide a kind of safety and protected space for many learners. However, many of the questions (e.g., about technical support) are often asked by multiple people and are therefore of corresponding interest to the course as a whole. In addition, answering frequently asked questions individually ties up personnel resources that are no longer available for individually necessary clarification and support. Therefore, it is also advisable to prepare a FAQ from the questions, which is permanently available to the participants on the teaching-learning platform. Emails or the content of telephone calls that affect the entire course can be shared anonymously on the teaching-learning platform in the forum or announced for the next regular support meeting (e.g., as an audio or video conference). In this way, teachers guide and steer learners, which contributes to the development of interdisciplinary competencies required in healthcare.

Conclusion

Teachers must agree clear rules with learners on the form in which support can, should, and must take place during the online phases if necessary. Learners help shape the learning process accordingly.

4.3.1.5 Special Challenges in Online Phases

Courses in the blended learning format combine the advantages of strongly structured and mandatory à la carte events and more optional and facultative events based on the cafeteria principle. Especially in the online phases of guided self-learning, participants can use offerings to compensate for identified weaknesses. Online phases are also suitable as preparation for modules in the sense of a propaedeutic or zero module. In addition, online phases can be used to prepare continuously for the examination that regularly concludes a module and can exert particular pressure on learners. Examination anxiety can be countered in this way. The additional content can be dynamically expanded by the teachers by responding to the learning levels shown in the tests, applications and exercises and by exploring and selecting the available information, podcasts and explanatory videos (e.g., on the Internet) and databases (e.g., papers in Medline®) and, for example, posting them with links for low-threshold access on the teaching-learning platform. In the evaluation, participants often reflect that they perceive these options as individually enriching, feel personally addressed, are motivated by them and benefit accordingly, even if no directly personalized information is provided by the teachers.

Online cooperation between learners also makes it possible to leave educational offerings with smaller numbers of participants in an institution's portfolio in a way that makes didactic sense and is economically viable. Online cooperation is not limited to a single cohort. Digitization also offers the opportunity to link different institutions or locations. Participants can form groups or tandems and work together on tasks and exercises in breakout rooms, as well as document, share, process, and optimize their results in shared documents (e.g., Etherpad). In addition to professional competence, such events aim at social, personal, and interdisciplinary competence development. The motivation to participate in group work is analogous to group work in the analog setting. Social loafing has to be taken into account by the teachers, e.g., in the size of the group or the composition of the groups. It is advisable to specify certain selection criteria for the group constellation (e.g., size, different professions, different qualification levels) and to transfer the responsibility for the group composition to the participants within this framework. The tasks must be developed by the teachers in such a way that they promote and challenge the motivation of the group and tell a story, i.e., they can also be broken down into several subtasks. Work results developed jointly in the groups can be incorporated into the overall concept of the module, including the test and examination phase. The work results can be mutually evaluated according to participatively developed or predefined criteria. Results, such as a wiki (Jonietz 2005), a glossary, didactic miniatures or podcasts, can be taken up in the course or, for example, be made available to subsequent courses and expanded or maintained by them (e.g., updating). The groups can keep online learning diaries for orientation and structuring, in which progress is reflected in the sense of a target-performance analysis and weaknesses and their compensation or success strategies are also documented (Baumgartner et al. 2004; Draheim and Beuschel 2005; Baumgartner 2005).

4.3.2 Course Planning

4.3.2.1 Outcome-Oriented Learning Goals

Online teaching is first and foremost a methodological approach. The methodology is not an end in itself, but the selection and implementation is determined by various factors. Depending on the goal of the event to be planned and the framework conditions on the part of the teachers and the learners, the decision of the teaching scenario must first be made. In view of the above, a mix of enrichment and integration approach in the blended learning format of exclusively online teaching should be preferred. As courses progress, experience is gained and adjustments may be necessary. This agility contributes to the optimization of the teaching concept. The detailed design follows the principle: from general aspects to the concrete teaching unit, i.e., first the general framework, e.g., regulations, curricula, timeline, is collected, which is decisive for the course. Within this framework, the entire course is subsequently mapped and subdivided into teaching units.

The learning content and forms of examination follow the outcome-oriented learning objectives (Lammerding-Köppel and Baatz 2013). The rough learning objectives of a module are derived from the overarching guideline objective of the educational program, taking into account the overall curriculum. In this way, redundancies are to be avoided or deliberately set. In order to develop learning objectives for a module and later on detailed objectives for an individual course in the module, it is helpful to use Bloom's learning objectives taxonomy, according to which different qualification levels are mapped in gradations (Bloom 1976; Gershon 2015). Learning objectives can be classified according to cognitive (knowing, understanding, applying, analyzing, synthesizing, and evaluating), affective (emotional states such as interest, attentiveness, attitudes, appreciations, values, and attitudes), and psychomotor (related to the performance of actions such as intuition, manipulation, and imitation) aspects (Euler 1992). Competencies include the individual potentials that have not yet been used, i.e., in order to develop competencies, a status quo must be collected to assess existing competencies (Heyse 2007).

▶ **Important** The learning objectives or their achievement are reflected in particular in competence-oriented examinations during or at the end of the module. Learning objectives are not the same as learning content and didactic methods.

Teachers can specify competency-oriented learning goals or set an impulse for a joint goal development process by asking the learners for their expectations. This can be an initial team-building approach for the teaching-learning group. This process often takes place in the first classroom session, but does not necessarily require it. It is possible, for example, to plan an online phase in preparation for a module, in which the learners, supported by media (e.g., virtual whiteboard, remote brainstorming session), exchange expectations, cluster and derive rough learning objectives moderated by the teacher (e.g., video conference). The learning objectives or their achievement are reflected in particular in a competency-based exam at the end of the module. Outcome-oriented learning objectives are not the same as learning content and methods. In order to achieve the broad goals (distant goals), the individual courses pursue sub-goals or fine goals (proximate goals) (Terhart 1997). Accordingly, the learning content can be further structured and the appropriate methods can be chosen. It is possible to pursue sub-goals and learning content over several events within an entire module, or to pursue these, in one event at a time. This structuring into units that are self-contained in terms of content and didactics also lends itself to learning progress checks or to business games in which the following unit requires the successful completion of the predecessor.

With regard to the learning objectives and contents of the entire module, it must be weighed up what is suitable for the online phase or what requires the presence of the participants on an optional or mandatory basis. Which contents can be offered as knowledge acquisition with suitable tests and exercises, which contents require interaction in the group, which applications can be carried out independently and which require a tandem constellation or learning pairs. Which equipment is mandatory (e.g., stable and fast Internet connection, virtual reality, and augmented reality) and thus represents an exclusion criterion. If an existing face-to-face course is to be converted to blended learning, it can be helpful to start planning by mapping the analog face-to-face course completely in tabular form (e.g., in Excel®) (course name, prerequisites, learning objectives, learning content, didactic methods, social form, test/examination form, technical equipment, tandem teaching, scope/workload, etc.). With this overview it is easy to identify which of the courses or which parts of them can also be realized online. It is also possible to define the parts that are offered synchronously or asynchronously. This also refers to the choice of methods. Methods follow the same principles in the online format as they do in analog teaching, but in the online format they are more often known by an English-language designation and, due to the lack of direct interaction, implementation errors, and organizational weaknesses emerge more dominantly. The content and methods filtered in this way can now be transferred to the online format. For this purpose, the table set up can be further developed.

As in analog face-to-face courses buffers should also be planned for online teaching, e.g., to take up current developments or to be able to offer learners an extension of the processing period in the event of unplanned learning obstacles. Such buffers require that teachers know from the course planning of the entire educational program which of the contents are required in subsequent modules, for example.

As already mentioned, the teaching-learning platform should be enriched with material during the course of the module. For this purpose, various registers can be created on the teaching-learning platform, e.g., according to the date of the event, according to phases, and according to topic blocks. Content that is thematized later or tasks to be solved should only be opened at this time, and content that is possibly only temporarily relevant should be closed accordingly. The "Hide content" function is used for this purpose. In this way, the concentration can be directed and an overload of the participants can be avoided.

The structure of the individual registers can be created by the teachers themselves based on the tabular overview created previously. For structuring purposes, it makes sense to present the structure to the learners (e.g., online in a welcome video or as a structured introductory text that can be enriched with the learning objectives and rules of the game after they have been coordinated) and to keep it for all registers.

Conclusion

A tabular overview of module planning supports teachers in planning blended learning. The table structure is used to structure the teaching-learning platform, which is enriched with material and tasks in the course of the module.

4.3.2.2 Didactic Methods and Associated Social Forms

In terms of didactic methods, activating forms of teaching are also preferable to passive ones (e.g., frontal lectures) in online teaching. In the meantime, analog media (e.g., metaplan wall, flipchart, whiteboard, and blackboard) have been transferred to digitally available software and can be used accordingly in both phases of blended learning. It is essential that the method in educational programs is not an end in itself, but follows outcome-oriented learning goals and content (Hallet 2006). It is not mandatory to master a wide range of methods (including the software). In general, and in both analog and online settings, conditions will lead to constraints and there will be instructor preferences. Learners often show less enthusiasm for activating forms of teaching. This is due, among other things, to the facts that they fall back on a learning biography of rote memorization and that the forms of examination are not competency-oriented, but focus exclusively on the reproduction of knowledge. University didactic centers offer a variety of method training courses for online teaching as well.

In the tabular overview already recommended above for planning (row Teaching methods), in the teaching units that have already been identified as relevant for online teaching, it is necessary to critically review which of the methods are suitable with regard to the entire setting. Closely related to this is the choice of social form, or optimally implemented methods require the social form of individual work, learning pair, small group work, plenary (Meyer 2009). The decision for a method and social form is connected with the support resources of the teachers, which have to be planned in the preparation. It may be necessary to make further adjustments to real-life conditions (Bremer 2005a).

In the health care sector, educational programs are application- and action-oriented with regard to the competencies to be developed and the necessary performance in health care (Jilg et al. 2015; Frank 2005). In addition to the expansion of knowledge, the independent development of content, case work, and interaction with other participants or the teachers are decisive. Common methods that can also be implemented in online teaching include problem-based learning, research-based learning, simulation training, project and workshop work, and role plays.

The assignment, which also transparently shows the framework conditions (e.g., duration, milestones, dates and type of supervision, and documentation of results), takes place via the teaching-learning platform. Figure 4.10 provides an overview of the aspects to be considered when setting tasks in online phases of the educational program.

Conclusion
Outcome-oriented learning goals require specific methods to be achieved, which in turn require a corresponding social form. Educational measures for the optimization of health care are usually strong application- and action-oriented.

4.3.2.3 Target Group, Communication, and Cooperation Orientation

Regardless of whether online or face-to-face phases are involved, the different learning types (Schrader 1994) and, accordingly, motivation, prior knowledge and experience, level of activity, quality and quantity of participation, willingness to experiment, helpfulness, and self-organization skills must be taken into account for a successful course. Especially in online phases, media competence, equipment (technical and personnel), and infrastructure (learning location) also play a greater role. Educational programs are often structured in such a way that, in addition to presence (in online mode or face-to-face), there are also self-learning phases that are comparable to the conditional requirements of online phases. In these self-learning phases, learners research online in databases, carry out evaluations on the PC using statistics programs or prepare texts and presentations on the PC using materials available online. Therefore, the difference in the necessary personnel and technical requirements is relatively

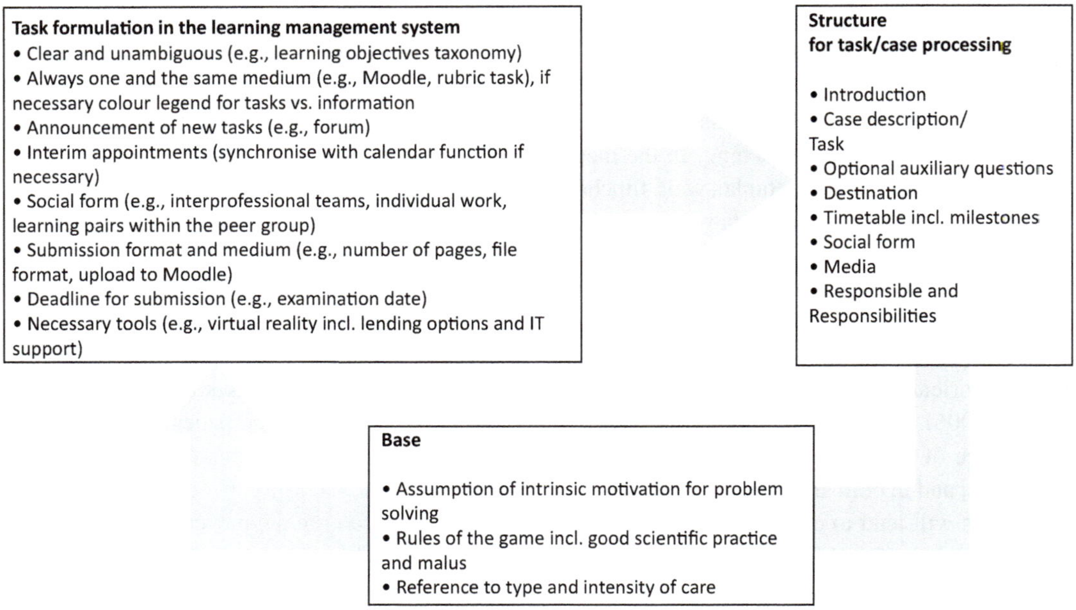

Fig. 4.10 Overview of the main aspects of the online mode and phase. (Winkelmann, C.)

small. An exception may be newcomers and those returning to the field who have gained their educational experience in an analog setting and have had relatively little contact with online tools and PC programs in practice or at work or in their private lives. It is important to identify this group and make all available resources available to them at a low threshold. For this group, tutorials from the educational institution's IT support or freely available explanatory videos and educational offerings that have previously been explored and selected by the teachers, as well as learning mentorships, can already represent support options for closing the gap.

► **Important** Complete satisfaction of the needs of all learning types in one course is unrealistic. An approximation can be achieved by varying content access, didactic methods, social forms, and scenarios.

For successful online teaching the learning location is essential in that the equipment and environment of the teachers and the learners can differ greatly compared to face-to-face events. Learning locations can be the workplace (e.g., office), the home office, mobile workplaces (e.g., park, restaurant, and hotel), the library, the educational institution (e.g., PC lab), and others. Depending on this, the conditions differ, e.g., with regard to ambient noise, consideration for others, distraction possibilities, stability and speed of the Internet connection, access options, and PC usage rights.

► **Important** The target group orientation applies to both online teaching and face-to-face events. Online teaching benefits from optimal technical and infrastructural conditions. To ensure these, it is advisable to inform participants about the necessary technical requirements before the event, if possible.

For social and interdisciplinary competence development according to the CanMEDS-roles framework, suitable methods and social forms are to be planned. The seven roles differentiated herein; Professional, Communicator, Collaborator, Health Advocate, Scholar, Manager, and Expert and their interrelationships are nowadays determinant for curricula development in education and training in health professions and health care professionals (Frank 2005; Jilg et al. 2015; MFT 2015; Flaiz et al. 2019). Conferencing systems that also allow for breakout rooms to be set up for small group work and return to the main session, chats and forums controlled by the teaching-learning platform, or etherpads can help to promote communication and cooperation skills in addition to technical skills in conjunction with individual assignments up to business games. A distinction is made between synchronous and asynchronous offerings. Synchronous offers take place for everyone at a fixed time. The simultaneous dial-in to the conference or the simultaneous processing of documents by the participants are characteristic of this. The associated structure, e.g., of the learners' daily routine, is advantageous. They can plan the time for the course. For the teachers it is an opportunity for joint reflection and status quo determination or for setting important impulses, especially for obligatory appointments. Synchronous offerings benefit from spontaneous interaction among participants. Therefore, contributions may be intuitive, impulse-giving, and provide, for example, a technical overview rather than deepening. Working together on the surface (also through low-threshold methods such as brainstorming) creates a high level of participation. Asynchronous offerings potentiate the advantage of local and temporal independence of online teaching by giving participants more flexibility. At the same time, they require a high degree of personal competence from the learners in terms of self-discipline and self-directed learning. What is also challenging in this format is that there is a time extension of information and communication processes. A question is usually answered with a time delay and a topic is discussed with a time delay (Bremer 2005a). This requires learners to select questions and topics according to importance and urgency, as well as to make an effort to find their own solution and to take responsibility for the solution. Accordingly, the quality of answers and contributions by other participants can be significantly increased in asynchronous formats compared to synchronous formats and the associated spontaneity. Reliability and trust are essential for cooperative teamwork, especially in asynchronous formats. It can therefore be crucial for the successful collaboration of the teaching-learning group to start the event with synchronous formats and only plan asynchronous formats in the course of the event.

4.3.2.4 Expansion of the Didactic Scope Through Tests and Examinations

In the blended learning format, all common forms of assessment can be implemented. With a view to the outcome-oriented learning objectives, the tests should be primarily competency-oriented. Knowledge tests are to be offered asynchronously in the online phase, e.g., as multiple-choice tasks.

It is advisable to create an examination or test section on the teaching/learning platform and to store all information relevant to examinations there, including links to higher-level pages such as professional laws, regulations of chambers or examination regulations of institutions, and to corresponding structures (e.g., examination office). The forms of examination should be defined, the necessary forms archived on the teaching/learning platform, and the respective assessment criteria transparent.

Tests, exercises, and examinations serve on the one hand to measure and evaluate competencies and on the other hand to expand knowledge and competencies (Roediger and Karpicke 2006). Therefore, it can be didactically valuable to choose a form of examination that consists of different partial examinations to be completed in the course of the entire module. This lends itself to problem-based learning, case work, or combinations of knowledge reproduction, practical applications (e.g., simulation), and reflective reports (e.g., OSCE, portfolio, and learning diary). The option of repeated, reflective practice in a protected space (also individually and asynchronously in the skills lab) promotes action-oriented competencies of learners (Timmermann et al. 2007; Ahlers et al. 2009). Tasks with different levels of difficulty, varying complexity, peer teaching and assessment as well as supplementary lectures are suitable didactic instruments to broaden the view, to promote empathy and to carry out structured self- and peer assessment.

Conclusion

Tests and examinations should be defined and planned as part of the overall didactic concept congruent with outcome-oriented learning objectives, content, activating teaching methods, and social forms.

4.3.3 PakT

4.3.3.1 Interindividual Differences of Active Tactile Sensations

Palpation is a basic competence of medical and physiotherapeutic professionals, especially for clinical diagnostics and manually performed therapy. Studies show strong interindividual variations of the haptic threshold (see also Sect. 3.2), but valid, practicable testing, and training systems of active tactile performance are not used for qualification. Testing of haptic thresholds, training of active perceptual skills, and integration of PakT into existing curricula can optimize the quality of patient care. A PakT module can complement existing curricula via self-study, peer teaching, and blended learning with comparatively large online phases. The basic process, content, scope, and possible mode of PakT in each case is shown in Fig. 4.11.

Manual intervention for diagnostics and therapy focuses on dedicated skills and abilities in key exploration. In Germany, there are various concepts for manual therapy education and training, which are also aimed at different professions and educational levels, such as trainees, students, and graduates. Accordingly, the knowledge base and existing competencies are heterogeneous (Winkelmann 2020).

The structure of the curricula always includes practical teaching units in addition to theoretical ones. The aim of practice is to impart practical

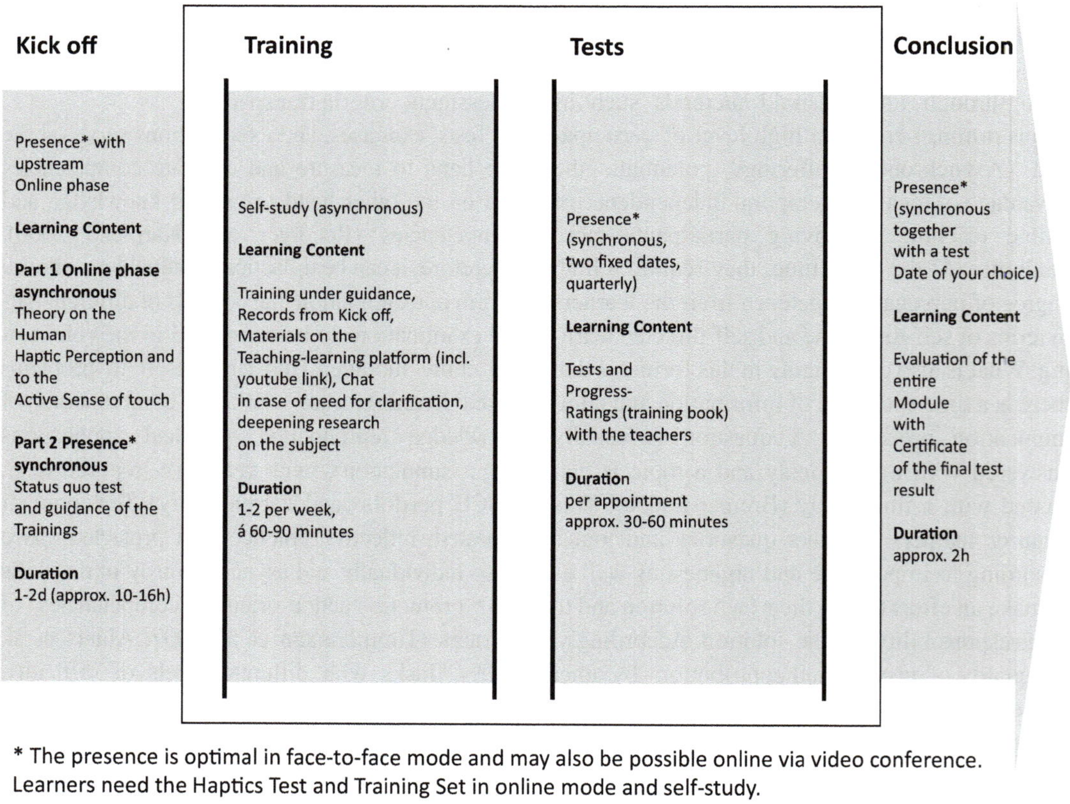

Fig. 4.11 Schematic representation of the PakT module. (Winkelmann, C.)

skills and knowledge (MPhG 1994; PhysTh-APrV 1994; MFT 2015). The curricula identify theoretical lectures, practical demonstrations, and practice sessions, among others, as methods, but without further differentiating them (Beyer et al. 2017). In particular, feeling, sensing a movement, and localizing a change are understood to be focal points of clinical diagnostics and manually executed therapy. With the developing tactile senses, it should be possible to collect findings quickly and reliably (Brokmeier 2009; Thalhamer 2017; Streeck et al. 2017). In praxi, however, the haptic abilities necessary for this are not examined in the participants. These are assumed to be present by the teachers. In the course of medical, physical, and manual therapy education and training, courses on palpation of findings or manually performed therapy focus almost exclusively on anatomy, physiology as well as grip techniques, hand and body positions of the learners in the context of the body region to be examined or treated. Area-wide valid and practicable tests, in which the active haptic tactile threshold could be determined analogous to a vision or hearing test at the beginning and in the course of the education and training, as well as in the professional life cycle, are not used even rudimentarily. The same is true for the standardized training of active haptic tactile performance, although inexpensive, practicable, valid and reliable test, and training sets are available and, moreover, recommended in the context of qualification in the health care profession (Grunwald 2010; Mueller and Grunwald 2013; Mueller et al. 2014c).

Conclusion
To compensate for differences in haptic abilities in prerequisites and to support manual therapy education and training that ensures results without reducing their previous quality standards, a propaedeutic course in a blended learning format and also through the use of valid test and training sets can promote active tactile performance (Winkelmann et al. 2019).

4.3.3.2 Qualification Goals with Special Consideration of Manual Therapy and Diagnostics

Knowledge and skills taught in manual therapy modules should also be reflected through application in practice (Timmermann et al. 2007; Walber and Jütte 2015). The methodological competence and performance coupled with other competencies should contribute to improving the quality of treatment and, last but not least, ensure patient safety.

The competence development of the learners requires their confrontation in and with real problem situations, which are usually extremely complex. For this, the learners, accompanied by the teachers, have to develop solution approaches step by step (Frank 2005; Timmermann et al. 2007; Erpenbeck and Heyse 2010; Meyer 2013; Jilg et al. 2015; Walber and Jütte 2015). It is significant that unambiguous, correct answers do not exist in scientific self-understanding, but coping with the complexity of situation and person requires a certain standardization of structures and processes. For this purpose, heuristic models (e.g., learning pyramid according to Miller 1990) can provide a framework for the use of simulations in educational programs with the indicative goal of optimizing health care. Figure 4.12 shows the ideal-typical process from knowledge to competence to performance.

Explicitly in simulations such as those made possible for learners in the Skills Lab (e.g., mobile haptics lab), the complexity of the real healthcare situation (Sopka et al. 2013), in which those affected and their relatives, as well as in some cases the professionals, find themselves in a situation that is unique for them, can only be simulated approximately. This applies in particular to the reactions of patients and their relatives. Profiling and professionalization in this regard is also regularly based on experience. The measurement and assessment of competencies is associated with corresponding difficulties when it takes into account the various competency classes relevant in health care (e.g., professional-methodical, activity- and implementation-oriented, personal, and social-communicative competencies).

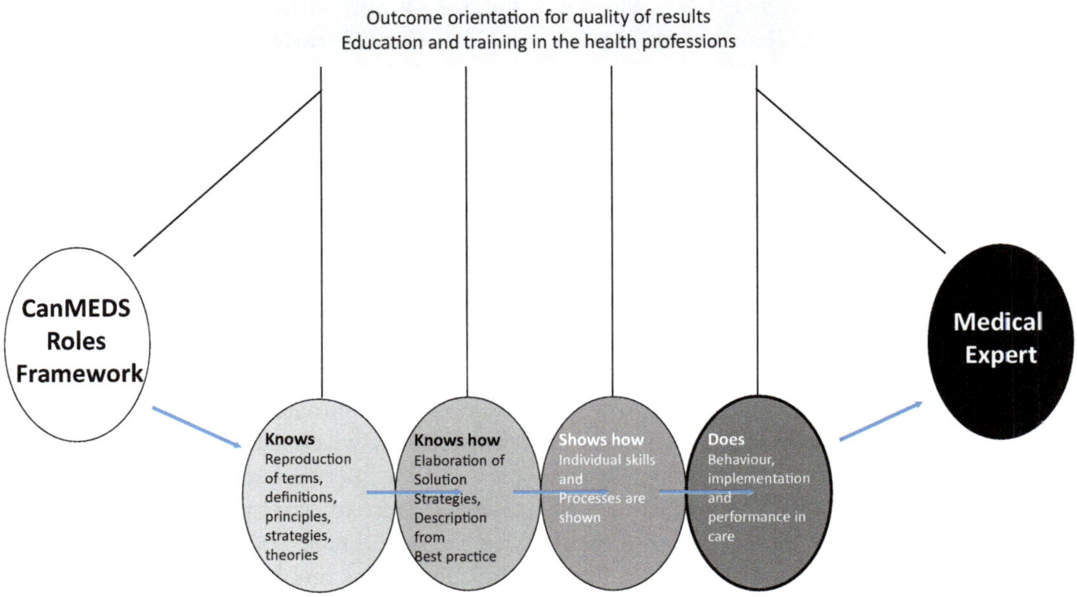

Fig. 4.12 From knowledge to performance in health care. (Winkelmann, C.)

> **Important** Competencies are compellingly distinct from learning content. Essential for optimal health care is the performance in the real requirement.

Professionals in manual diagnostics and therapy are expected to have competencies that can be assigned to different areas and qualification goals (Calonder Gerster 2007; Erpenbeck and Heyse 2010; Jilg et al. 2015; Klemme and Siegmann 2015):

Expertise

Knowledge and understanding of graduates builds on and substantially exceeds the level of their respective credentials for entry into manual therapy education and training.

Graduates demonstrate a broad and integrated knowledge and understanding of the scientific basis of manual therapy. The knowledge and understanding corresponds to the state of the relevant professional literature and at the same time includes some in-depth knowledge at the current state of research in manual therapy.

The problems are recorded in their situational context and in appropriate complexity. They critically analyze which influencing factors must be taken into account in order to solve the problem. Graduates assess the extent to which individual theoretical models can contribute to solving the problem.

Specific aspects of expertise include:

- Comprehensive factual knowledge
- Critical understanding of the subject content
- Reflection on the applicability of theories in practice
- Reference to situations from own practical experience
- Deepened understanding of organizational contexts
- Appropriate assessment of problems
- Consideration of interfaces to adjacent areas of responsibility
- Understanding at various system levels on organizational structures, measures, processes, and legal foundations

Methods Expertise

Relevant information is identified using scientific methods. Scientific findings are interpreted in a case-related manner. Graduates apply a broad spectrum of techniques and methods in diagnostics and therapy to solve complex patient- or client-centered problems. They select the appropriate methods and techniques from this spectrum and apply them in a solution-oriented manner. From this, they develop new question and therapy objectives.

The techniques, methods, and concepts established in manual diagnostics and therapy and commonly used in the respective discipline and profession are known. The respective strengths and weaknesses are assessed so that the independent selection is made appropriately and according to the situation.

Techniques and methods including sound care planning, documentation, and other aspects of quality management are successfully implemented, even in the face of frequently changing requirements due to individual patient findings as well as changing external conditions. Theoretical knowledge as well as professional technical experience is built upon.

Specific aspects of methodological competence include:

- Assessing the relevance of the techniques and methods in manual diagnostics and therapy and in the direct professional field of application
- Assess the practicality and limitations of techniques and methods
- Experiential knowledge in the use of different techniques and methods
- Prudence and structured
- Accuracy and conscientiousness
- Systematic approach

Personal Competence

Graduates demonstrate a high degree of reflexivity and deal with change even in complex situations. They independently transfer their own knowledge and skills to the respective existing requirements.

They learn implicitly and explicitly and have an open attitude to change. They establish clear responsibilities for their area of activity. They take responsibility for the tasks that lie with them, with which they also personally identify and contribute to the care team.

Specific aspects of personal competence include:

- Ability to learn
- Perseverance and persistence
- Independent search for situationally appropriate solutions
- Creativity and impetus for further developments and innovations
- Independence and personal responsibility
- Time management and ability to prioritize
- Self-management, resilience
- Diligence and sense of duty
- Sense of responsibility
- Commitment and reliability
- Support for innovations and new developments
- Solution-oriented action
- Openness to criticism and willingness to learn
- Sovereignty in dealing with mistakes and failures
- Experience your own work-life flow

Overarching Action Competence

Graduates of manual therapy education and training use their theoretical expertise and reflected experiential knowledge to act appropriately, authentically, and successfully in various professional practice situations.

Specific aspects of the overarching action competency are:

- Action appropriate to the situation
- Understanding of overarching contexts and processes
- Critical judgment
- Foresight and prudence
- Personal responsibility and initiative
- Reflection and shaping of one's own life plan
- Able to act even in the context of a globalized working world
- Reflective attitude towards societal, social, and ecological implications of one's own actions
- Assessment of the applicability and usefulness of theories for practice
- Reflection of practice against a theoretical background

4.3.3.3 Requirements for Palpation

Manual medical diagnostics and therapy per se uses the hand, hands and fingers in a special quality and quantity (Brokmeier 2009; Gautschi 2015; Beyer et al. 2017). In addition to anamnesis, inspection, grip techniques, pressure, traction and others, the palpation of tissues, such as muscles, nerves, bones, ligaments, tendons, blood vessels, connective tissue, and skin plays a central role. The assessment is carried out in a side-by-side comparison. The aim of palpation is the perception of tissue changes and their evaluation with regard to a possible connection to the patient's problem (Klemme and Siegmann 2015; Streeck et al. 2017).

Palpation is generally understood to mean feeling and, in the medical context, palpation. Palpation can be performed in very different ways. In some cases, only a small part of the fingertip is used to palpate a nerve. To palpate large structures, several fingers are also used. In addition, depending on the nature and location of the structure, different palpation pressure is applied (Laekeman and Kreutzer 2009). Superficial palpation to assess skin, and with light pressure of subcutaneous tissue in terms of temperature, moisture, skin quality, edema, can be distinguished from deep palpation. Deep palpation is used on fascia, muscle, bone, ligaments in relation to tissue response to transverse stretch and pressure. Consistency, change, and resistance are also assessed (Brokmeier 2009). (For more in-depth information on the perceptual dimensions of the haptic systems also Chap. 1.)

Palpation prerequisites and action orders are (Brokmeier 2009; Laekeman and Kreutzer 2009):

- The starting position must ensure that the structure to be palpated is optimally accessible.
- By using bedding material, a bedding can be created that contributes to the relaxation of the relevant body region or overall physical and mental relaxation.
- Do not apply too much pressure with the palpation finger.
- Hands should be clean, well-groomed, and warm; fingernails filed short.
- The hand and finger joints should have good mobility and muscular stabilization.
- Since patients may respond differently to stimuli associated with palpation, information about the reason for and technique of palpation and the possible body reactions to which the patient should be prepared is valuable prior to initial physical contact (see also Sects. 5.1 and 5.2).

To train the sense of touch, the perceptual and palpation processes are trained to make proprioceptive information and structural differences conscious. This requires the greatest concentration with cognitive open-mindedness. Possibilities for error can be rooted in the individual and must be taken into account in the teaching-learning scenario. Common errors are according to Brokmeier (2009):

- Learner is tense and focused on wanting to find something specific.
- Fingertips and/or finger tips are applied with too much pressure.
- Only one local point is palpated without, for example, using comparative information from surrounding, superficial or deeper tissues.
- It is unclear to the learner in which tissue layer the palpating finger is currently moving.
- The didactic concept of the teachers in the various training and further education institutions serves to ensure quality. The theoretical content taught can be reproduced by the learners in oral examinations, among other things. What is challenging, on the other hand, is the verification of correct practical performance. In the learning process as well as in the examination setting, a group of four persons (test person, learner, observer, and expert) is usually necessary for this. The proband receives stimuli about the grip technique of the expert versus the learner and gives appropriate feedback to the learner. The observer follows the movements performed by the expert versus the learner and provides appropriate feedback (ÄMM 2021). It is also common for the expert to place his or her hands on top of the learner's to guide movement and direction.

4.3.3.4 Test and Training Sets for Active Tactile Performance

Palpation results that can lead to therapeutic consequences are based on active tactile perception. A healthy person is able to detect elevations of only 1 μm on a smooth surface with his fingertips during active palpation (Louw et al. 2000, 2002; see also Sect. 1.1.3). The performance of active tactile perception shows large interindividual differences in scientific studies (see also Sect. 3.2). Among other things, individual disposition, exercise, age, occupation and activity as well as diseases of the kidneys, liver, thyroid gland have an influence on this (Mueller and Grunwald 2013). However, the related performance quality is not tested in a standardized way with the beginning and in the course of medical, physical, and manual therapy education and training. Similarly, although training to increase perceptual ability in the haptic area is implicitly provided through practice in medical, physical, and manual therapy courses and in patient-related practical application, it is not explicit (Brokmeier 2009).

A haptic threshold test set evaluated in several application studies and the haptic figures test and training set with special stimulus pads are available for both testing and training purposes (see also Sect. 4.2.3.ff). Both sets are strongly oriented towards exploratory occupational situations. Thus, it is possible to choose the starting position individually, as well as to perform the exploration with open eyes. At the same time, the scientific quality of a reproducible test situation is guaranteed. The sets are particularly suitable for self-study as well as peer teaching and assessment. Provided that the sets can be borrowed, for example, from a Skills Lab coordination office or via the institution-specific library, the sets are also suitable for the blended learning format. The implementation of a haptic threshold measurement with the Haptic Threshold Test is presented in an educational film on the YouTube portal under the search term "Haptic Threshold Test." The respective implementation manual including the test forms is part of the test and training inventory and is also available as a pdf file on the websites of the haptics laboratory (Mueller et al. 2014c).

The average execution time for the haptic threshold test is between 15 and 30 min, depending on the person performing the test (Mueller and Grunwald 2013; Mueller et al. 2014c).

The Haptic Figure Test and Training Set consists of the Haptic Figure Test Set and the Haptic Figure Training Set. The stimuli used consist of two-dimensional height reliefs of various geometric figures that differ in terms of their complexity.

The aim of haptic training is to improve both the haptic thresholds and the haptic recognition performance of healthy individuals. The haptic thresholds as well as the haptic recognition performance are recorded by pre-measurement as an input test before the start of the training phase and post-measurement after the end of the training phase (post-measurement) (Grunwald 2010; Mueller et al. 2014c).

4.3.3.5 Implementation of a PakT Module in Existing Curricula

Due to the strong interindividual variations of the haptic threshold, the use of valid, practicable test and training systems is relevant, especially for the preparation for and during medical, physiotherapeutic, and manual therapy education and training (Mueller and Grunwald 2013; Winkelmann and Grunwald, 2018; Winkelmann et al. 2018).

The areas of competence form overlaps and transitions and are partly fluid (Erpenbeck and Heyse 2010). Nevertheless, with regard to active tactile perception in the context of a preparatory and/or accompanying course, it is comprehensible that the quality of active tactile performance lies clearly in the area of methodological competence against the background of application in a concrete action situation, as well as critical result reflection and evaluation (Winkelmann et al. 2019). De facto, palpation is primarily anchored in the area of technical competence (anatomy, physiology) in existing curricula, and secondarily in the area of methodological competence (grip technique), but neither teachers nor learners are aware of the potential of active touch (haptic threshold). Table 4.4 shows the relevant didactic aspects in PakT (see also Fig. 4.11).

Table 4.4 Didactic aspects in the propaedeutic course PakT

Didactic aspect	Basic course		Advanced course	
	Theory	Practice	Theory	Practice
Focus on application	The participants understand the scientific findings on haptic perception. They independently research, record and interpret relevant information	They perform the haptic test and training procedure in a standardized manner. In relation to the patient-specific situation, they are aware of the strengths and weaknesses of the procedure	The participants select effective techniques for testing and training haptic perceptual performance and apply them efficiently to develop new questions and solutions. Contextually, they have in-depth anatomical knowledge	They adequately assess the possibilities, practicability, and limitations of the haptic test and training procedure. The participants independently establish the practical transfer
	They have anatomical expertise	You will know other techniques for training active tactile perception and apply them in a selected manner		
Evident didactic methods and social forms	Seminars and lectures also online and asynchronous, individual work, self-study aimed at knowledge enhancement	Seminars, exercises, teaching supervision, presence, synchronous, partly asynchronous self-study, peer teaching	Seminars, exercises, projects, group work, including online and asynchronous, some self-study	Seminars, exercises, processing of cases also from own professional practice, problem-based group work also online, synchronous and asynchronous
Tests, competence assessment	Knowledge tests (e.g., multiple choice), cloze, quiz	Peer teaching and evaluation possible according to defined criteria (e.g., operating instructions in the test and training set)	Reflection as documentation of the learning process and knowledge gain, self-assessment, and assessment by others	Reflection as documentation of the learning process and knowledge gain (e.g., learning diary), self-assessment and assessment by others, reflection report, study design, exposé

▶ **Important** Medical, physiotherapy, and manual therapy curricula do not address training and testing of the active sense of touch. Basic palpation skills for clinical diagnosis and therapy are developed primarily through anatomy, physiology, and grip technique.

This approach is comparable to the driver's license, which is issued only on the knowledge of rules and signs, as well as driving a vehicle in traffic, but would not require an eye test.

Anchoring a module outside of legally prescribed, nationally coordinated and institution-specific accredited curricula is a challenge. Through PakT, the goal of medical, physical, and manual therapy education and training—optimization of health care—is not jeopardized; on the contrary, it is more likely to be achieved through PakT (Winkelmann et al. 2017). It is significantly more difficult to justify the workload in this regard. If there is conviction and will on the part of those responsible, this motivation can be used to find options for anchoring it in existing curricula. These options must include relevant logistical and organizational aspects (e.g., procurement of the test and training sets for a mobile haptics lab or for the library collection, decision of the lending structures and procedure, and teaching load) (Ahlers 2013; Vollmer and Mönk 2013).

In order to optimize the learning success of the participants in the context of the outcome-oriented learning goals, adequate planning of the module and the implementation of suitable teaching-learning methods as well as test and examination forms are the prerequisites. The following conditions and didactic methods positively influence the success of simulation and are recommended for PakT (Issenberg 2005; Meyerhoff and Brühl 2015; Walber and Jütte 2015):

- Clearly defined learning objectives for each task
- Option for repeated, reflective practice under relatively stable conditions (e.g., consistency of tissue, skin drawing)
- Integration of the simulation in the skills lab into the curriculum and consideration in the workload
- Different and individually adapted difficulty levels
- Presentation of various clinical images and cases
- Safe learning environment that protects participants and tolerates mistakes
- Option to practice individually, also as an asynchronous offer
- Structured feedback
- Self-test

The experiences and insights gained by the learners should also be constructively reflected on together with other learners, in tandem with teachers or alone according to a previously known and discussed grid, e.g., in a learning diary, in order to secure the results. Constructive also means that the demonstrated action and application is not commented in a teaching manner, but that the participants are accompanied by the teachers. Successful performance should be made conscious and experienced as success (Timmermann et al. 2007; Meyer 2013; Meyerhoff and Brühl 2015). For this purpose, the assessment criteria should be made transparent, e.g., on the teaching-learning platform. In learning pairs or small group work, the guidelines for assessment and feedback rules must be clear and attention must be paid to their compliance. Reminders in this regard by the teachers reinforce the correct use and motivational handling of assessments for all participants and map their affective and cognitive competencies.

4.3.3.6 Essence

The haptic performance of learners should be continuously assessed in the course of education and training and, if necessary, trained accordingly. The implementation of valid haptic testing and training systems can be an approach to improve the quality of education and training standards and to optimize patient care. The presented test and training systems make it possible to measure and train the haptic perception ability of healthy persons under objective and reproducible conditions. In doing so, the presented test and training procedures are oriented as closely as possible to explorative professional situations and also ensure the scientific quality of a reproducible test situation. Under certain conditions, the application is also possible in self-study. However, the securing of results requires adequate planning, clear task definition and reflection of the performance. The simulation in the skills lab should be integrated into the curriculum. The test and training sets can be borrowed from the library or the skills lab by the participants as needed, so that the training can be designed in online mode, for example, independent of location and time.

References

Aboutorabi A, Arazpour M, Bahramizadeh M, Farahmand F, Fadayevatan R. Effect of vibration on postural control and gait of elderly subjects: a systematic review. Aging Clin Exp Res. 2018;30(7):713–26. https://doi.org/10.1007/s40520-017-0831-7.

Ahissar M, Hochstein S. Attentional control of early perceptual learning. Proc Natl Acad Sci U S A. 1993;90(12):5718–22. https://doi.org/10.1073/pnas.90.12.5718.

Ahlers O. Der richtige Rahmen entscheidet: Curriculare Implementierung der Simulation. In: St Pierre M, Breuer G, editors. Simulation in der Medizin. Grundlegende Konzepte – klinische Anwendung. Berlin: Springer; 2013. p. 77–81.

Ahlers O, Spies C, Brau C, Georg W, Hanfler S, Bubser F, de Grahl C, Senf R, Schlosser HG, Kerner T. Theoretische und praktische notfallmedizinische Kompetenz Studierender vor dem Praktischen Jahr – ein Vergleich verschiedener Studiengänge an der Berliner Charité. Anaesth Intensive Med. 2009;50:627.

Ahn M-C, Song C-H. Immediate effects of local vibration on ankle plantarflexion spasticity and clonus of both the gastrocnemius and soleus in patients with spinal cord injury. J Korean Soc Phys Med. 2016;11(2):1–11. https://doi.org/10.13066/kspm.2016.11.2.1.

Aman JE, Elangovan N, Yeh I-L, Konczak J. The effectiveness of proprioceptive training for improving motor function: a systematic review. Front Hum Neurosci. 2014;8:1075. https://doi.org/10.3389/fnhum.2014.01075.

Aminian-Far A, Hadian M-R, Olyaei G, Talebian S, Bakhtiary AH. Whole-body vibration and the prevention and treatment of delayed-onset muscle soreness. J Athl Train. 2011;46(1):43–9. https://doi.org/10.4085/1062-6050-46.1.43.

ÄMM – Ärztevereinigung für Manuelle Medizin Ärzteseminar Berlin (ÄMM) e.V. Universitäre Standards – interdisziplinäres Lehren, Lernen & Denken! Online verfügbar unter. 2021. https://www.dgmm-aemm.de/index.php?id=117. abgerufen am 01.01.2021.

Ayres AJ. Southern California sensory integration tests manual. Los Angeles: Western Psychological Services; 1972.

Bachmann G, Dittler M, Lehmann T, Glatz D, Rösel F. Das Internetportal LearnTechNet der Uni Basel: Ein Online Supportsystem für Hochschuldozierende im Rahmen der Integration von E-Learning in die Präsenzuniversität. In: Haefeli O, Bachmann G, Kindt M, editors. Campus 2002 – Die Virtuelle Hochschule in der Konsolidierungsphase. Münster: Waxmann; 2001. p. 87–97.

Baltaci G, Harput G, Haksever B, Ulusoy B, Ozer H. Comparison between Nintendo Wii Fit and conventional rehabilitation on functional performance outcomes after hamstring anterior cruciate ligament reconstruction: prospective, randomized, controlled, double-blind clinical trial. Knee Surg Sports Traumatol Arthrosc. 2013;21(4):880–7. https://doi.org/10.1007/s00167-012-2034-2.

Baumgartner P. Eine neue Lernkultur entwickeln. Kompetenzbasierte Ausbildung mit Blogs und E-Portfolios. In: Hornung-Prähauser V, editor. ePortfolio Forum Austria. Salzburg: Österreich; 2005. p. 33–8.

Baumgartner P, Bergner I, Pullich L. Weblogs in education—a means for organisational; 2004.

Beets IAM, Macé M, Meesen RLJ, Cuypers K, Levin O, Swinnen SP. Active versus passive training of a complex bimanual task: is prescriptive proprioceptive information sufficient for inducing motor learning? PLoS One. 2012;7(5):e37687. https://doi.org/10.1371/journal.pone.0037687.

Beyer L, Nisser J, Harke G, Loudovici-Krug D. Ärztliche Zusatzweiterbildung „Manuelle Medizin/Chirotherapie" unter besonderer Beachtung des motorischen Lernens. Man Med. 2017;55:34–9.

Bliss TV, Lomo T. Long-lasting potentiation of synaptic transmission in the dentate area of the anaesthetized rabbit following stimulation of the perforant path. J Physiol. 1973;232(2):331–56. https://doi.org/10.1113/jphysiol.1973.sp010273.

Bloom BS, editor. Taxonomie von Lernzielen im kognitiven Bereich. Weinheim und Basel: Beltz; 1976.

Bogaerts A, Verschueren S, Delecluse C, Claessens AL, Boonen S. Effects of whole body vibration training on postural control in older individuals: a 1 year randomized controlled trial. Gait Posture. 2007;26(2):309–16. https://doi.org/10.1016/j.gaitpost.2006.09.078.

Bremer C. Chats im eLearning. Rollenspiele und andere didaktische Elemente in der netzgestützten Hochschullehre. In: Beißwenger M, Storrer A, editors. Chat-Kommunikation in Beruf, Bildung und Medien: Konzepte - Werkzeuge - Anwendungsfelder. Stuttgart: Ibidem-Verlag; 2005a. p. 89–100.

Bremer C. Handlungsorientiertes Lernen mit Neuen Medien. In: Bloh E, editor. Online-Pädagogik. Bd. 2. Baltmannsweiler: Schneider Lehmann B; 2005b. p. 175–97.

Brokmeier AA. Kursbuch Manuelle Therapie. OMT - Orthopaedic Manipulative Therapy: Biomechanik, Neurologie, Funktionen. 4. Aufl, Books on Demand; 2009.

Brox E, Konstantinidis ST, Evertsen G, Fernandez-Luque L, Remartinez A, Oesch P, Civit A. GameUp: exergames for mobility – a project to keep elderly active. In: Kyriacou E, Christofides S, Pattichis CS, editors. XIV Mediterranean conference on medical and biological engineering and computing 2016, Bd. 57 (IFMBE proceedings). Cham: Springer International Publishing; 2016. p. 1225–30.

Brunetti O, Filippi GM, Lorenzini M, Liti A, Panichi R, Roscini M, et al. Improvement of posture stability by vibratory stimulation following anterior cruciate ligament reconstruction. Knee Surg Sports Traumatol Arthrosc. 2006;14(11):1180–7. https://doi.org/10.1007/s00167-006-0101-2.

Bush JA, Blog GL, Kang J, Faigenbaum AD, Ratamess NA. Effects of quadriceps strength after static and dynamic whole-body vibration exercise. J Strength Cond Res. 2015;29(5):1367–77. https://doi.org/10.1519/JSC.0000000000000709.

Calonder Gerster AE. Das CH-Q Kompetenz-Management-Modell. Ein integriertes Gesamtangebot zur Kompetenzentwicklung und zur Schaffung einer Kompetenzkultur in Bildung und Arbeitswelt. In: Erpenbeck J, von Rosenstiel L, editors. Handbuch Kompetenzmessung. Erkennen, verstehen und bewerten von Kompetenzen in der betrieblichen, pädagogischen und psychologischen Praxis. 2., überarb u erw Aufl. Stuttgart: Schäffer-Poeschel; 2007. p. 719–36.

Camerota F, Celletti C, Suppa A, Galli M, Cimolin V, Filippi GM, et al. Focal muscle vibration improves gait in Parkinson's disease: a pilot randomized, controlled trial. Mov Disord Clin Pract. 2016;3(6):559–66. https://doi.org/10.1002/mdc3.12323.

Camerota F, Celletti C, Di Sipio E, de Fino C, Simbolotti C, Germanotta M, et al. Focal muscle vibration, an effective rehabilitative approach in severe gait impairment due to multiple sclerosis. J Neurol Sci. 2017;372:33–9. https://doi.org/10.1016/j.jns.2016.11.025.

Carey LM, Matyas TA, Oke LE. Sensory loss in stroke patients: effective training of tactile and proprioceptive discrimination. Arch Phys Med Rehabil. 1993;74(6):602–11. https://doi.org/10.1016/0003-9993(93)90158-7.

Carrico C, Chelette KC, Westgate PM, Powell E, Nichols L, Fleischer A, Sawaki L. Nerve stimulation enhances task-oriented training in chronic, severe motor deficit after stroke: a randomized trial. Stroke. 2016;47(7):1879–84. https://doi.org/10.1161/STROKEAHA.116.012671.

Carrico C, Westgate PM, Powell ES, Chelette KC, Nichols L, Pettigrew LC, Sawaki L. Nerve stimulation enhances task-oriented training for moderate-to-severe hemiparesis 3-12 months after stroke: a randomized trial. Am J Phys Med Rehabil. 2018;97(11):808–15. https://doi.org/10.1097/PHM.0000000000000971.

Casadio M, Morasso P, Sanguineti V, Giannoni P. Minimally assistive robot training for proprioception enhancement. Exp Brain Res. 2009;194(2):219–31. https://doi.org/10.1007/s00221-008-1680-6.

Celnik P, Hummel F, Harris-Love M, Wolk R, Cohen LG. Somatosensory stimulation enhances the effects of training functional hand tasks in patients with chronic stroke. Arch Phys Med Rehabil. 2007;88(11):1369–76. https://doi.org/10.1016/j.apmr.2007.08.001.

Collins JJ, Imhoff TT, Grigg P. Noise-enhanced tactile sensation. Nature. 1996;383(6603):770.

Conforto AB, Anjos D, Monteiro S, Bernardo WM, da Silva AA, Conti J, Machado AG, Cohen LG. Repetitive peripheral sensory stimulation and upper limb performance in stroke: a systematic review and meta-analysis. Neurorehabil Neural Repair. 2018;32(10):863–71. https://doi.org/10.1177/1545968318798943.

Conrad MO, Scheidt RA, Schmit BD. Effects of wrist tendon vibration on arm tracking in people poststroke. J Neurophysiol. 2011;106(3):1480–8. https://doi.org/10.1152/jn.00404.2010.

Cordo P, Lutsep H, Cordo L, Wright WG, Cacciatore T, Skoss R. Assisted movement with enhanced sensation (AMES): coupling motor and sensory to remediate motor deficits in chronic stroke patients. Neurorehabil Neural Repair. 2009;23(1):67–77. https://doi.org/10.1177/1545968308317437.

Costantino C, Galuppo L, Romiti D. Short-term effect of local muscle vibration treatment versus sham therapy on upper limb in chronic post-stroke patients: a randomized controlled trial. Eur J Phys Rehabil Med. 2017;53(1):32–40. https://doi.org/10.23736/S1973-9087.16.04211-8.

Cuppone AV, Squeri V, Semprini M, Masia L, Konczak J. Robot-assisted proprioceptive training with added vibro-tactile feedback enhances somatosensory and motor performance. PLoS One. 2016;11(10):e0164511. https://doi.org/10.1371/journal.pone.0164511.

de Santis D, Zenzeri J, Casadio M, Masia L, Riva A, Morasso P, Squeri V. Robot-assisted training of the kinesthetic sense: enhancing proprioception after stroke. Front Hum Neurosci. 2014;8:1037. https://doi.org/10.3389/fnhum.2014.01037.

Dinse HR, Kleibel N, Kalisch T, Ragert P, Wilimzig C, Tegenthoff M. Tactile coactivation resets age-related decline of human tactile discrimination. Ann Neurol. 2006;60(1):88–94. https://doi.org/10.1002/ana.20862.

Dinse HR, Wilimzig C, Kalisch T. Learning effects in haptic perception. In: Grunwald M, editor. Human haptic perception: basics and applications. Basel: Birkhäuser; 2008. p. 165–82. Online verfügbar unter. https://link.springer.com/chapter/10.1007/978-3-7643-7612-3_13.

Doyle S, Bennett S, Fasoli SE, McKenna KT. Interventions for sensory impairment in the upper limb after stroke. Cochrane Database Syst Rev. 2010;6:CD006331. https://doi.org/10.1002/14651858.CD006331.pub2.

DQR - Bund-Länder-Koordinierungsstelle für den Deutschen Qualifikationsrahmen für lebenslanges Lernen (DQR). Liste der zugeordneten Qualifikationen. Online verfügbar unter. 2017. https://www.dqr.de/media/content/Liste%20der%20zugeordneten%20Qualifikationen_01082017.pdf. abgerufen am 07.01.2021.

Draheim S, Beuschel W. Social not technological? Funktionalitäten und Szenarien für neue Lehr-und Lernformen am Beispiel Weblogs. In: Tavangarian D, Nölting K, editors. Auf zu neuen Ufern! E-Learning heute und morgen. New York: Waxmann; 2005. p. 27–36. URN: urn:nbn:de:0111-pedocs-117465.

Duregon F, Vendramin B, Bullo V, Gobbo S, Cugusi L, Di Blasio A, et al. Effects of exercise on cancer patients suffering chemotherapy-induced peripheral neuropathy undergoing treatment: a systematic review. Crit Rev Oncol Hematol. 2018;121:90–100. https://doi.org/10.1016/j.critrevonc.2017.11.002.

Ebersbach G, Edler D, Kaufhold O, Wissel J. Whole body vibration versus conventional physiotherapy to improve balance and gait in Parkinson's disease. Arch Phys Med Rehabil. 2008;89(3):399–403. https://doi.org/10.1016/j.apmr.2007.09.031.

Edwards JH, Reilly GC. Vibration stimuli and the differentiation of musculoskeletal progenitor cells: review of results in vitro and in vivo. World J Stem Cells. 2015;7(3):568–82. https://doi.org/10.4252/wjsc.v7.i3.568.

Eickhof C. Das systematische repetitive Basistraining. In: Minkwitz K, Platz T, editors. Armmotorik nach Schlaganfall: Neue Ansätze für Assessment und Therapie. Idstein: Schulz-Kirchner Verlag GmbH; 2001. p. 97–111.

Elbert T, Pantev C, Wienbruch C, Rockstroh B, Taub E. Increased cortical representation of the fingers of the left hand in string players. Science. 1995;270(5234):305–7. https://doi.org/10.1126/science.270.5234.305.

Erpenbeck J, Heyse V. Aktualisierter KompetenzAtlas. In: Heyse V, Erpenbeck J, Ortmann S, editors. Grundstrukturen menschlicher Kompetenzen Praxiserprobte Konzepte und Instrumente. Waxmann: Münster; 2010. p. 123–55.

Esculier J-F, Vaudrin J, Bériault P, Gagnon K, Tremblay LE. Home-based balance training programme using Wii Fit with balance board for Parkinsons's disease: a pilot study. J Rehabil Med. 2012;44(2):144–50. https://doi.org/10.2340/16501977-0922.

Euler D. Didaktik des Computerunterstützten Lernens. Praktische Gestaltung und theoretische Grundlagen, Band 3 der Reihe Multimediales Lernen in der Berufsbildung, Nürnberg: BW Bildung und Wissen; 1992.

Feldman DE, Brecht M. Map plasticity in somatosensory cortex. Science. 2005;310(5749):810–5. https://doi.org/10.1126/science.1115807.

Filippi GM, Brunetti O, Botti FM, Panichi R, Roscini M, Camerota F, et al. Improvement of stance control and muscle performance induced by focal muscle vibration in young-elderly women: a randomized controlled trial. Arch Phys Med Rehabil. 2009;90(12):2019–25. https://doi.org/10.1016/j.apmr.2009.08.139.

Findlater SE, Dukelow SP. Upper extremity proprioception after stroke: bridging the gap between neuroscience and rehabilitation. J Mot Behav. 2017;49(1):27–34. https://doi.org/10.1080/00222895.2016.1219303.

Fisher G, Quel de Oliveira C, Verhagen A, Gandevia S, Kennedy D. Proprioceptive impairment in unilateral neglect after stroke: a systematic review. SAGE Open Med. 2020;8:1–11. https://doi.org/10.1177/2050312120951073.

Flaiz B, Winkelmann C, Simon A. On the development of the competence profile for the master program "advanced practice in health care". In: Application-oriented higher education research (AOHER), 2019, vol 4(4). p. 77–84. CN34-1326/G4, ISSN2096-2045.

Frank JR. The CanMEDS 2005 physician competency framework. Better standards. Better physicians. Better care. Ottawa: The Royal College of Physicians and Surgeons of Canada. Online verfügbar unter. 2005. http://www.ub.edu/medicina_unitateducaciomedica/documentos/CanMeds.pdf. abgerufen am 01.01.2021.

Freyler K, Krause A, Gollhofer A, Ritzmann R. Specific stimuli induce specific adaptations: sensorimotor training vs. reactive balance training. PLoS One. 2016;11(12):e0167557. https://doi.org/10.1371/journal.pone.0167557.

Garcia-Agundez A, Folkerts A-K, Konrad R, Caserman P, Tregel T, Goosses M, et al. Recent advances in rehabilitation for Parkinson's disease with exergames: a systematic review. J Neuroeng Rehabil. 2019;16(1):17. https://doi.org/10.1186/s12984-019-0492-1.

Gautschi R. Triggerpunkt-Therapie. In: Böhni U, Lauper M, Locher H, editors. Manuelle Medizin 1: Fehlfunktion und Schmerz am Bewegungsorgan verstehen und behandeln. Stuttgart: Thieme; 2015. p. 296–302.

Gershon M. How to use bloom's taxonomy in the classroom: the complete guide. CreateSpace Independent Publishing Platform; 2015.

Gibson EJ. Improvement in perceptual judgments as a function of controlled practice or training. Psychol Bull. 1953;50(6):401–31. https://doi.org/10.1037/h0055517.

Gilbert CD, Sigman M, Crist RE. The neural basis of perceptual learning. Neuron. 2001;31(5):681–97. https://doi.org/10.1016/s0896-6273(01)00424-x.

Gioftsidou A, Vernadakis N, Malliou P, Batzios S, Sofokleous P, Antoniou P, et al. Typical balance exercises or exergames for balance improvement? J Back Musculoskelet Rehabil. 2013;26(3):299–305.

Golden CJ, Hammeke TA, Purisch AD. Diagnostic validity of a standardized neuropsychological battery derived from Luria's neuropsychological tests. J Consult Clin Psychol. 1978;46(6):1258–65.

Golden CJ, Purisch AD, Hammeke TA. Manual of the Luria-Nebraska neuropsychological battery: forms I & II. Los Angeles: Western Psychological Services; 1985.

Gorman P, Krummel T, Webster R, Smith M, Hutchens D. A prototype haptic lumbar puncture simulator. Stud Health Technol Inform. 2000;70:106–9.

Grunwald M. Haptic Pad's: Eine neue Methode zur Messung und zum Training haptischer Wahrnehmungsleistungen. Man Med. 2010;6:474–6.

Grunwald M, Gertz H-J. Störung Der Haptischen Wahrnehmung Bei Anorexia Nervosa. In: Grunwald M, Beyer L, editors. Der bewegte Sinn. Grundlagen und Anwendungen zur haptischen Wahrnehmung. Basel: Birkhäuser; 2001. p. 135–50.

Grunwald M, Mueller SM. Chapter 22 Scientific principles of palpation In: Mayer J, Standen C, editors. Textbook of Osteopathic Medicine. 1st Edition. Munich: Elsevier; 2017. p. 251–63. ISBN: 9780702052651.

Grunwald M, Weiss T. Inducing sensory stimulation in treatment of anorexia nervosa. QJM. 2005;98(5):379–80.

Grunwald M, Busse F, Hensel A, Riedel-Heller S, Kruggel F, Arendt T, et al. Theta-power differences in patients with mild cognitive impairment under rest condition and during haptic tasks. Alzheimer Dis Assoc Disord. 2002a;16(1):40–8. https://doi.org/10.1097/00002093-200201000-00006.

Grunwald M, Ettrich C, Busse F, Assmann B, Dähne A, Gertz H-J. Angle paradigm: a new method to measure right parietal dysfunctions in anorexia nervosa. Arch Clin Neuropsychol. 2002b;17(5):485–96.

Haas CT, Turbanski S, Kessler K, Schmidtbleicher D. The effects of random whole-body-vibration on motor symptoms in Parkinson's disease. NeuroRehabilitation. 2006;21(1):29–36. Online verfügbar unter. http://fox.leuphana.de/portal/de/publications/the-effects-of-random-wholebodyvibration-on-motor-symptoms-in-parkinsons-disease(1c7770a4-dfe3-4417-a3ff-31ba4af349c1).html.

Hallet W. Didaktische Kompetenzen. Lehr- und Lernprozesse erfolgreich begleiten. 1. Aufl. Stuttgart: Klett Lernen und Wissen; 2006.

Han J, Waddington G, Adams R, Anson J, Liu Y. Assessing proprioception: a critical review of methods. J Sport Health Sci. 2016;5(1):80–90. https://doi.org/10.1016/j.jshs.2014.10.004.

Harrar V, Spence C, Makin TR. Topographic generalization of tactile perceptual learning. J Exp Psychol Hum Percept Perform. 2014;40(1):15–23. https://doi.org/10.1037/a0033200.

Herzog MH, Fahle M. The role of feedback in learning a vernier discrimination task. Vis Res. 1997;37(15):2133–41. https://doi.org/10.1016/s0042-6989(97)00043-6.

Heyse V. KODE®X-Kompetenz-Explorer. In: Erpenbeck J, von Rosenstiel L, editors. Handbuch Kompetenzmessung. Erkennen, verstehen und bewerten von Kompetenzen in der betrieblichen, pädagogischen und psychologischen Praxis. 2., überarb u erw Aufl. Stuttgart: Schäffer-Poeschel; 2007. p. 504–14.

Hijmans JM, Geertzen JHB, Dijkstra PU, Postema K. A systematic review of the effects of shoes and other ankle or foot appliances on balance in older people and people with peripheral nervous system disorders. Gait Posture. 2007;25(2):316–23. https://doi.org/10.1016/j.gaitpost.2006.03.010.

Hilkens PH, van den Bent MJ. Chemotherapy-induced peripheral neuropathy. J Peripher Nerv Syst. 1997;2(4):350–61.

Höffken O, Veit M, Knossalla F, Lissek S, Bliem B, Ragert P, et al. Sustained increase of somatosensory cortex excitability by tactile coactivation studied by paired median nerve stimulation in humans correlates with perceptual gain. J Physiol. 2007;584(Pt 2):463–71. https://doi.org/10.1113/jphysiol.2007.140079.

Ikuno K, Kawaguchi S, Kitabeppu S, Kitaura M, Tokuhisa K, Morimoto S, et al. Effects of peripheral sensory nerve stimulation plus task-oriented training on upper extremity function in patients with subacute stroke: a pilot randomized crossover trial. Clin Rehabil. 2012;26(11):999–1009. https://doi.org/10.1177/0269215512441476.

Issenberg SB. Features and uses of high-fidelity medical simulations that lead to effective learning: a BEME systematic review. Med Teach. 2005;27(1):10–28.

Itzcovich E, Riani M, Sannita WG. Stochastic resonance improves vision in the severely impaired. Sci Rep. 2017;7(1):12840. https://doi.org/10.1038/s41598-017-12906-2.

Jeon M-J, Jeon H-S, Yi C-H, Kwon O-Y, You S-H, Park J-H. Block and random practice: a wii fit dynamic balance training in older adults. Res Q Exerc Sport. 2020;92(3):352–60.

Jilg S, Möltner A, Berberat P, Fischer MR, Breckwoldt J. How do supervising clinicians of a University Hospital and Associated Teaching Hospitals rate the relevance of the key competencies within the CanMEDS roles frame work in respect to teaching in clinical clerkships? GMS Z Med Ausbild. 2015;32(3):Doc 33.

Jöbges EM, Elek J, Rollnik JD, Dengler R, Wolf W. Vibratory proprioceptive stimulation affects Parkinsonian tremor. Parkinsonism Relat Disord. 2002;8(3):171–6. https://doi.org/10.1016/s1353-8020(01)00016-5.

Johnson KO, Phillips JR. Tactile spatial resolution. I. Two-point discrimination, gap detection, grating resolution, and letter recognition. J Neurophysiol. 1981;46(6):1177–92. https://doi.org/10.1152/jn.1981.46.6.1177.

Jones MT. Progressive-overload whole-body vibration training as part of periodized, off-season strength training in trained women athletes. J Strength Cond Res. 2014;28(9):2461–9. https://doi.org/10.1519/JSC.0000000000000571.

Jones MT, Parker BM, Cortes N. The effect of whole-body vibration training and conventional strength training on performance measures in female athletes. J Strength Cond Res. 2011;25(9):2434–41. https://doi.org/10.1519/JSC.0b013e31822817cf.

Jonietz D. Ein Wiki als Lernumgebung? Überlegungen und Erfahrungen aus schulischer Sicht. In: Haake JM, Lucke U, Tavangarian D, editors. DeLFI 2005: 3. Deutsche e-Learning Fachtagung Informatik, 13-16, September 2005 in Rostock, Germany. Bonn: Gesellschaft für Informatik e.V.; 2005. p. 35–44.

Kaas AL, van de Ven V, Reithler J, Goebel R. Tactile perceptual learning: learning curves and transfer to the contralateral finger. Exp Brain Res. 2013;224(3):477–88. https://doi.org/10.1007/s00221-012-3329-8.

Kaelin-Lang A, Sawaki L, Cohen LG. Role of voluntary drive in encoding an elementary motor memory. J Neurophysiol. 2005;93(2):1099–103. https://doi.org/10.1152/jn.00143.2004.

Kalisch T, Tegenthoff M, Dinse HR. Improvement of sensorimotor functions in old age by passive sensory stimulation. Clin Interv Aging. 2008;3(4):673–90. https://doi.org/10.2147/cia.s3174.

Kalisch T, Ragert P, Schwenkreis P, Dinse HR, Tegenthoff M. Impaired tactile acuity in old age is accompanied by enlarged hand representations in somatosensory cortex. Cereb Cortex. 2009;19(7):1530–8. https://doi.org/10.1093/cercor/bhn190.

Kang H, Lu J, Xu G. The effects of whole body vibration on muscle strength and functional mobility in persons with multiple sclerosis: a systematic review and meta-analysis. Mult Scler Relat Disord. 2016;7:1–7. https://doi.org/10.1016/j.msard.2016.02.008.

Kattenstroth JC, Kalisch T, Sczesny-Kaiser M, Greulich W, Tegenthoff M, Dinse HR. Daily repetitive sensory stimulation of the paretic hand for the treatment of sensorimotor deficits in patients with subacute stroke: RESET, a randomized, sham-controlled trial. BMC Neurol. 2018;18(1):2. https://doi.org/10.1186/s12883-017-1006-z.

Kaut O, Allert N, Coch C, Paus S, Grzeska A, Minnerop M, Wüllner U. Stochastic resonance therapy in Parkinson's disease. NeuroRehabilitation. 2011;28(4):353–8. https://doi.org/10.3233/NRE-2011-0663.

Kepplinger B, Baran H, Sedlnitzky-Semler B, Badawi N-R, Erhart H. Stochastic resonance activity influences serum tryptophan metabolism in healthy human subjects. Int J Tryptophan Res. 2011;4:49–60. https://doi.org/10.4137/ijtr.s7986.

Kerres M, Jechle T. Betreuung des Lernens in telemedialen Lernumgebungen. Unterrichtswissenschaft. 2000;28(3):257–77.

Kiese-Himmel C. TAKIWA. Göttinger Entwicklungstest der Taktil-Kinästhetischen Wahrnehmung; Manual. Göttingen: Beltz Test; 2003.

Klemme B, Siegmann G. Clinical Reasoning: Therapeutische Denkprozesse lernen. Stuttgart: Thieme; 2015.

Kluding PM, Bareiss SK, Hastings M, Marcus RL, Sinacore DR, Mueller MJ. Physical training and activity in people with diabetic peripheral neuropathy: paradigm shift. Phys Ther. 2017;97(1):31–43.

Krakauer JW, Shadmehr R. Consolidation of motor memory. Trends Neurosci. 2006;29(1):58–64. https://doi.org/10.1016/j.tins.2005.10.003.

Krewer C. Die Rolle der Somatosensorik beim motorischen Lernen. Neuroreha. 2019;11(3):112–6. https://doi.org/10.1055/a-0980-2191.

Laekeman M, Kreutzer R. Großer Bildatlas der Palpation: Anatomische Strukturen gezielt lokalisieren und begreifen. Heidelberg: Springer; 2009.

Lam FMH, Lau RWK, Chung RCK, Pang MYC. The effect of whole body vibration on balance, mobility and falls in older adults: a systematic review and meta-analysis. Maturitas. 2012;72(3):206–13. https://doi.org/10.1016/j.maturitas.2012.04.009.

Lammerding-Köppel M, Baatz C. Auch Lehrende lernen dazu: Grundkonzepte der Didaktik. In: St Pierre M, Breuer G, editors. Simulation in der Medizin. Grundlegende Konzepte – klinische Anwendung. Berlin: Springer; 2013. p. 93–103.

Legge GE, Madison C, Vaughn BN, Cheong AMY, Miller JC. Retention of high tactile acuity throughout the life span in blindness. Percept Psychophys. 2008;70(8):1471–88. https://doi.org/10.3758/PP.70.8.1471.

Lim C. Multi-sensorimotor training improves proprioception and balance in subacute stroke patients: a randomized controlled pilot trial. Front Neurol. 2019;10:157. https://doi.org/10.3389/fneur.2019.00157.

Lissek S, Wilimzig C, Stude P, Pleger B, Kalisch T, Maier C, et al. Immobilization impairs tactile perception and shrinks somatosensory cortical maps. Curr Biol. 2009;19(10):837–42. https://doi.org/10.1016/j.cub.2009.03.065.

Liu W, Lipsitz LA, Montero-Odasso M, Bean J, Kerrigan D, Casey; Collins, James J. Noise-enhanced vibrotactile sensitivity in older adults, patients with stroke, and patients with diabetic neuropathy. Arch Phys Med Rehabil. 2002;83(2):171–6. https://doi.org/10.1053/apmr.2002.28025.

Lo AC, Guarino PD, Richards LG, Haselkorn JK, Wittenberg GF, Federman DG, et al. Robot-assisted therapy for long-term upper-limb impairment after stroke. N Engl J Med. 2010;362(19):1772–83. https://doi.org/10.1056/NEJMoa0911341.

Louw S, Kappers AML, Koenderink JJ. Haptic detection thresholds of Gaussian profiles over the whole range of spatial scales. Exp Brain Res. 2000;132:369–74.

Louw S, Kappers AML, Koenderink JJ. Haptic discrimination of stimuli varying in amplitude and width. Exp Brain Res. 2002;146:32–7.

Marconi B, Filippi GM, Koch G, Giacobbe V, Pecchioli C, Versace V, et al. Long-term effects on cortical excitability and motor recovery induced by repeated muscle vibration in chronic stroke patients. Neurorehabil Neural Repair. 2011;25(1):48–60. https://doi.org/10.1177/1545968310376757.

Mehrholz J. Effekte sensomotorischen Trainings auf die Sensorik des Armes nach Schlaganfall. Neuroreha. 2019;11(3):99. https://doi.org/10.1055/a-0980-2253.

Meyer H. Unterrichts-Methoden I: Theorieband. Berlin: Cornelsen Verlag Scriptor; 2009. p. 136 ff.

Meyer O. Simulators don't teach – Lernprozesse und Simulation. In: St Pierre M, Breuer G, editors. Simulation in der Medizin. Grundlegende Konzepte – klinische Anwendung. Berlin: Springer; 2013.

Meyer S, Karttunen AH, Thijs V, Feys H, Verheyden G. How do somatosensory deficits in the arm and hand relate to upper limb impairment, activity, and participation problems after stroke? A systematic review. Phys Ther. 2014;94(9):1220–31. https://doi.org/10.2522/ptj.20130271.

Meyerhoff J, Brühl C. Fachwissen lebendig vermitteln. Das Methodenhandbuch für Trainer und Dozenten. Wiesbaden: Springer; 2015.

MFT - Medizinischer Fakultätentag der Bundesrepublik Deutschland e. V. NKLM. Nationaler Kompetenzbasierter Lernzielkatalog Medizin (NKLM). Online verfügbar unter. 2015. http://www.nklm.de/files/nklm_final_2015-07-03.pdf. abgerufen am 01.01.2021.

Miller GE. The Assessment of clinical skills/competence/performance. Academic Medicine. 65, Bd. 9. Online verfügbar unter. 1990. http://winbev.pbworks.com/f/Assessment.pdf. abgerufen am 01.01.2021.

Mizrahi D, Broderick C, Friedlander M, Ryan M, Harrison M, Pumpa K, Naumann F. An exercise intervention during chemotherapy for women with recurrent ovarian cancer: a feasibility study. Int J Gynecol Cancer. 2015;25(6):985–92.

Moezy A, Olyaei G, Hadian M, Razi M, Faghihzadeh S. A comparative study of whole body vibration training and conventional training on knee proprioception and postural stability after anterior cruciate ligament reconstruction. Br J Sports Med. 2008;42(5):373–8. https://doi.org/10.1136/bjsm.2007.038554.

Montagu A. Touching. The human significance of the skin. 3rd ed. New York, NY: Harper & Row; 1986.

Morrison S, Simmons R, Colberg SR, Parson HK, Vinik AI. Supervised balance training and wii fit-based exercises lower falls risk in older adults with type 2 diabetes. J Am Med Dir Assoc. 2018;19(2):185.e7–185.e13.

Moss F, Ward LM, Sannita WG. Stochastic resonance and sensory information processing: a tutorial and review of application. Clin Neurophysiol. 2004;115(2):267–81. https://doi.org/10.1016/j.clinph.2003.09.014.

MPhG - Masseur- und Physiotherapeutengesetz vom 26. (BGBl. I S. 1084), das zuletzt durch Artikel 21 des Gesetzes vom 15. August 2019 (BGBl. I S. 1307) geändert worden ist. Online verfügbar unter. 1994. https://www.gesetze-im-internet.de/mphg/BJNR108400994.html. abgerufen am 01.01.2021.

Mueller SM, Grunwald M. Haptische Wahrnehmungsleistungen: Effekte bei erfahrenen und unerfahrenen Physiotherapeuten. Man Med. 2013;51:473–8.

Mueller SM, Habermann S, Dudda J, Grunwald M. Observation of own exploration movements impairs haptic spatial perception. Exp Brain Res. 2013;231(4):415–23. https://doi.org/10.1007/s00221-013-3706-y.

Mueller S, Winkelmann C, Krause F, Grunwald M. Occupation-related long-term sensory training enhances roughness discrimination but not tactile acuity. Exp Brain Res. 2014a;232(6):1905–14.

Mueller SM, Stengler K, Jahn I, Grunwald M. Sensory integration capacity is diminished in obsessive compulsive disorder patients with poor insight but not in patients with intact insight. Int Neuropsychiatri Dis J. 2014b;2(4):141–52. https://doi.org/10.9734/INDJ/2014/8102.

Mueller S, Winkelmann C, Grunwald M. Messung und Training der haptischen Wahrnehmung. Vorstellung des Haptik-Schwellen-Tests sowie des Haptik-FigurenTest und Trainingssets. Zeitschrift für Physiotherapeuten. 2014c;66(10):91–5. https://doi.org/10.1007/s00221-014-3882-4.

Murillo N, Kumru H, Vidal-Samso J, Benito J, Medina J, Navarro X, Valls-Sole J. Decrease of spasticity with muscle vibration in patients with spinal cord injury. Clin Neurophysiol. 2011;122(6):1183–9. https://doi.org/10.1016/j.clinph.2010.11.012.

Nelles G, et al. Rehabilitation von sensomotorischen Störungen. Leitlinien für Diagnostik und Therapie in der Neurologie. Hg. v. Kommission Leitlinien der Deutschen Gesellschaft für Neurologie. Online verfügbar unter. 2018. https://www.awmf.org/uploads/tx_szleitlinien/030-123l_S2k_Rehabilitation_sensomotorische_St%C3%B6rungen_2018-04-verlaengert.pdf. zuletzt geprüft am 21.06.2020.

Nicholson VP, McKean M, Lowe J, Fawcett C, Burkett B. Six weeks of unsupervised Nintendo Wii Fit gaming is effective at improving balance in independent older adults. J Aging Phys Act. 2015;23(1):153–8. https://doi.org/10.1123/JAPA.2013-0148.

Nitz JC, Kuys S, Isles R, Fu S. Is the Wii Fit a new-generation tool for improving balance, health and well-being? A pilot study. Climacteric. 2010;13(5):487–91.

Novak P, Novak V. Effect of step-synchronized vibration stimulation of soles on gait in Parkinson's disease: a pilot study. J Neuroeng Rehabil. 2006;3:9. https://doi.org/10.1186/1743-0003-3-9.

Paoloni M, Mangone M, Scettri P, Procaccianti R, Cometa A, Santilli V. Segmental muscle vibration improves walking in chronic stroke patients with foot drop: a randomized controlled trial. Neurorehabil Neural Repair. 2010;24(3):254–62. https://doi.org/10.1177/1545968309349940.

Patton JL, Kovic M, Mussa-Ivaldi FA. Custom-designed haptic training for restoring reaching ability to individuals with poststroke hemiparesis. J Rehabil Res Dev. 2006;43(5):643–56.

Pereira MP, Gobbi LTB, Almeida QJ. Freezing of gait in Parkinson's disease: evidence of sensory rather than attentional mechanisms through muscle vibration. Parkinsonism Relat Disord. 2016;29:78–82. https://doi.org/10.1016/j.parkreldis.2016.05.021.

PhysTh-APrV - Ausbildungs- und Prüfungsverordnung für Physiotherapeuten vom 6. (BGBl. I S. 3786), die zuletzt durch Artikel 22 des Gesetzes vom 15. August 2019 (BGBl. I S. 1307) geändert worden ist. Online verfügbar unter. 1994. https://www.gesetze-im-internet.de/physth-aprv/PhysTh-APrV.pdf. abgerufen am 01.01.2021.

Platz T, Eickhof C, van Kaick S, Engel U, Pinkowski C, Kalok S, Pause M. Impairment-oriented training or Bobath therapy for severe arm paresis after stroke: a single-blind, multicentre randomized controlled trial. Clin Rehabil. 2005;19(7):714–24. https://doi.org/10.1191/0269215505cr904oa.

Pleger B, Foerster AF, Ragert P, Dinse HR, Schwenkreis P, Malin JP, et al. Functional imaging of perceptual learning in human primary and secondary somatosensory cortex. Neuron. 2003;40(3):643–53. https://doi.org/10.1016/s0896-6273(03)00677-9.

Pollock A, Farmer SE, Brady MC, Langhorne P, Mead GE, Mehrholz J, van Wijck F. Interventions for improving upper limb function after stroke. Cochrane Database Syst Rev. 2014;11:CD010820. https://doi.org/10.1002/14651858.CD010820.pub2.

Pompeu JE, Mendes FADS, da Silva KG, Lobo AM, de Paula Oliveira T, Zomignani AP, Piemonte MEP. Effect of Nintendo Wii™-based motor and cognitive training on activities of daily living in patients with Parkinson's disease: a randomised clinical trial. Physiotherapy. 2012;98(3):196–204.

Prioreschi A, Makda MA, Tikly M, McVeigh JA. In patients with established RA, positive effects of a randomised three month wbv therapy intervention on functional ability, bone mineral density and fatigue are sustained for up to six months. PLoS One. 2016;11(4):e0153470. https://doi.org/10.1371/journal.pone.0153470.

Priplata AA, Niemi JB, Harry JD, Lipsitz LA, Collins JJ. Vibrating insoles and balance control in elderly people. Lancet. 2003;362(9390):1123–4. https://doi.org/10.1016/s0140-6736(03)14470-4.

Priplata AA, Patritti BL, Niemi JB, Hughes R, Gravelle DC, Lipsitz LA, et al. Noise-enhanced balance control in patients with diabetes and patients with stroke. Ann Neurol. 2006;59(1):4–12. https://doi.org/10.1002/ana.20670.

Quasthoff S, Hartung HP. Chemotherapy-induced peripheral neuropathy. J Neurol. 2002;249(1):9–17. https://doi.org/10.1007/pl00007853.

Ragert P, Schmidt A, Altenmüller E, Dinse HR. Superior tactile performance and learning in professional pianists: evidence for meta-plasticity in musicians.

Eur J Neurosci. 2004;19(2):473–8. https://doi.org/10.1111/j.0953-816x.2003.03142.x.
Reitan RM, Davison LA. Clinical neuropsychology: current status and applications. Wiley, NY: Halsted Press Division; 1974.
Reitan RM, Wolfson D. The Halstead-Reitan neuropsychological test battery. Theory and clinical interpretation. 2nd ed. South Tucson, AR: Neuropsychology Press; 1993.
Reitan RM, Wolfson D. Using the Tactile Form Recognition Test to differentiate persons with brain damage from control subjects. Arch Clin Neuropsychol. 2002;17(2):117–21.
Roediger HL, Karpicke JD. The power of testing memory: basic research and implications for educational practice. Perspect Psychol Sci. 2006;1(3):181–210.
Schmitt AC, Repka CP, Heise GD, Challis JH, Smith JD. Comparison of posture and balance in cancer survivors and age-matched controls. Clin Biomech. 2017;50:1–6. https://doi.org/10.1016/j.clinbiomech.2017.09.010.
Schrader J. Lerntypen bei Erwachsenen. Weinheim: Deutscher Studien Verlag; 1994. p. 25.
Seo NJ, Kosmopoulos ML, Enders LR, Hur P. Effect of remote sensory noise on hand function post stroke. Front Hum Neurosci. 2014;8:934. https://doi.org/10.3389/fnhum.2014.00934.
Severini G, Delahunt E. Effect of noise stimulation below and above sensory threshold on postural sway during a mildly challenging balance task. Gait Posture. 2018;63:27–32. https://doi.org/10.1016/j.gaitpost.2018.04.031.
Sharififar S, Coronado RA, Romero S, Azari H, Thigpen M. The effects of whole body vibration on mobility and balance in Parkinson disease: a systematic review. Iran J Med Sci. 2014;39(4):318–26.
Shih M-C, Wang R-Y, Cheng S-J, Yang Y-R. Effects of a balance-based exergaming intervention using the Kinect sensor on posture stability in individuals with Parkinson's disease: a single-blinded randomized controlled trial. J Neuroeng Rehabil. 2016;13(1):78. https://doi.org/10.1186/s12984-016-0185-y.
Sitjà Rabert M, Rigau Comas D, Fort Vanmeerhaeghe A, Santoyo Medina C, Roqué i Figuls M, Romero-Rodríguez D, Bonfill Cosp X. Whole-body vibration training for patients with neurodegenerative disease. Cochrane Database Syst Rev. 2012;(2):CD009097. https://doi.org/10.1002/14651858.CD009097.pub2.
Smith PS, Dinse HR, Kalisch T, Johnson M, Walker-Batson D. Effects of repetitive electrical stimulation to treat sensory loss in persons poststroke. Arch Phys Med Rehabil. 2009;90(12):2108–11. https://doi.org/10.1016/j.apmr.2009.07.017.
Sopka S, Simon M, Becker SK. "Assessment drives Learning": Konzepte zur Erfolgs- und Qualitätskontrolle. In: St Pierre M, Breuer G, editors. Simulation in der Medizin. Grundlegende Konzepte – klinische Anwendung. Berlin: Springer; 2013. p. 83–92.
Stefani L, Galanti G, Klika R. Clinical implementation of exercise guidelines for cancer patients: adaptation of ACSM's guidelines to the Italian Model. JFMK. 2017;2(1):4.
Stevens JC, Foulke E, Patterson MQ. Tactile acuity, aging, and braille reading in long-term blindness. J Exp Psychol Appl. 1996;2(2):91–106. https://doi.org/10.1037/1076-898x.2.2.91.
Stolzenberg N, Belavý DL, Rawer R, Felsenberg D. Whole-body vibration versus proprioceptive training on postural control in post-menopausal osteopenic women. Gait Posture. 2013;38(3):416–20. https://doi.org/10.1016/j.gaitpost.2013.01.002.
Streckmann F, Zopf EM, Lehmann HC, May K, Rizza J, Zimmer P, et al. Exercise intervention studies in patients with peripheral neuropathy: a systematic review. Sports Med. 2014;44(9):1289–304. https://doi.org/10.1007/s40279-014-0207-5.
Streeck U, Focke J, Melzer C, Streeck J. Manuelle Therapie und komplexe Rehabilitation. Berlin: Springer; 2017.
Stubblefield MD, Burstein HJ, Burton AW, Custodio CM, Deng GE, Ho M, et al. NCCN task force report: management of neuropathy in cancer. J Natl Compr Cancer Netw. 2009;7(Suppl 5):1–26. https://doi.org/10.6004/jnccn.2009.0078.
Sutherland C, Hashtrudi-Zaad K, Sellens R, Abolmaesumi P, Mousavi P. An augmented reality haptic training simulator for spinal needle procedures. IEEE Trans Biomed Eng. 2013;60(11):3009–18. https://doi.org/10.1109/TBME.2012.2236091.
Terhart E. Lehr-Lernmethoden. 2. Aufl. München: Juventa; 1997.
Thalhamer C. Probleme des klinischen Wiederbefunds. Man Med. 2017;55:29–33.
Timmermann A, Eich C, Russo SG, Barwing J, Hirn A, Rode H, Heuer JF, Heise D, Nickel E, Klockgether-Radke A, Graf BM. Lehre und Simulation: Methoden, Anforderungen, Evaluation und Visionen. Anaesthesist. 2007;56:53–62.
Toulotte C, Toursel C, Olivier N. Wii Fit® training vs. adapted physical activities: which one is the most appropriate to improve the balance of independent senior subjects? A randomized controlled study. Clin Rehabil. 2012;26(9):827–35.
Tremblay F, Backman A, Cuenco A, Vant K, Wassef MA. Assessment of spatial acuity at the fingertip with grating (JVP) domes: validity for use in an elderly population. Somatosens Motor Res. 2000;17(1):61–6.
Tulodziecki G, Herzig B. Handbuch Medienpädagogik. Band 2: Mediendidaktik. Stuttgart: Klett-Cotta Verlag; 2004.
Tyson SF, Hanley M, Chillala J, Selley AB, Tallis RC. Sensory loss in hospital-admitted people with stroke: characteristics, associated factors, and relationship with function. Neurorehabil Neural Repair. 2008;22(2):166–72. https://doi.org/10.1177/1545968307305523.
van Boven RW, Johnson KO. The limit of tactile spatial resolution in humans: grating orientation dis-

crimination at the lip, tongue, and finger. Neurology. 1994;44(12):2361–6. https://doi.org/10.1212/wnl.44.12.2361.

van Dijk R, Kappers AML, Postma A. Haptic spatial configuration learning in deaf and hearing individuals. PLoS One. 2013;8(4):e61336. https://doi.org/10.1371/journal.pone.0061336.

van Nes IJW, Latour H, Schils F, Meijer R, van Kuijk A, Geurts ACH. Long-term effects of 6-week whole-body vibration on balance recovery and activities of daily living in the postacute phase of stroke: a randomized, controlled trial. Stroke. 2006;37(9):2331–5. https://doi.org/10.1161/01.STR.0000236494.62957.f3.

Veerbeek JM, van Wegen E, van Peppen R, van der Wees PJ, Hendriks E, Rietberg M, Kwakkel G. What is the evidence for physical therapy poststroke? A systematic review and meta-analysis. PLoS One. 2014;9(2):e87987. https://doi.org/10.1371/journal.pone.0087987.

Verschueren SMP, Roelants M, Delecluse C, Swinnen S, Vanderschueren D, Boonen S. Effect of 6-month whole body vibration training on hip density, muscle strength, and postural control in postmenopausal women: a randomized controlled pilot study. J Bone Miner Res. 2004;19(3):352–9. https://doi.org/10.1359/JBMR.0301245.

Voelcker-Rehage C, Godde B. High frequency sensory stimulation improves tactile but not motor performance in older adults. Mot Control. 2010;14(4):460–77. https://doi.org/10.1123/mcj.14.4.460.

Vollmer J, Mönk S. Blick nach vorne: Was bringt die Zukunft? In: St Pierre M, Breuer G, editors. Simulation in der Medizin. Grundlegende Konzepte – klinische Anwendung. Berlin: Springer; 2013. p. 343–8.

Walber M, Jütte W. Entwicklung professioneller Kompetenzen durch didaktische Relationierung in der wissenschaftlichen Weiterbildung. In: Hartung O, Rumpf M, editors. Lehrkompetenzen in der wissenschaftlichen Weiterbildung: Konzepte, Forschungsansätze und Anwendungen. Wiesbaden: Springer; 2015.

Warlow C, van Gijn J, Dennis M, Wardlaw J, Bamford J, Hankey G, et al. Stroke: practical management. 3rd ed. Oxford: Blackwell Publishing Ltd.; 2008.

Weiss T. Plastizität im somatosensorischen System. In: Grunwald M, Beyer L, editors. Der bewegte Sinn. Grundlagen und Anwendungen zur haptischen Wahrnehmung. Basel: Birkhäuser Verlag; 2001. p. 53–60.

Wells C, Ward LM, Chua R, Timothy Inglis J. Touch noise increases vibrotactile sensitivity in old and young. Psychol Sci. 2005;16(4):313–20. https://doi.org/10.1111/j.0956-7976.2005.01533.x.

Winkelmann C. Qualifikationsziele in Aus- und Weiterbildungsprogrammen der manuellen Therapie. Therapie lernen Bildung Forschung Praxis. 2020;9(9):32–9. ISSN 2195-058X.

Winkelmann C, Grunwald M. Preparatory course to haptic sensory discrimination skills. Ann Phys Rehabil Med. 2018;61:e526.

Winkelmann C, Beyer L, Grunwald M. Propädeutikum zur aktiven Tastsinnesleistung (PakT). Man Med. 2017;55(4):197–204. https://doi.org/10.1007/s00337-017-0281-5.

Winkelmann C, Grunwald M, Beyer L. Konzeption eines Propädeutikums zur aktiven Tastsinnesleistung im Rahmen der manualtherapeutischen Ausbildung. Physikalische Medizin, Rehabilitationsmedizin, Kurortmedizin. 2018;28(4):43.

Winkelmann C, Beyer L, Mueller SM, Grunwald M. Fühlen lernen - Test und Training aktiver Tastsinnesleistungen in Physio- und Manualtherapie. P02.08. Der Schmerz. 2019;33(Suppl 1):43–4.

Wong JD, Wilson ET, Gribble PL. Spatially selective enhancement of proprioceptive acuity following motor learning. J Neurophysiol. 2011;105(5):2512–21. https://doi.org/10.1152/jn.00949.2010.

Wong M, Peters RM, Goldreich D. A physical constraint on perceptual learning: tactile spatial acuity improves with training to a limit set by finger size. J Neurosci. 2013;33(22):9345–52. https://doi.org/10.1523/JNEUROSCI.0514-13.2013.

Yang J-D, Liao C-D, Huang S-W, Tam K-W, Liou T-H, Lee Y-H, et al. Effectiveness of electrical stimulation therapy in improving arm function after stroke: a systematic review and a meta-analysis of randomised controlled trials. Clin Rehabil. 2019;33(8):1286–97. https://doi.org/10.1177/0269215519839165.

Yardley L, Bishop FL, Beyer N, Hauer K, Kempen GIJM, Piot-Ziegler C, et al. Older people's views of falls-prevention interventions in six European countries. Gerontologist. 2006;46(5):650–60. https://doi.org/10.1093/geront/46.5.650.

Zarkou A, Lee SCK, Prosser LA, Hwang S, Jeka J. Stochastic resonance stimulation improves balance in children with cerebral palsy: a case control study. J Neuroeng Rehabil. 2018;15(1):115. https://doi.org/10.1186/s12984-018-0467-7.

Social Touch and Touching Patients

5

Stephanie Margarete Mueller

Contents

S. M. Mueller (✉)
Haptic Research Lab, Paul-Flechsig-Institute for Brain Research, Leipzig University, Leipzig, Germany
e-mail: s.mueller@medizin.uni-leipzig.de

S. M. Mueller et al., *Human Touch in Healthcare*, https://doi.org/10.1007/978-3-662-67860-2_5

5.1 Ethical Aspects

5.1.1 Touching Patients

5.1.1.1 Necessary Touches to Health Care

In diagnostic, therapeutic, and nursing contexts, touch is a prerequisite for successful treatment. Compared to other everyday touches, these touches represent exceptional situations in the lives of both patients and the professionals performing the touches in several respects:

1. Strangers often perform the touches. Specifically, touches often take place independently of a personal relationship between the patient and professional (for example, during the application of massage therapy or the transfer of the patient from their bed) or between patients (for example, during group interventions or partner exercises).
2. The touches are sometimes painful or unpleasant. Therefore, they are in strict contrast to most social touches, which are usually associated with positive connotations.
3. Taboo zones (see Sect. 5.1.2) cannot always be maintained.

Patients expect and tolerate appropriate and necessary physical contact in medical contexts, which often results in tacit consent. However, from an ethical perspective, with touching, a transgression of physical and possibly emotional boundaries occurs despite the necessity of touch. Practicing healthcare professionals are, thus, required to reflect intensively on the **manner of touching** and to act in **agreement with the patient**. This also applies to interactions with sedated patients. Patients should be empowered to make informed decisions regarding therapy. Furthermore, any physical contact with patients is subject to the same medical ethics guidelines as all other interventions. The main points of these guidelines are as follows:

- The prohibition of causing harm physically, psychologically, or socially.
- Respecting and promoting the well-being of the individual.
- Respecting the patient's self-determination.
- Protecting human dignity.

5.1.1.2 Communicative/Social Touches

Social touches can be distinguished from necessary touches that serve a medical or nursing purpose. These social touches, which often occur spontaneously, fulfill social or emotional functions. Interpersonal touches can have a calming, comforting, or stress-reducing effect. It is possible to use such touches specifically for these purposes in medical and nursing contexts. For example, nonverbal gestures can convey and strengthen closeness, trust, and affection. In addition, a brief touch can highlight the urgency and importance of a statement. However, the prerequisites for such touches are that the relationship between the individuals involved is positive, the status of both individuals allows it, and the situation is perceived as appropriate (see Sect. 5.2.2). If one or more of these prerequisites are not met, there is a risk that even with the best of intentions, the social touch may have the opposite effect and be perceived as unpleasant or even threatening.

▶ **Important** Physical contact in health care always has a social aspect that affects the relationship level of the individuals involved. There are no non-social acts of contact.

In both medically necessary and social touch, the integrity of the toucher and the individual being touched is important. Specifically, it is critical that all parties feel comfortable with the actions performed and feel safe enough to articulate what they are comfortable with and what they dislike. Therefore, an atmosphere should be created in which the patient's autonomy is preserved without fear of negative consequences. This also applies to well-intentioned non-therapy-related touching. The patient's right to self-determination must be respected and their independent decisions accepted, and to ensure this, appropriate questions and agreements can be implemented. Healthcare representatives must not, under any circumstances, harm patients emotionally, sexually, or physically through touching or other actions, and this includes that patients must not be touched to satisfy own needs (Scheel 2019; Davidzar and Giger 1997).

▶ **Definition** Types of touches:

- *Medically necessary touching:*
  - All touches that serve to provide health care
- *Social touches*:
  - Communicative touch: nonverbal gestures (e.g., to attract attention and to greet or to say goodbye to someone).
  - Emotional touch: all empathic and affectionate touches intended to have a comforting, strengthening, or calming effect.
  - Playful touches (e.g., in the context of sports, dance, and theater).
  - Protective/defensive touches: holding or defensive touches to protect oneself or another person.
  - Physically damaging touches.
  - Erotic touches.

5.1.2 Acceptable Body Areas and Situations

5.1.2.1 Body Areas

Physical contact is an integral part of social relationships and nonverbal communication. In everyday life, body touching occurs mainly between people who know each other personally. Body touching also occurs in public settings and between strangers (e.g., on the train), but research findings show that an interpersonal emotional bond is the best predictor of social touching. Accordingly, an individual's social connectedness in a social network can be deduced from the frequency with which social touches occur between individuals (Willis and Briggs 1992; Hill and Dunbar 2003).

Accordingly, the frequency of touching between individuals strongly depends on their **emotional attachment to** each other. This relationship is assumed to be a cross-cultural phenomenon. According to a multicultural observational and survey study involving 1368 individuals from five different countries, including Finland, Italy, Russia, France, and the United Kingdom (Suvilehto et al. 2015), intimate partners have the highest contact rate, followed by close friends, parents, and siblings. Conversely, more distant relatives and acquaintances are touched less often, and strangers hardly at all.

The parts of the body that may be touched are also related to the strength of the emotional bond (Fig. 5.1; Suvilehto et al. 2015). While spouses and life partners are usually allowed to touch all parts of the body, distant relatives and acquaintances are generally only allowed to touch the hands and arms and, possibly, the shoulders or back. Women tend to allow more touching of the shoulders and back by distant relatives and acquaintances, while men tend to reject this. Close friends and close family members occupy an intermediate position in terms of touching areas.

Except in relation to partners, taboo zones are the intimate areas, breasts, and buttocks. For strangers, the legs, and especially the thighs, are also taboo. Most people act intuitively according to these principles and know which touches are appropriate in everyday life. Interestingly, in the study, very similar statements were made by the participants of the different nations regarding which parts of the body may be touched by whom (Suvilehto et al. 2015).

▶ **Important** All interpersonal touches transmit social and emotional information that is interpreted and evaluated by the recipient of the touch. As with all other types of communication, four factors are critical to interpreting touch: the message, the sender, the receiver, and the situation (Ellis 1995).

5.1.2.2 Situations

Whether and on which body parts a person agrees to be touched depends not only on the personal relationship between the individuals but also on the situation. One study compiled different situa-

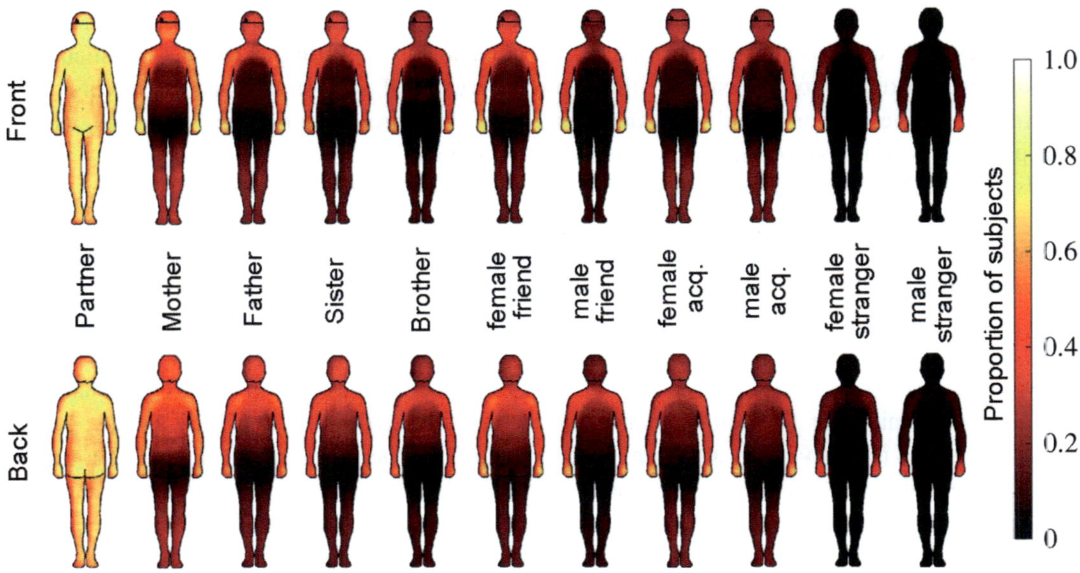

Fig. 5.1 Social touching by family, strangers, and distant acquaintances. Whether people agree to be touched and on which parts of their body depends on the situation and their relationship with the person touching them. Strangers and distant acquaintances are usually allowed to touch only very limited areas of the body. Lighter colors in the image indicate regions where body touching is more likely to be tolerated. (Fig. from Suvilehto et al. 2019)

tions in which touching is perceived as appropriate (Suvilehto et al. 2015). Most often, touching hands and arms takes place in the context of greetings and goodbyes. Indeed, touch gestures for **greetings/goodbyes** were the only ones tolerated by almost the whole sample, regardless of emotional attachment, and these gestures were tolerated even with distant acquaintances and strangers. However, touches often differ in the extent of physical contact (e.g., hug vs. handshake) depending on the emotional attachment between the individuals. In contrast, almost all the respondents in the study indicated that they would accept touching regardless of the personal relationship if it occurred **to provide assistance.**

The duration and intensity of touch are also relevant for its acceptance. For example, a quick tap on the arm or shoulder to attract someone's attention (e.g., as a warning or hint) is usually tolerated. Conversely, the evaluation of stroking or holding touches strongly depends on the situation and the touching person.

For some types of touch, a strong emotional bond and an appropriate situation are prerequisites. Accordingly, affectionate touch used solely to bring pleasure to the other person (even without sexual intent) is accepted almost exclusively from the partner. Comforting touch also requires a close emotional bond or a medical or pastoral relationship of trust. Consistent with this, in a previous survey, almost all the patients indicated that compassionate touch from their physician on the arm would be appropriate and desired, especially in situations of **emotional distress and loss** (e.g., the announcement of a serious diagnosis or the impending death of a loved one) (Cocksedge et al. 2013).

In addition to emotional attachment, **social or occupational status** also plays a role in touch (Henley 1973). This is especially relevant when physical contact occurs between individuals with different social statuses. For example, according to observational studies, praising, or supportive touches are more often performed by individuals with higher status toward those with lower status, and this usually involves touching the arm or shoulder. In contrast, lower-status individuals are more likely to perform formal touches, such as a handshake, on higher-status individuals. This status-dependent behavior can be observed between bosses and employees, between patients and healthcare professionals, and sometimes also within heterogeneous patient groups.

5.1.3 Cultural/Religious Differences

Cultural and religious differences in the acceptability of touch must also be considered (Mujallad and Taylor 2016; Sorajjakool et al. 2017; Ilkilic and Takim 2007). For example, physical gestures between strangers, which are considered to show polite manners in many cultural circles (e.g., shaking hands to greet someone or seal an agreement), may be perceived as unpleasant or even intrusive by individuals of other cultural backgrounds. In medical or nursing care, having consideration for all people of all backgrounds is paramount. This consideration also applies to the behavior rules and codes of conduct between men and women in the Islamic and Orthodox faiths.

Some Muslims, for example, experience intense feelings of shame in response to the physical touch of strangers. Therefore, to maintain privacy, the body is covered with special clothing, and physical contact with individuals of the opposite sex who are not family members is avoided. Consequently, physical contact between unrelated and unmarried men and women can be perceived as a violation of privacy. For this reason, a Muslim may refuse a handshake, a medical or nursing examination, or treatment by someone of the opposite sex. However, illness as an emergency is recognized in Islamic ethics as a state of exception and may, under certain circumstances, temporarily override some social rules between men and women. Accordingly, necessary physical contact in the context of medical examinations or nursing procedures is an exceptional situation that cannot be equated with touching in everyday life. However, different families may have different approaches. For example, some Muslims living in Germany accept the handshake as a form of greeting and may feel offended if it is omitted. To prevent misunderstandings and avoid offending feelings and principles, it is, thus, advisable to discuss the values of the patient and relatives during the first contact. If desired and organizationally possible, Muslim patients should be cared for by same-sex medical staff. The same consideration and sensitivity should be applied when dealing with people of any faith, especially if specific religious rules of contact exist (Mujallad and Taylor 2016; Sorajjakool et al. 2017; Ilkilic and Takim 2007).

▶ **Important** Touch can be experienced differently depending on cultural/religious background, sex, environmental conditions, and body region.

5.2 Short Touches and Their Consequences

This section considers the effects of brief or fleeting social touches, which are usually performed by strangers. Regarding the effects of relaxation massages and other therapeutic touches lasting several minutes, see Chap. 8. Regarding the emotion-regulating and anxiety-regulating effects of physical contact with close individuals, see Sect. 5.5.3.

5.2.1 Expectation and Sex Effects

Social touch has the potential to have calming and stress-reducing effects, alleviate anxiety, and lower the heart rate, respiratory rate, and blood pressure. However, these effects, which are desirable in the medical context, are not an unconditional consequence of every touch. Instead, the physiological, cognitive, and behavioral consequences of touch can range from **neutral to strongly positive or negative**. From an evolutionary perspective, any touch requires immediate attention to evaluate whether it poses a danger (Wilhelm et al. 2001). Depending on the result of this evaluation, a stress reaction (fight/attack, flight, freeze) or a relaxation reaction will follow. Beyond the initial responses, touches can transmit substantially more complex meanings and consequences. Depending on the perceived function and meaning (e.g., warn, comfort, erotically stimulate, restrict movement), touch can trigger very different physical reactions.

For touch to have a calming and stress-reducing effect, several conditions must be met, and these are largely identical to those described in Sect. 5.1. These conditions include that only selected body parts may be touched and that the touching should be performed by people who are either close to the person or are assisting them in a critical situation. Furthermore, the situation and the context play a central role in determining whether touch is perceived as appropriate and pleasant or not.

5.2.1.1 Expectation Effects

Various research projects have been conducted to determine the factors that influence the **physiological effects of brief touches by strangers.**

In most studies, heart rate has been used as a physiological measure. In this context, some authors have reported that short touches result in an increase in heart rate (Lynch et al. 1974; Edens et al. 1992; Williams and Kleinke 1993), while others have reported decreases in heart rate (Drescher et al. 1980, 1985). For a long time, it remained unexplained why opposite results were found in studies with apparently similar experimental situations. In retrospect, it is apparent that the experiments that identified a reduction in heart rate had a crucial difference; specifically, in those experiments, the participants were **fully informed beforehand by whom and why they would be touched.** Conversely, in the studies in which an increase in heart rate was observed, the touching occurred unexpectedly and without justification. Therefore, the decisive factor in determining the participants' reactions was whether (a) they expected the touch and perceived it to be part of the experiment or (b) they perceived it as a nonspecific, potentially inappropriate social gesture. By transferring these findings to the context of health care, it should be understood that it is important to inform patients in advance about action steps involving the body (e.g., taking blood, palpation, and washing), including in intensive care contexts for sedated or comatose patients. Although most patients generally expect to be touched in a medical context for diagnostic and treatment purposes, many patients cannot anticipate the required action steps. In addition, most patients in these contexts are anxious and uncertain about their health status and the meaning of examinations and results. Accordingly, sudden touches can appear threatening, trigger the fear of pain, and cause a sense of incapacitation. These effects are further amplified if the person is undressed, if the touching occurs on the trunk, intimate areas, or legs, or if the patient cannot visually follow the actions. These processes likely cause the increase in heart rate and changes in patients' heart rhythms frequently observed during interactions with healthcare workers (Lynch et al. 1974).

> ▶ **Important** By announcing, justifying, and describing the actions of *medically necessary* touching, stress and anxiety reactions in patients can be prevented and reduced.

However, using heart rate as a sole measure does not allow reliable conclusions to be drawn regarding the complex processes of the autonomic nervous system (Wilhelm et al. 2001). For example, reductions in heart rate can be observed not only during relaxation processes but also in the context of orientation reactions (turning toward a sudden stimulus). In this case, the heart rate decreases for only a few seconds while the individual evaluates the stimulus. Paradoxically, on occasion, in response to a **persistent perceived threat, a slowing of the heart rate can also occur**. For example, one study investigated the response of individuals with social phobia to an announced touch on the wrist. The authors found that the participants had a decreased heart rate while waiting for the touch and during the touch itself. Concurrently, however, the authors observed an increase in other physiological markers (blood pressure, skin conductance, and respiratory rate). In addition, the participants reported feeling uncomfortable and anxious in anticipation of and during touch. This is an unusual finding in terms of the fact that heart rate and blood pressure typically respond in unison in stressful and relaxing situations. In contrast, in these **individuals with social phobia,** a form of autonomic coactivation was observed (the parasympathetic *and* sympathetic nervous systems were activated). This coactivation process may occur when a situation is perceived as threatening but there is no possibility of escape or fighting

(Wilhelm et al. 2001). In this case, the person freezes in place and remains in a situation perceived as threatening.

Consequently, it is not sufficient to assess physiological relaxation solely based on the heart rate. The individual's subjective perception of the meaning of the touch is crucial to correctly interpreting the physiological response. Therefore, professionals in health care who wish to perform social touch on patients should closely observe patient reactions during social touch (e.g., sudden sweating) and obtain verbal consent if necessary.

> **Important** Even an announced and well-intentioned *social* touch can trigger stress, depending on how the patient perceives the touch.

5.2.1.2 Sex Effects

The way in which individuals react to touch also depends on the sex of the individuals involved as well as the expectations and experiences associated with touch. Currently, studies on sex effects exist only for males and females but not for non-binary or trans individuals.

In one study examining sex effects, patients were briefly touched while being prepared for surgery (Whitcher and Fisher 1979). During patient education (going through informational materials together), the nurse providing the education touched the patients on the arm for about 1 min. Subsequently, the patients were asked by another independent person how anxious and worried they were about the surgery and possible complications. After the surgery, the patients' blood pressure was measured several times in the recovery room. The results showed different effects for female and male patients. Specifically, women who were touched before surgery reported lower anxiety and apprehension scores on the survey than women in the no-touch control group. In addition, the touched women had systematically lower postoperative blood pressure scores. In contrast, the men who were touched showed higher anxiety and blood pressure scores than the men in the no-touch control group. These results suggest that touch during preoperative patient education may benefit some individuals' preoperative and postoperative physiologic status. In this case, women benefited from touch by a female nurse. Given the fact that this study showed negative results in relation to touch for the male patients, preoperative touch may not be recommended for this group. The study dates from 1979, so the results may also be influenced by generational or age effects. Therefore, more recent studies in similar settings are required.

In addition to the sex of the toucher, **expectancy and context effects** play a major role in the perception and outcomes of touch. In a previous study that conducted laboratory experiments, males showed particularly strong reactions when an unwarranted and unjustified touch was performed on the shoulder during a cognitive task. In this study, unjustified touch resulted in poorer test performance by men on mental tasks (Digit Symbol Substitution Test) and lower sympathy toward the touching person (Sussman and Rosenfeld 1978). Interestingly, touching was perceived less strongly as a transgression by the participating men when a prior explanation for the touching was given (Sussman and Rosenfeld 1978). Fewer effects were found overall for the participating women. The reported effects are in line with those of studies on perceived personal distance. Again, sex differences were reported for violations of personal distance; specifically, on average, women tended to tolerate crowded spaces better than men (Hartnett et al. 1970; Pedersen and Heaston 1972).

Further experiments have confirmed that the context in which touch occurs also plays a crucial role in sex effects. In those studies, it was found that social touch led to an increase in heart rate, whereas manual pulse measurement at the wrist led to a decrease in heart rate (Nilsen and Vrana 1998; Drescher et al. 1985). Furthermore, particularly strong physiological reactions (increases in heart rate and blood pressure) were observed in women who were touched by a male experimenter without announcement or justification. Conversely, when the touch was announced and justified (pulse measurement), the reactions of men and women did not differ, regardless of whether the experimenter was male or female (Nilsen and Vrana 1998; Drescher et al. 1985).

► **Important** Sex effects occur primarily during social touching. In the case of professionally justified and announced bodily touching (e.g., medical examination), no sex effects are usually observed.

The reasons why women and men react differently to the touch of strangers have not yet been conclusively explained. Theoretical considerations assume the reasons include cultural and learned causes as well as archaic conflict patterns. Additionally, the influence of sexual orientation or gender on reactions to touch has not yet been investigated. Some studies suggest that homophobic attitudes underpin the contradictory and sometimes negative effects when a man is touched by another man (cf. Sect. 5.2.3) (Dolinski 2010).

► **Important** In everyday life, social touching occurs most frequently between women and comparatively rarely between men. However, in experimental settings, it has been shown that the effects of social touching between men and women and between men are strongly dependent on the situation and the intention of the person performing the touching.

5.2.2 Perception of Emotions and Intentions

5.2.2.1 Nonverbal Expression of Feelings

Feelings and emotions are communicated and perceived in everyday life via several sensory channels. However, scientific studies have primarily examined verbal and facial expressions of emotions. Interestingly, people can recognize different emotions in others even when only isolated information is available. For example, if only photographs of facial expressions are shown or only vocal utterances are played, people can recognize the emotions with great accuracy (Ekman 1993; Scherer et al. 2003). However, in everyday life, not only verbal and facial expressions but also body posture and touch play a role in communicating emotions. A previous experiment, thus, investigated which physical expressions people use to convey emotions when they are not allowed to use voice or speech (App et al. 2011). It was found that a combination of body posture and facial expression represented most emotions. Therefore, observing body posture and facial expressions provides sufficient information to reliably recognize emotions (e.g., sadness or anger). However, three specific feelings had more distinctive communication features, including shame, love, and affection:

- **Shame** was communicated primarily through body posture and less through facial expression.
- Intimate and trusting feelings, such as **love and affection**, were predominantly conveyed through touch and physical contact.
- Touch and physical contact were used considerably less to convey other feelings.
- Similarly, observers could confidently identify affection and love when these were expressed through physical touch. In contrast, observers found it difficult to recognize affection and love when expressed only through facial expressions and body posture.

In another experiment, older adults were shown 30-s videos in which a nurse was shown listening to a nursing home resident. The caregiver touched the resident on the arm in half of the videos. In the other videos, the nurse leaned toward the resident but did not touch them. In all the videos, the individuals indicated that the caregiver showed affection and immediacy. However, the ratings were significantly higher for those videos with a brief touch (Moore and Gilbert 1995).

► **Important** Love and affection, or sympathy, are best comprehensible when expressed through body contact. Conversely, other feelings, such as shame, pride, joy, or sadness, are conveyed more through body posture and facial expressions than through touch.

5.2.2.2 Intention and Mood of the Touching Person

In the previous section, the nonverbal ways in which feelings can be expressed were discussed. In everyday life, however, people analyze touch primarily in terms of the possible **intention of the person touching them**. Every physical touch is immediately evaluated in terms of its meaning for the organism. This process likely has evolutionary origins and is designed to protect the body from injury. An unexpected touch immediately focuses attention on the touched body part as well as the source of the touch. This response occurs without exception and is independent of whether an object, animal, or another human triggered the touch. Depending on the result of the intention and **danger assessment**, the touch is followed by a certain biological reaction (including a drop/rise in heart rate and blood pressure, cf. Sect. 5.2.1) and a certain behavioral response (e.g., avoiding the touch orwithdrawing the hand in the case of accidental touch) (Nilsen and Vrana 1998; Drescher et al. 1985; Wilhelm et al. 2001). Affectionate, comforting, and praising actions that involve physical contact, for example, are usually only tolerated if trustworthy people carry them out and if the touch is appropriate for the situation. Otherwise, there may be a defensive reaction following the unappreciated touch.

Interestingly, although the characteristics of the person and the situation play a role in the danger assessment following touch, the **characteristics of the touch** itself are also important. The characteristics of a touch (e.g., speed, pressure, duration, skin moisture) depend on the intention and emotional mood with which the touch is performed. For example, a nursing activity can be performed anxiously, gently, gruffly, or with sexual connotations. The same applies to medical examinations or physiotherapy. Accordingly, the warmth or moisture of the touching hands may differ depending on the individual's intentions. For example, the touches of an anxious or insecure person would be characterized by moist, cold hands, and careful touches with low pressure. The subtle differences in skin temperature, moisture, pressure, and speed of the actions can be perceived with great accuracy by the person being touched due to the high sensitivity of the haptic system (Sect. 1.1).

Similarly, **moods or aversions** can influence actions on the patient's body in the medical context, even if this is not intended. Private conversations with the patient or the patient's relatives or immersion in one's own thoughts may also lead to actions on the patient's body being influenced by the respective mood. For example, stimulating conversations and thoughts can cause an intensification of the applied pressure and an acceleration of the movements. Attention diverted in this way can also impair the diagnostic process, cause the healthcare professional to inadvertently inflict pain on the patient, or not perceive signals from the patient.

Despite these significant effects, few studies on these phenomena exist to date. The lack of studies on this topic can be explained by the fact that experimental studies on intention recognition are difficult to implement. However, in one study, participants were stroked on the forearm at two different speeds (3 cm/s and 18 cm/s; cf. also Sect. 1.1.5). All other variables (skin moisture, skin temperature, and pressure) were unchanged. The authors found that even an isolated change in stroking speed led to a change in perceived intention. Accordingly, slower stroking was perceived as praising, supportive, familiar, or intimate. Conversely, the faster stroking was perceived as a warning or a sign of aggression (Kirsch et al. 2018). This study result indicates the high sensitivity of the underlying evaluation system in interpreting the slightest differences in touch, even when environmental conditions and the touching individual are held constant.

▶ **Important** The intention and mood of the toucher can be recognized with high certainty by the touched person based on the characteristics of a touch (speed, pressure, and duration).

5.2.3 Influencing Attitudes: Evaluation of a Person or the Setting

A brief touch on the hand, arm, or shoulder can positively influence attitudes toward the person performing the touch and toward the environment (Gallace and Spence 2010; Huisman 2017). One of the best-known studies on this topic was conducted in a library (Fisher et al. 1976). When returning their library card, some students were "accidentally" touched on the hand by the library employee (<1 s), whereas the comparison group received their library card without hand contact. Shortly after that, the students were asked by another person to participate in a quality survey about the library and the staff. The students who had been touched gave more positive ratings than those who had not been touched, and this was true regardless of whether they remembered being touched. In addition, the touched individuals rated their state of mind more positively than the untouched individuals. Sex effects may also influence these results; specifically, touch tended to produce larger effects in the female students than in the male students. However, the sex of the librarian showed no influence in this study, possibly because the touch was perceived as accidental by all the students.

The results have been confirmed by several later studies. In one study, students were briefly (<5 s) touched on the arm by a lecturer during a consultation (Steward and Lupfer 1987). In the consultation, the student and lecturer sat next to each other while the lecturer gave the student constructive criticism about their test performance and offered suggestions for improvement. In a subsequent survey, the students who had been touched rated the lecturer as friendlier, more understanding, more interesting, and more capable than the students who had not been touched. In addition, touch positively affected the students' academic performance; in particular, the students who had been touched showed better test scores on subsequent exams than the students in the control group. Sex effects were not found in this study. The authors interpreted the results to mean that touch **was a reinforcing nonverbal expression of sympathy**.

A study of student teachers who completed a mandatory hour of psychological counseling about their career aptitude yielded similar results. Half of the participants were given a handshake as a greeting and, when saying goodbye, were touched on the arm during the consultation. In contrast to the control group, students who had been touched rated the counselor more positively and as more competent (Hubble et al. 1981).

In the context of customer service, it has also been shown that brief touches can lead to stronger positive evaluations. In one study, customers rated a bookstore more positively and spent more time in the store if they were touched briefly on the arm at the entrance (when handed a flyer) (Hornik 1992). Additionally, in another study, prospective customers at a used car lot rated the used car salespeople who briefly touched them on the arm as friendlier, more honest, more open, more pleasant, and more courteous (Erceau and Guéguen 2007). Guests of a restaurant (Hornik 1992) and of an airline (Wycoff and Holley 1990) also rated the waiter/restaurant or flight attendants/airline significantly better if they had been touched briefly by the waiter or flight attendant. Additionally, servers who briefly touched their guests received more tips. The study in the restaurant additionally examined the influence of attractiveness on the touch effect (Hornik 1992). As may be expected, physical attractiveness was shown to enhance the touch effect; specifically, more attractive servers who touched their customers received more positive ratings and more tips than less attractive ones. Attractive female servers received the best ratings and the most tips from female restaurant customers, whom they briefly touched during their visit.

Analogous to the previous explanations, the perceived **meaning of touch** has also been found to have a decisive influence in studies such as this. Touch can always be perceived positively or negatively depending on its appropriateness, its level of intimacy, and the message it conveys (Steward and Lupfer 1987). If touch is perceived as inappropriate, too intimate, or condescending/oppressive, it will most likely be interpreted negatively. In this case, the positive effects on the evaluation of the person and the environment may fail to materialize, or there may even be negative effects instead. The same applies to the effects of touch on fairness and willingness to participate, which are reported in the next chapter.

5.2.4 Influencing Behavior: Prosocial Behavior & Willingness to Participate

In addition to influencing attitudes and evaluations, casual touch may also affect certain behaviors, and these influences are assumed to be related. As described in the previous chapter (Sect. 5.2.3), a brief touch may cause the toucher to be evaluated as friendlier, more open, and more sharing. It is known from altruism research that individuals are more likely to engage in prosocial and helping behavior when they evaluate those in need positively (Kelley and Byrne 1976; Takemura 1993). Consistent with this effect, touch from a physically attractive person has been shown to cause stronger prosocial behaviors in the individual being touched (e.g., greater tipping and stronger altruism).

However, it can be assumed that touch alone is insufficient to increase prosocial behavior. Instead, other nonverbal signals, such as smiling and eye contact, must accompany the touch (Kleinke 1977; Lewis et al. 1997), as these nonverbal signals play an essential role in individuals' assessments of the credibility and meaning of the situation.

Contrary to popular belief, the effects of brief touch are not transmitted by C-tactile nerve fibers (see Sect. 2.1.8) (Rosenberger et al. 2018). Instead, these highly specialized nerve pathways selectively respond to slow, caressing touch (3 cm/s). Given the intense intimacy conveyed by such touches, caressing touch between strangers is generally discouraged. Without consent, there is a risk that the touch could be perceived as a form of assault or sexual harassment and that the person may react accordingly (attack, stare, and flight).

▶ **Important** The influence of brief touch on behavior relies on the following factors:
- The brief touch or eye contact increases attention and arousal.
- The person and situation are evaluated as credible and relevant.

5.2.4.1 Prosocial Behavior

The phenomenon of a brief touch leading to increased helpfulness, honesty, and generosity in the touched individual is also known as the **Midas effect** (Crusco and Wetzel 1984). The effects have been observed in various situations and field experiments. Some of the best-known experiments indicated a positive relationship between touching and tipping amount in a restaurant or bar (Hornik 1992; Guéguen and Jacob 2005). Other experiments have shown that people who are briefly touched on the arm are more likely to comply with a request or demand; for example, in one experiment, people who had just found money in a phone booth were asked to give it back, and both eye contact and a brief touch significantly improved the likelihood of return (Kleinke 1977; Brockner et al. 1982). In other studies, a brief touch on the forearm also increased the likelihood and speed of helping to pick up dropped documents (Guéguen and Fischer-lokou 2003), as well as the likelihood of the touched individual to watch a large, very active dog while the owner went into a pharmacy (Guéguen and Fischer-lokou 2002).

In all the experiments, larger effects tended to occur when opposite-sex pairs were observed, with participants showing stronger prosocial behavior when they were touched by a person of the opposite sex. One study explicitly investigated this (Dolinski 2010) using an experiment in which passersby were asked to put a stamped letter in a mailbox. The reason given for the request was that the individual with the letter urgently needed to catch a train. It was observed that men who had been touched by men were less willing to comply with the request than men who were not touched. However, with all other sex combinations, the likelihood of posting the letter increased with a brief touch. In a more in-depth study, male sports students were asked if they would volunteer as referees for a sports festival. The students had previously completed various questionnaires, including one to determine homophobic attitudes. Again, in this experiment, the men who were briefly touched by men were, on average, less willing to help than those who were not touched. An in-depth analysis showed that the intensity of homophobia explained this difference; of the men who had been touched, those who had reported higher homophobia scores were the most reluctant to help. However, replications of this study in diverse cultural samples are currently not available.

5.2.4.2 Willingness to Participate

Whether a brief touch increases a person's willingness to participate in an activity is related to the perceived magnitude of the request (Huisman 2017). If a person is asked to do something that requires very little (e.g., give directions) or considerable (e.g., donate blood) effort, the influence of a touch on their decision is minimal (Guéguen et al. 2011). Conversely, for medium-level demands, a short touch can increase the willingness to engage in the activity. For example, studies have reported that passersby and students were more likely to participate in a survey or to complete a questionnaire with a brief touch (Gallace and Spence 2010; Hornik 1987; Willis and Hamm 1980). Furthermore, when people who were already participating in a survey or seminar were briefly touched, this increased the intensity of their participation. For example, in one study, students who had been briefly touched on the arm were more likely to volunteer to explain something on the whiteboard (Guéguen 2004). Additionally, other studies showed that individuals who were touched persisted for longer with repetitive and prolonged tasks (Patterson et al. 1986; Nannberg and Hansen 1994).

▶ **Important** Social touches lasting only a few seconds can influence the evaluation of individuals or situations and promote prosocial behavior and willingness to participate. These effects are most reliably documented for opposite-sex individuals or when women perform the touch. However, between two men, homophobic attitudes can prevent or reverse the positive effects.

5.3 Placebo Effects, Adherence, and Competence

Touching patients is a fundamental prerequisite for health care. For students and trainees, the focus of their work is on learning diagnostic procedures and treatment techniques. In contrast, lessons in which the manner of appropriate touching is taught or practiced only occur as an exception. The ethical rules of conduct for dealing with patients indirectly include appropriate physical contact, but whether social touching is carried out in addition to necessary touching (cf. Sect. 5.1.2. Touching patients) depends heavily on the example set by superiors and the individual's courage to touch.

Inhibitions regarding touching patients are often observed in students and trainees. Additionally, fears of being viewed as unprofessional, too intimate, too dominant, or even sexually inappropriate may influence students' and trainees' willingness to engage in social touching. Furthermore, status, age, sex, and culture influence the way in which interpersonal touch is interpreted. Touching is a complex social behavior that cannot be defined by strict guidelines and is highly contextual. Nevertheless, appropriate touch is central to effective and compassionate care in the medical context (Davin et al. 2019). For this reason, there is an urgent need to reflect on the interpersonal and cultural meanings as well as the beneficial and harmful effects of touch as early as during training. Therefore, learning content should answer the following questions: What is acceptable professional behavior? To what extent do the needs of the patient influence what is acceptable? What forms of touch exist? In which situations are they appropriate, beneficial, or possibly harmful?

▶ **Important** Situations in which touch may be relevant in a medical context include the following:

- Physical examinations.
- Physical treatments.
- Nursing activities.
- Greetings and farewells.
- Comfort/sympathy/support.
- Nonverbal communication.

5.3.1 Nonverbal Communication in the Practitioner–Patient Relationship

A handshake marks the beginning and end of an encounter in many cultures. In medical settings, it has been shown that physicians who perform this brief hand contact are perceived as more empathetic and compassionate than those who do not perform it (Sklansky et al. 2014). In an experimental setting, individuals who shook hands at the beginning of a meeting were found to achieve better joint solutions to problems. These studies show that the handshaking ritual can reinforce both parties' cooperative behaviors and adherence to agreements (Schroeder et al. 2019). Even without verbal input, a handshake is tantamount to a cooperative agreement, which positively **affects the patient's adherence** and, consequently, the healing process.

▶ **Definition** **Compliance** describes a patient's tendency to follow medical advice.

Adherence describes the patient's motivation to follow therapy specifications that the practitioner and the patient have jointly defined.

Due to hygiene regulations and concerns about the transmission of pathogens through hand-to-hand contact, handshakes are now no longer performed by many healthcare professionals (Sklansky et al. 2014; Kramer and Heidecke 2016). Regulations restricting handshakes in medical contexts and implementing stricter hand hygiene programs can help reduce disease transmission and curb the spread of hospital germs.

In addition, patient attitudes toward handshakes as a form of greeting and farewell are also changing. For example, in a 2004 survey, 80% of respondents stated that they would like the physician to shake their hand in greeting (Makoul et al. 2007). However, in a recent survey from 2019, only 58% stated that this type of gesture was important to them. In this survey, patients older than 65 years were more likely to value handshakes as a greeting (68% of this age group) as opposed to 47% of respondents in the 18–44 age group (Savageau et al. 2020).

The long-term impact on greeting culture of the COVID-19 pandemic containment rules cannot currently be estimated. One possible consequence of the containment rules is that people's awareness of the risk of infection via hand contact may be increased, and in the future, more people may reject this greeting gesture due to hygiene concerns. This possibility speaks in favor of using alternative nonverbal communication techniques to establish and maintain rapport. For cases in which rapport is lacking and the patient rejects the handshake out of fear of infection or performs it with mixed feelings despite concerns, the handshake could have a negative impact on the relationship and adherence. For example, in one study, a handshake offered by a person with a cold was shown to decrease the other person's willingness to cooperate; such an offer—especially by a healthcare professional—may be interpreted as showing indifference or even harmful intent (Schroeder et al. 2019). Accordingly, it is not recommended to force a handshake if either party is uncomfortable with it. Forced physical touch can give the impression of inconsiderate or even malicious behavior, which could undermine the practitioner's competence and inhibit the patient's willingness to cooperate. This example illustrates the effect of the handshake: **a cooperative alliance (an agreement)** is obtained to reach a set of goals. In cases of doubt, the individuals' attitude toward handshakes should be clarified during the initial contact.

For many patients, doctor visits and hospitalizations are associated with emotional uncertainty, fear, and anxiety. This uncertainty is accompanied by a **particular sensitivity to nonverbal cues**, which occurs to gain additional information about the practitioner or their disease

(Crane and Crane 2010). Therefore, it is crucial that the body language (posture, facial expression) of the practitioner promotes a positive practitioner–patient relationship. In some cases, nonverbal communication influences patients more than verbal content (Pensieri et al. 2018), and the nonverbal communication of the practitioner can have either a beneficial or harmful effect on the progress of the patient's disease (Crane and Crane 2010). The underlying mechanisms of these effects are multifaceted:

- Unfavorable body language on the part of the professional may cause the patient not to ask questions if there are problems with understanding or not to feel confident enough to describe unpleasant symptoms.
- A lack of or contradictory nonverbal communication (see Table 8) can lead to the patient not understanding the professional's recommendations, underestimating or overestimating their importance, and following them incorrectly or not at all.
- On the psychological level, negative nonverbal signals can increase the patient's insecurities and fears about their disease.

Appropriate nonverbal communication is an important factor in preventing these negative effects. This is particularly important in health care because a good relationship and perceived empathy can positively influence patient satisfaction and adherence as well as strengthen the intrinsic therapeutic effects and self-healing powers (Pensieri et al. 2018; Benedetti 2013) (see also Sect. 5.3.2). Table 5.1 compares positive and negative nonverbal communication tools for clinical practice (Crane and Crane 2010; Pensieri et al. 2018).

The severe time constraints of patient contact may lead to more emphasis on hygiene than nonverbal communication through handshakes, eye contact, and posture. However, to **establish rapport and build trust,** it is necessary to reflect on the nonverbal signals that are being sent. This is especially true when ritualized gestures such as handshakes are prevented, whether for hygienic, cultural, or disease-related reasons. In principle, it is possible to establish and maintain rapport, for example, by smiling appropriately and maintaining a posture facing toward the patient (active listening) (Fine and Rajput 2020).

Table 5.1 Facilitating and hindering nonverbal communication during patient contact

Nonverbal gesture	Best expression	Worst expression
Facial expression	Smile (if appropriate)	Frown
View direction	Regular eye contact both when listening and speaking	No or constant eye contact
Nodding	Frequent affirmative nodding	No or few nods
Alignment of the body	Open posture	Crossed posture
	Turned toward the patient	Averted from the patient
	Upper body bent forward in sitting position	Reclined
	About 1 m distance during conversation	Too close or too far away
Language	Varied prosody and voice pitch	Monotone
	Medium volume and reasonable speed	Too quiet (or loud), too fast (or slow)
	Explaining (or not using) technical terms	Technical language
	Adapting to the patient	Inappropriate for the patient
Handshake	Confident with medium power	Very soft or painful

Table by Crane and Crane (2010) and Pensieri et al. (2018)

▶ **Definition Rapport** refers to the trusting relationship between the medical professional and the patient.

Additionally, in light of the use of digital patient records, it is prudent for physicians to consider their nonverbal signals to the patient; indeed, physicians look at the computer screen for approximately 30–60% of the limited consultation time. While the physicians look at the screen, **less emotional responsiveness and fewer psychosocial exchanges** occur with the patient (Roter et al. 2006). Consequently, the physician looking at the screen can weaken communication with the patient and make misunderstandings more likely, which may reduce the patient's satisfaction and preparedness to follow instructions. In the worst case, this poor communication could lead to serious treatment errors (Pensieri et al. 2018; Roberts 2002) (for more details, see Sect. 5.3.2).

5.3.2 Compliance, Adherence, and Self-Healing Processes

5.3.2.1 Treatment Adherence

To date, few systematic studies exist on promoting adherence and self-healing through social touch. However, adequate communication and positive relationships with patients contribute to better adherence to treatment plans, more regular medication use (Zolnierek and DiMatteo 2009), and reduced duration of hospital stays (Halbesleben and Rathert 2008b). Conversely, an inappropriate relationship between the healthcare professional and the patient may trigger uncertainty and dissatisfaction with treatment in the patient and lead to low treatment adherence. For example, a qualitative analysis examining the association between the **practitioner-patient relationship and medication adherence** in patients with HIV (Roberts 2002) found that patients who reported a low fit between their expectations and physician behavior took their medications irregularly, discontinued their medications, or changed physicians, resulting in treatment delays. Negative perceptions of physician behavior included physician haste, low scheduling flexibility in urgent cases, low emotional accessibility, and low social/private involvement. Similarly, the relationship with the patient takes a central role in physical therapy and occupational therapy.

Furthermore, negative relationships with patients can have a detrimental effect on the health and well-being of healthcare workers by **promoting stress and exhaustion**. This, in turn, can result in a vicious cycle of uninvolved, detached, and jaded behavior on the part of the healthcare worker, deterioration of the relationship with the patient and the quality of care, and, finally, increased stress levels and the risk of burnout among healthcare staff (Halbesleben and Rathert 2008a; Groth and Grandey 2012).

As described in the previous section (Sect. 5.3.1), the body language of the practitioner can have a positive influence on patient satisfaction (Roter et al. 2006). In one study, regardless of the medical diagnosis, those practitioners who used open-minded and affectionate nonverbal gestures were rated more positively. The patients' satisfaction was even more strongly influenced by the nonverbal cues than by the quality of the medical information in the conversation.

> ▶ **Important** Open, compassionate body language and active listening foster a positive relationship with the patient, which can increase compliance, adherence, and patient satisfaction.

Physician-patient meetings are well-suited for experimental studies of treatment adherence because they are limited in time and nonverbal techniques can be experimentally varied. However, the results are also relevant for representatives of other healthcare professions and should inform their behavior toward patients.

One study examined whether brief touch influenced whether patients with pharyngitis took antibiotics as prescribed (Guéguen et al. 2010). A total of 326 patients (aged 20–30 years) were treated by six different physicians, and the physicians were instructed to look their patients in the eye and say, "It is essential that you take your medication to prevent the recurrence of symptoms." Half of the patients were touched lightly on the forearm for 1–2 s. After 7 days, the patients were visited at home, told about the study, and asked to show how many pills were left. The patients who had been touched on the arm took the medication more regularly and, consequently, had fewer tablets left. This effect occurred for both female and male patients and was independent of the sex of the physician. This result suggests that through a targeted, brief touch, the **urgency and importance of a statement can be reinforced**. In addition, the patients who were touched rated their physician as more **competent**

and more sympathetic than the patients in the control group who were not touched (cf. Sect. 5.2.3).

Another group of researchers studied the effect of touch on children aged 4 to 10 years old during a screening visit to the dentist (Greenbaum et al. 1993). During the study, the children were encouraged twice by the dentist, and the participants in the experimental group were simultaneously encouragingly touched on the upper arm. The results showed that touching reduced anxiety and avoidance during the dental examination. After the examination, the children who were touched assessed the visit to the dentist more positively than the children in the control group.

▶ **Important** A brief social touch can enhance the impact of a statement (e.g., urgency, comfort, encouragement, and reassurance).

5.3.2.2 Placebo Effects and Self-Healing

Placebos are usually understood as medications that do not contain a pharmacologically active ingredient but nevertheless produce an objective reduction in symptoms compared with no therapy at all. However, the mere ingestion of a tablet without an active ingredient does not lead to healing effects; instead, for a placebo effect to be triggered, various advantageous environmental conditions must be met (Benedetti 2013; Olshansky 2007; Breidert and Hofbauer 2010). In contrast, unfavorable conditions can have hindering effects on the healing process. This is known as the nocebo effect. The **crucial factors for placebo effects** are as follows:

- The psychosocial context in which treatment takes place.
- The behavior of the practitioner.
- The patient's expectations of a treatment.

All three factors are closely interrelated. The psychosocial context is mainly determined by the cultural significance of the physician/therapist as a healer and the relationship with the patient (Howe et al. 2019). Therefore, one prerequisite for placebo effects is that the patient is fundamentally convinced of the competence of the person treating them and trusts them. For a positive placebo effect, the behavior of the practitioners should be confident, demonstrating that they are convinced of the effectiveness of the treatment. The practitioner should attend to the patient in a compassionate, approachable, and understanding manner, give the patient space to express their complaints and feelings, and take the patient seriously. These prerequisites underline that placebo effects are not exclusively limited to medications but can enhance the effect of any treatment (Langewitz 2017), such as surgical or manual therapies.

Another relevant factor for the placebo effect is the expectations of the patient, which are formed both from the **practitioner's behavior** and the **patient's previous experiences and beliefs**. For example, a long-term study covering 20 years examined the risk factors that contributed to death from myocardial infarction in women (Eaker et al. 1992) and found that women with stronger beliefs about being prone to heart attacks were significantly more likely to suffer a heart attack. This effect was independent of age, blood pressure, cholesterol level, diabetes, smoking, and body mass index. Therefore, among individuals with similar objective risk factors for cardiovascular disease, patient expectations explained differences in disease progression. Patients' expectations are partly influenced by what their practitioner says about their prognosis and disease progression. Moreover, in today's information society, reports from Internet articles and blogs likely also play an important role. In principle, opinions and expectations can be influenced by any person who is perceived as an expert (whether through their own medical history or qualifications).

▶ **Important** The relationship with the patient plays an influential—albeit difficult to measure—role in the healing process. Confidence, prognosis, and cues from a practitioner can significantly influence a patient's expectations regarding disease progression.

The underlying mechanisms of placebo and nocebo effects are complex and difficult to evaluate. For example, minor lifestyle changes can partly explain **placebo effects** (healthier diets, more or better sleep, more harmonious social contacts) (Howe et al. 2019). In addition, positive expectations and **the practitioner's confidence have a** calming effect on the patient. Calm patients are less anxious and sleep better, which improves their immune function. In the opposite case, worry and uncertainty about one's health are stress factors that can negatively affect the immune system and, thus, impair self-healing processes. In line with the complexity of the influencing factors, it is not surprising that the size and duration of placebo effects vary between studies, ranging from placebo having no effect to having the same efficacy as standard treatment.

Interestingly, however, some findings show that certain conditions can magnify placebo effects. For example, a recent study suggested that **personality traits such as anxiety or optimism** may influence placebo effects (Zhou et al. 2019). Participants applied a cream to their arm and were told that the cream either (a) had a minimal analgesic effect, (b) reduced but did not eliminate pain, or (c) completely prevented pain. Subsequently, pain stimuli were applied through electric pulses to the arm, and the individuals who were more optimistic and less anxious showed lower pain sensations than the anxious and pessimistic individuals. The study also showed that those participants who perceived the pain stimuli as the least painful were those who were told that the cream would reduce pain but not eliminate it. In other words, a **realistic and credible expectation** promotes confidence in a treatment, which results in the largest placebo effects.

A close relationship with the patient may also enhance placebo effects (Benedetti 2013; Howe et al. 2019), and the previously described better adherence to treatment when the practitioner has a close relationship with the patient may be a key contributor to this. Moreover, the **intensity of care and attention** also has an influence on the placebo effect. Indeed, various studies have shown larger placebo effects when patients are given more care and attention. For example, placebo acupuncture treatments were found to be significantly more successful in reducing arm pain than placebo tablets (Kaptchuk et al. 2006), and the pain-reducing effects remained stable over the entire treatment period of 8 weeks. The unique feature of placebo acupuncture is that the needles do not penetrate the skin but only adhere to it. Nevertheless, tactile stimuli are triggered by the adhesions. In addition, the attachment of the placebo needles requires several minutes of attention and **gentle touch by the practitioner** (Kerr et al. 2011; Chae and Olausson 2017). In contrast, a placebo pill is only prescribed and subsequently taken by the patient independently (Chae et al. 2018).

In another study, the same group of researchers investigated whether the way in which placebo acupuncture was performed influenced the placebo effect (Kaptchuk et al. 2008). For this purpose, 262 patients with irritable bowel syndrome were randomized into three groups: (a) a waiting control group without treatment, (b) placebo acupuncture during which the practitioner and patient were not allowed to talk to each other, and (c) placebo acupuncture with warm, empathic interaction, active listening, and supportive expressions by the practitioner. As expected, the patients who received empathic interaction showed the greatest improvement in their symptoms and quality of life. In addition, both the placebo acupuncture groups reported significantly better outcomes than the individuals in the control group.

▶ **Important** The following factors likely underpin placebo effects, and they are partly determined by the behavior of the practitioner and the relationship with the patient:

- Reduction of anxiety and stress.
- An increase in positive feelings.
- Release of endogenous neurotransmitters, hormones, and immune regulators.
- Greater treatment adherence.
- Higher motivation to lead healthier lifestyles.
- Expectancy and conditioning effects.

5.3.3 Tips for Teaching

The impact of touch as a therapeutic tool goes far beyond the practical action during the physical examination and treatment. As a means of communication, touch overcomes language and cultural barriers. Touch is also the basis for forming and maintaining relationships and provides comfort in painful and fearful situations. In the company of close acquaintances and relatives, people use touch to communicate intuitively and without great shyness. However, in the context of professional healthcare occupations, the focus of touch is often on necessary care, partly because of the fear of crossing boundaries, being misinterpreted, or being misunderstood due to social touching. The authors of this book believe that consciously addressing touch and physical contact is an important foundation for all health professions and should, thus, be addressed as a central topic early in training (Davin et al. 2019).

It is important that trainees and students learn what **an unusual situation medical touch is in a person's everyday life** (cf. Sect. 5.1.2). A touch by a stranger is a transgression for any person. Moreover, many patients do not have sufficient medical training to anticipate diagnostic or therapeutic processes. Curiosity or the desire to help can cause healthcare professionals to act on the patient's body without notice, while the patient, as a feeling, thinking person, is pushed into the background. The resulting feelings of insecurity, tension, and fear can permanently disrupt the practitioner's relationship with the patient, resulting in noncompliance, therapy discontinuation, or a change of practitioner. These outcomes, in turn, can have negative consequences on the healing process.

Conversely, all healthcare professionals should be aware of the situations in which touch, as a means of communication, can improve patient well-being. This requires knowing what kinds of touch are appropriate and how social touch can be performed intentionally and effectively in a professional context (Davin et al. 2019; Kelly et al. 2014). Problem-based learning, casework, and simulation in small groups are suitable for addressing the topic of touch in the context of education, training, and postgraduate education.

Possible topics for portfolio or discussion sessions include the following:

- When is social touch appropriate/not appropriate in a medical/therapeutic/nursing context?
- How does it feel to be examined?
- What can I do to reassure a patient?
- Which fears and insecurities do I have about touching a patient?
- Report positive and negative experiences with social and professional touch in a medical context.
- When is consent required, and how do I obtain it?
- How are superiority, power, and touch associated?
- When is a guardian required, and for what purpose?
- How can touch be misunderstood, and how do I deal with it?
- How can I tell that a patient is uncomfortable?
- How can I deliver bad news?
- How do I deal with terminally ill patients and their families?
- What can I do when patients are assaultive?

5.4 Embodiment

Embodiment is a field of social and cognitive psychology research that examines how the body influences and is influenced by thought, speech, and feelings. Intuitively, actors and other performers use the physical manifestation of feelings and thoughts to represent and capture various mental states. The central aspect of embodiment is that body postures, as well as tactile, haptic, or proprioceptive stimuli, can affect cognitive and emotional processes. In this way, the findings of embodiment research are in strict contrast to traditional cognitive science. For example, in traditional cognitive research, thoughts are regarded as purely mental processes that occur in the brain and, consequently, occur largely independently of the rest of the body. However, in recent years, research has shown that learning, feelings, and thoughts can be altered by body posture, movement, and other bodily sensations. The research approaches to embodiment are predominantly descriptive, and the explanatory approaches so far are almost exclusively theoretical.

In the present chapter, some phenomena are presented as examples of how physical states can change feelings, thoughts, or attitudes. This chapter aims to create awareness of this mind–body connection. This knowledge can be used to influence one's own mood, attitude, or outlook and to understand patients better.

▶ **Definition Embodiment** describes the interaction between the psyche and the body:

1. Mental states affect posture, voice, facial expressions, gestures, and physiology.
2. Physical conditions can influence feelings, thoughts, and attitudes (Pschyrembel Klinisches Wörterbuch 2020).

5.4.1 Facial Feedback Hypothesis

One of the best-known studies on facial feedback examined how facial expressions influence emotional responses. For this purpose, participants held a pencil transversely between their teeth so that the muscles that are active during laughter were activated. In the control condition, participants were asked to enclose the pen longitudinally with their lips, creating a facial expression more similar to sadness and preventing laughter. The authors found that in the laughing condition, cartoons and short movies were rated as funnier than in the condition that suppressed smiling (Strack et al. 1988; Soussignan 2002).

Another study investigated how contracted eyebrows affect mood and found that an angry or sad facial expression led to a more negative evaluation of images (Larsen et al. 1992). Similarly, in another study, perceived self-confidence changed in participants who recounted autobiographical experiences of success, either smiling or with their eyebrows furrowed in anger (Stepper and Strack 1993). Participants who recounted success with an angry look **felt less confident** than participants who recounted success with a smile. Furthermore, participants in the smiling condition reported being in a better general mood than participants in the angry condition.

5.4.2 Body Posture

5.4.2.1 Hero Pose (Power Posing)

Similarly to facial expressions, body postures can affect the mental state. Experiments investigating these effects usually disguise the experimental body postures to prevent the participants from guessing what is being studied. For example, one study explained to the participants that the aim was to investigate the effects of different ergonomic work postures on productivity (Stepper and Strack 1993). Participants were seated in a simple chair at a table, and the table and chair heights were varied, which resulted in either a straight, upright sitting position or a slumped, bent-over posture. The participants performed various tasks in these sitting positions, and at the end of the experiment, all participants received positive feedback about their performance. The authors found that the participants who received the feedback **sitting upright felt the most pride about their performance**. Therefore, positive feedback may be perceived most positively when the posture corresponds to the content of the feedback.

The results of a study investigating whether the effects persist after the posture has already been abandoned are even more notable (Riskind and Gotay 1982). In this study, the participants completed a series of experiments, and again, the goal of the study was masked. The participants were invited to take part in the validation of a test of spatial reasoning. After the first round of testing, they waited in the hallway, where another experimenter asked them to participate in another experiment while they were waiting. The participants were told that skin conductance would be studied as a function of muscle tension. For this purpose, the participants had to assume a specific body position and maintain that position for a period of time. The participants were fitted with electrodes at the neck, which were connected to measuring devices, and asked to adopt one of two positions: (a) seated, slightly bent forward, with the shoulders and head drooping, or (b) straight back, shoulders pulled back, with the head and gaze slightly tilted upward. The participants held their respective positions for 8 min. While the participants remained in the position, they filled out a questionnaire about their current mood (including sad, exhausted, joyful, and self-conscious). No differences were found in the reported mood states between the two postures. Eventually, the electrodes were removed, and the participants returned to their original experiment, where they performed a second spatial reasoning test. In truth, the test consisted of unsolvable puzzles that were used to investigate the participants' **persistence and perseverance**. The results showed that the participants who had sat leaning forward during the interim experiment were significantly less persistent in trying to solve the puzzles than the participants who had sat upright.

Crossing the arms in front of the chest (compared to other arm postures) can also lead to more perseverance during difficult tasks and, thus, contribute to better performance (Friedman and Elliot 2008).

A more in-depth study showed that adopting a high- or low-status posture can even cause hormonal changes (Fig. 5.2; Carney et al. 2010). The participants (both men and women) who had engaged in expansive postures for 2 min showed an **increase in testosterone levels and a decrease in cortisol (stress hormone) levels**. In addition, they reported feeling significantly more influential and powerful. Conversely, the participants who slumped and assumed low-status positions with their arms folded showed opposite changes in testosterone and cortisol. This study also demonstrated that the effects persisted for at least 15 min after the posture ended.

5.4.2.2 Posture of Depression

Given the findings reported above, it is not surprising that certain postures can also **maintain or intensify sad and negative emotions**. For example, the reduced stamina found in healthy participants following the adoption of a flexed, bent-over posture may suggest that this posture is interpreted as a behavioral cue of helplessness and depression (Riskind and Gotay 1982).

An experiment was conducted to specifically investigate the influence of posture on hospitalized patients with unipolar depression (major depression) (Michalak et al. 2014). The patients participated in a memory experiment in a bent or upright sitting position. They were asked to remember a series of positive (e.g., beautiful and enjoyable) and negative (e.g., depressed and exhausted) words. The patients who sat bent over showed a cognitive bias toward negative words; specifically, those patients remembered more negative words than positive words. The patients who had sat upright during the experiment did not show this bias; instead, they remembered the same number of negative and positive words. The results of another study involving patients with mild to moderate depression suggested that an upright posture could increase activity levels, **reduce fatigue, and reduce negative affect and tension** (Wilkes et al. 2017). It is not yet known how long such effects may last in patients with depressive disorders. However, it is clear that patients with depressive disorders are more likely to adopt hunched postures compared to healthy individuals (Wilkes et al. 2017). Perception training can help patients become aware of their posture and change it to counteract negative embodiment effects. In body therapy approaches, these and similar findings are already being applied in the psychiatric and psychosomatic fields (Wilda-Kiesel et al. 2011; Storch et al. 2017; Stolze 2002).

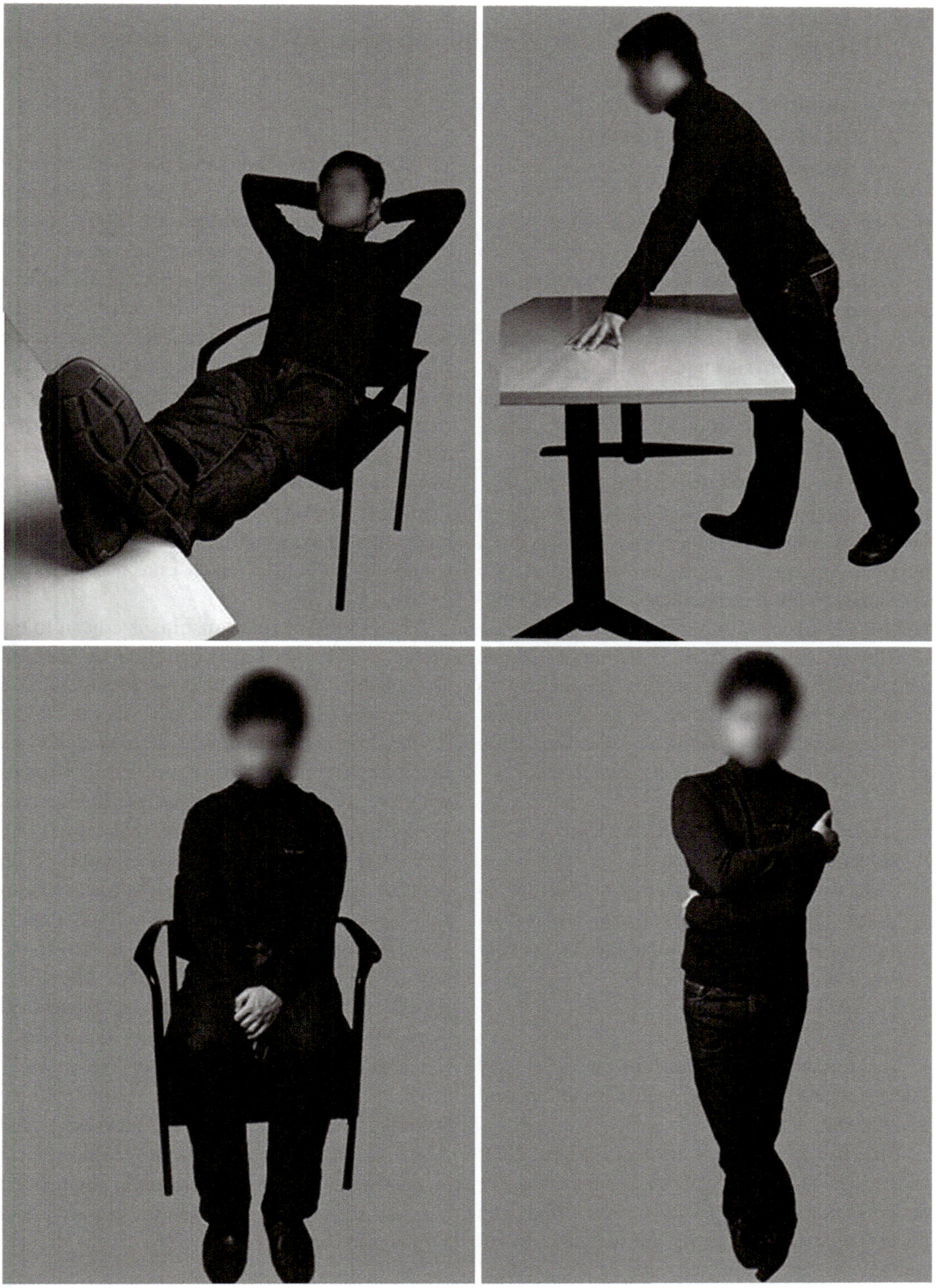

Fig. 5.2 Power posing. Postures of high (top) and low status (bottom). (Fig. from Carney et al. 2010)

5.5 Emotional and Social Aspects

5.5.1 Health Consequences of Loneliness and Social Isolation

In a survey conducted jointly by German public television (ZDF) and the Haptic Research Lab (University of Leipzig) with 763 participants living in their own homes, 32% reported "often" missing physical touch and 48% reported "sometimes" missing physical touch in the 70–85-year-old age group (Grunwald 2017). In contrast, in the younger groups, only 13%–15% of participants responded with "often," and as many as 34%–46% responded "never." Of the 61–85-year-old participants, 20% indicated that it had been months or even years since they had last been hugged. Among the younger participants, the percentage reporting that their last hug was several months ago was only 5%–8%.

Although this survey is not a representative sample and systematic surveys are lacking to date, it can be assumed that people over the age of 65 are least likely to be touched in their daily lives. Several factors may contribute to this:

- Death of the life partner/close friends.
- Relocation of adult children.
- Reduction of the social environment due to retirement and physical impairments, including declining sensory functions (especially seeing and hearing).
- Limited mobility.

The frequency of social touching is closely related to the extent of social isolation and loneliness.

Paradoxically, even in medical settings, older adults receive fewer social touches than younger patients (Barnett 1972; Schoenhofer 1989). The 66–100-year-old age group are touched significantly less than younger adults in the medical context. The most frequent social touches in the medical context are received by children under 5 years of age and adults aged 18–40 years. The reasons for this have not yet been determined.

▶ **Important** Lack of touch is particularly prevalent in people over 60 and is further exacerbated by severe illness and social isolation.

It is well known that social isolation and loneliness are **risk factors for poor health and premature death** (Holt-Lunstad 2017; Steptoe et al. 2013). A large meta-analysis that included 70 longitudinal studies with a total of 3.4 million participants showed that social isolation, loneliness, and living alone significantly shorten the lifespan (Holt-Lunstad et al. 2015). For social isolation and loneliness, the associated risk of dying younger is even greater than the mortality associated with severe obesity (BMI > 30) and physical inactivity (Flegal et al. 2013). Indeed, the risk is similar to the hazard potential associated with smoking and excessive alcohol consumption (see Fig. 5.3) (Holt-Lunstad et al. 2010; House et al. 1988).

The **quality of relationships** is crucial to the protective effect of social inclusion, as relationship quality, not the number of friends, affects feelings of loneliness (Victor et al. 2000; Routasalo et al. 2006). Several meta-analyses and longitudinal studies have shown that individuals who rate their social relationships as empathic, supportive, and responsive to their needs are 50%–91% more likely to survive than those with poor or inadequate social relationships (Holt-Lunstad et al. 2010). Furthermore, this effect is stable across covariates such as age, sex, initial health status, and cause of death. Therefore, regardless of a person's life situation and medical conditions, those with adequately close social relationships are more likely to survive.

▶ **Important** The effects of loneliness and social isolation on health are comparable to other risk factors such as smoking, high blood pressure, high cholesterol, obesity, and physical inactivity.

In children, especially in the youngest years of life, the consequences of social isolation are even more severe and even more closely associated with interpersonal contact (Andersen and

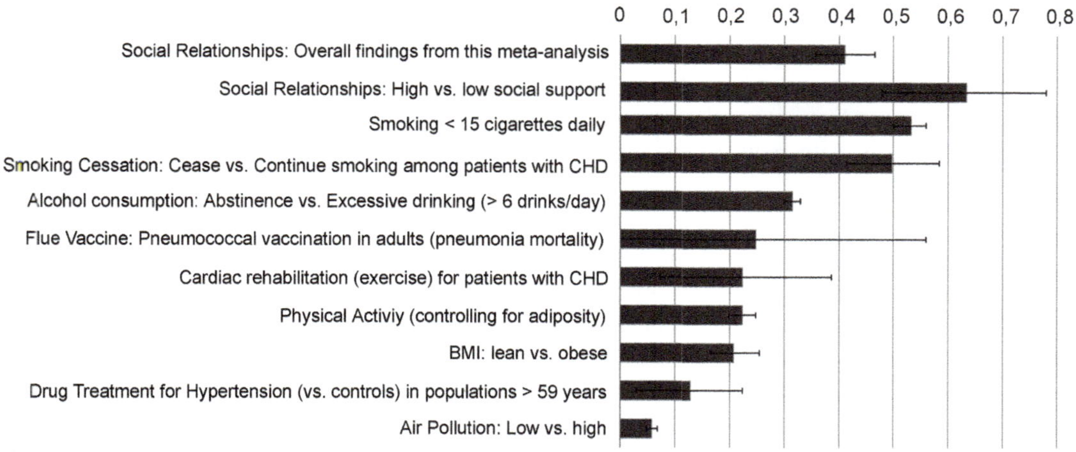

Fig. 5.3 Mortality risk under different conditions (Results of a meta-analysis.). Individuals with adequate social relationships are at least 50% more likely to survive than those with poor or inadequate social relationships. High social support can even increase this effect. This influence is comparable to the influence of known health risks due to lifestyle factors (e.g., smoking and obesity). (Fig. from Holt-Lunstad et al. 2010)

Guerrero 2008). In the first months of life, communication between the child and caregivers is based almost exclusively on various touch stimuli. Surviving without physical contact with other people is impossible in infancy and early childhood and usually leads to death. Even with adequate provision of nutrients and hygiene, children who grow up under social deprivation suffer lifelong impairments in their physical, cognitive, social, and psychological health. Evidence for the critical role of physical contact in emotional and physical development is based primarily on experiments with primates (Harlow 1958) and observations of orphans (Spitz 1949) (see Sect. 7.2.5).

5.5.2 Benefits of Social and Emotional Touch in Nursing Care

This section presents effects that can be triggered by communicative and emotional touch; for effects of therapeutic touch (e.g., hand and back massages), see Chap. 8.

Touch is especially important in geriatric and pediatric care, care for patients with cognitive impairment, care for patients with extended hospital stays, and acute, intensive, and palliative care. Uplifting, comforting touch can give the patient confidence and assurance, convey sympathy, reduce anxiety and loneliness, and, thus, improve the patient's mood. In addition, in medical and nursing environments in which the focus is often on physical care, social and emotional touch can help prevent feelings of dehumanization, both on the part of medical staff and patients.

The frequency and effects of touch in nursing care have been studied primarily in geriatric care. For these patients, physical and medical care require a significant amount of time and personnel. However, interpersonal conditions are at least as important for psychological well-being. The relationships with nurses and caregivers are a central part of the social network of patients under continuous care. Under these conditions, touch is an essential tool for non-verbal communication. Especially for patients with sensory or cognitive impairments or for those whose speech functions are limited, touch can support and complement verbal communication. Even when vision and hearing are impaired, the need for touch and closeness remains, just like the ability to feel emotions. Especially under stress, anxiety, and social isolation, social touch can help improve the well-being of the individuals concerned (Cho and Snyder 1996; Kim and Buschmann 1999; Gleeson and Timmins 2004).

> **Important** Chronic illness, reduced mobility, and declining sensory and cognitive abilities can result in anxiety, social isolation, sleep disturbances, and emotional disturbances. Social touch can help reduce these negative effects.

Significant staff shortages and the resulting overworking of nurses can lead to compromised social contact between nurses and patients/residents due to a lack of time. However, **even the omission of social touch can send subtle messages** if the omission is not justified. For example, care recipients who are exclusively touched in a nursing manner may feel that they are unattractive, a nuisance, or a burden, which can reinforce feelings of insecurity and low self-esteem (Cho and Snyder 1996).

In addition, social touch can also improve relationships and communication between family members and patients with cognitive impairment or under palliative care (Bush 2001). Even for loved ones, it is sometimes difficult to not just tend to the patient's physical needs. However, social touch can help individuals focus on the person being cared for—the human being behind the illness (Gleeson and Timmins 2004).

Knowledge of the social significance of touch is not new (Montagu 1978). Nevertheless, in the recent past, older adults in nursing homes had to be isolated in their rooms to protect them from infection with COVID-19, had to take their meals alone, and experienced strictly regulated or even prohibited access to relatives. This exceptional worldwide situation should be taken as an opportunity to reflect on the drastic consequences of a lack of interpersonal contact and social touch deprivation (cf. Sect. 5.5.1). Given the effects of touch described above, social isolation cannot be regarded as a long-term solution or a means of combating a pandemic. Even given the risk of infection, physical contact with close people must be enabled, such as by using protective suits and face masks. In cases where this is not possible, representatives of the healthcare professions, in their unique position, must have sufficient time to care for their clients to compensate for this serious social deprivation.

5.5.2.1 What Types of Social Touches Take Place in Healthcare?

Observational studies have shown that communicative and emotional touches occur between nurses and patients. However, those touches account for a much smaller proportion compared to nursing-related touches, and this discrepancy is partly explained by nurses' excessive workloads and time constraints. Additionally, the **definition of the nursing profession** as part of the healthcare system may also be a contributing factor. As defined by the International Council of Nurses (ICN; World Confederation of Nurses), the central role of nurses is "to promote health, prevent disease, and provide care and support for the sick, disabled, and dying" (ICN 2002). This definition encompasses the physical and psychological well-being of patients. Accordingly, nursing includes all activities necessary to maintain or promote physical and mental health. However, public awareness of how social touch can influence **psychological well-being, self-esteem, and self-efficacy is lacking.** Moreover, social touches are intuitively attributed to family and friends, which means that in everyday life, they are only carried out, tolerated, and desired by emotionally close people (cf. Sect. 5.1.1). Problematically, feelings of lack of touch are also hardly ever communicated, and few people are aware that diffuse **feelings of listlessness, loneliness, and hopelessness** can be caused by touch deprivation. In this context, the distancing rules during the COVID-19 pandemic resembled global self-awareness training regarding the frequency with which interpersonal touch occurs in everyday life. Many people became aware of their need for social touch for the first time, and this was triggered by the demand to keep their distance and reduce contact (e.g., during lockdown). This self-awareness can and should be used to practice empathic perspective-taking with patients in persistently socially isolated situations. Within this self-awareness lies an opportunity to integrate social touch into nursing activities, which has been called for repeatedly for many decades in the scientific literature (cf. Chap. 8) (Gleeson and Timmins 2004; Hollinger and Buschmann 1993; Montagu 1978).

▶ **Important** Feelings of listlessness, loneliness, and hopelessness are closely related to social isolation, loneliness, and a lack of touch.

The social touches that occur in care settings are often used in combination with verbal communication (Routasalo 1996; Gleeson and Timmins 2004). The touches can either complement verbal statements or provide an additional form of communication for patients who are language impaired. Examples of this communication are as follows:

- Indicating/pointing to things.
- Cheering up/encouraging.
- Soothing/comforting.
- Reprimanding/scolding.
- Being humorous/teasing.
- Hugging.
- Thanking.

Many of the social touches also occur in the context of nursing activities:

- Giving instructions/issuing a request.
- Giving an explanation.
- Bringing about decisions/letting decisions be made.
- Starting an action.
- Waking a patient.

However, there is evidence that social and emotional touch only occur when there is a good relationship between the patient and caregiver (Routasalo 1996). This finding suggests that touch is not used deliberately as a therapeutic tool but intuitively, by instinct.

5.5.2.2 Who Performs the Touches?

Several studies have shown that social touch is usually performed by caregivers (Schoenhofer 1989; Routasalo 1996). Only in the rarest cases are non-nursing touches stimulated by patients. This effect can be explained by the different statuses of the nurses and the patients, which result from the **dependent relationship of nursing care. The** status of the patients in their professional or social lives is of little relevance. Similarly, in other settings that social touches are usually initiated and carried out by the person with higher status (Henley 1973; Hall 1996; Watson 1975). The few touches that patients initiate are to attract a caregiver's attention or to show gratitude. Touching to show gratitude is rated by nurses as important and positive (Routasalo and Isola 1996), reflects a positive relationship between the patient and nurse, and positively impacts the work environment. Positive relationships, gratitude, and a positive work climate are protective factors that contribute to nurses being better protected from stressors and high workloads (Converso et al. 2015). Therefore, positive relationships with patients play a critical role in the health of healthcare workers, which can help protect against **exhaustion, depersonalization, and burnout.**

Similar to social touching in other contexts, different frequencies of touch have been found for male and female caregivers. Overall, female caregivers perform more social touching than male caregivers; some studies have also found that female patients are touched more than male patients (Barnett 1972; Routasalo 1996; Watson 1975; McCann and McKenna 1993). Some female caregivers perceive touching by male patients as having negative or sexual connotations (Routasalo and Isola 1996), whereas male patients perceive touch by female nurses as predominantly positive. In contrast, touching by male nurses is not perceived as pleasant by some female patients (McCann and McKenna 1993). Since more women are currently working in nursing professions than men, these perceptions are likely influenced by expectation effects. Specifically, experiences and memories of touch from other contexts may influence how patients perceive social touch by male nurses. However, the underlying factors are complex and have yet to be explored. Individual differences in attitudes toward touch among both patients and caregivers also play a role.

Physical violence such as hitting, pushing, or sexual assault is inadmissible in the medical context, just as in all other situations. Nevertheless, cases of assault by representatives of the healthcare profession do exist. In order to prevent possible cover-ups, protection concepts with zero-tolerance rules should be established, and persons of trust should be appointed as possible contacts in case of incidences of assault.

▶ **Further reading Tips** Hoffmann, U., Clemens, V., König, E., Brähler, E., & Fegert, J. M. (2020). Violence against children and adolescents by nursing staff: prevalence rates and implications for practice. Child and adolescent psychiatry and mental health, 14(1), 1–12.

d'Oliveira, A. F. P. L., Diniz, S. G., & Schraiber, L. B. (2002). Violence against women in healthcare institutions: an emerging problem. The Lancet, 359(9318), 1681–1685.

5.5.2.3 What Factors Influence Touch, and How Do Patients and Caregivers Perceive Touch?

Patients predominantly perceive caregivers' touch as warm, gentle, and soothing (Routasalo 1996). Whether social touch by caregivers is judged positively or negatively by patients is primarily related to the patients' perceived control. Indeed, touch is rated mostly positively (Hollinger and Buschmann 1993) in the following cases:

- If the touch is appropriate to the situation.
- If no greater intimacy is established than desired.
- If no condescending message is conveyed or resonates.

Conversely, negative evaluations arise if caregiving touch is perceived as **too intimate** or at odds **with the patient's abilities and needs**. This pattern is consistent with the finding that procedural support or a healthcare professional taking over activities of daily living that the patient is still able to manage by themselves can foster a **sense of loss of control and the development of learned helplessness** (Avorn and Langer 1982; Faulkner 2001). Time pressure and impatience on the part of caregivers can lead to unwanted assistance being provided, which may then promote the patient's insecurity and dependence. This insecurity and dependence, in turn, may lead to a faster deterioration of still-existing abilities as well as a loss of self-esteem and may also contribute to a further reduction in social touch. Indeed, some authors have reported that younger patients in good or stable condition receive more social touch than patients who are older or more severely ill (Barnett 1972; Watson 1975). In line with this, caregivers report that they feel more comfortable touching autonomous or marginally dependent patients than entirely dependent patients. That is, a **negative relationship between patients' health and the frequency of social touching** exists (Barnett 1972). Similar findings exist regarding patients with depression, as several authors have reported that depressed patients receive significantly fewer social touches than those who do not suffer from depression (Hollinger and Buschmann 1993; Watson 1975; Montagu 1978). However, severely ill individuals with high levels of dependency and great uncertainty about their condition would particularly benefit from social and emotional support. Consequently, in practice, those patients who require more social and emotional support receive less of it. Findings show that the severity of illness and the resulting risk of developing depression are moderated by social support. In particular, social support helps individuals cope with extreme life events or severe illnesses and manage them emotionally (Curtis et al. 2004; Greco et al. 2014), thus reducing the likelihood of the individual developing grief-related (reactive) depression. In addition, in individuals with reactive depression, adjustment disorder, or grief reaction, the need for physical contact (being held) increases (Stein and Sanfilipo 1985).

The findings regarding the lower frequency of social touching in individuals with higher care needs, dependency, and depression indicate that social touching does occur in nursing care but is rarely used deliberately in a therapeutic manner. Instead, **the social touches that occur arise spontaneously from patient interactions**. Patients in a positive mood and in better health communicate more with nursing staff, resulting in more opportunities for social touch. To counteract this paradox and fully exploit the health-promoting potential of social support, **social touch should be used more consciously as a therapeutic tool**. Standardized touch interventions lend themselves to this end. For example, hand massages, therapeutic touch, and hand holding with active listening have been incorporated into daily nursing care for several years (e.g., the Respectare® nursing concept). These standardized forms of touch can produce similar positive effects as spontaneous social touch, while being less dependent on the relationship with the patient.

► **Important** Older adults receive fewer social touches than younger patient groups. In addition, patients who are less independent, more seriously ill, or more depressed receive less social touch than patients in better health. However, these patient groups would particularly benefit from more touch and social support. Standardized touch interventions can compensate for this deficiency in the use of touch.

5.5.2.4 What Effects Can Social Touch Produce in Nursing?

Social touch contributes to patients' sense of safety and can have a **beneficial effect on self-esteem, security, and relaxation** (Routasalo and Isola 1996). Brief touches show seriously ill patients that the nurses are there for them and care about them (McCorkle 1974; Howard 1988). Particularly for patients under intensive care and artificial respiration, mindful physical contact (for example, according to the concept of **sensory stimulation**) can help reduce anxiety and restlessness, serve as a communication channel, and help patients to orient themselves in space and time. This type of touch may even help prevent **Post-Intensive Care Syndrome** (Kohler et al. 2019; Dyer 1995a, b).

In patients with dementia or other cognitive impairments, as well as patients just awakening from anesthesia (and those undergoing ventilator weaning), maintaining physical contact may increase **attentional focus** (Mallett 1990). For example, patients with Alzheimer's disease are more attentive and listen better when they are touched statically (e.g., by placing a hand on their arm or holding their hand) (Bartol 1979). Touch can also improve communication with confused patients (Langland and Panicucci 1982). For example, when a verbal prompt is combined with a light touch on the forearm, patients show significantly **more interactive behavior** in the form of positive verbal expressions and facial expressions than patients who receive only a verbal prompt (McCorkle 1974; Langland and Panicucci 1982).

There is also evidence that, in patients with dementia, social and compassionate touch can help patients exhibit **less challenging and aggressive behavior.** Accordingly, touch has a calming effect, protects patients from stress, and allows them to maintain regular behavior (Kim and Buschmann 1999; Marx et al. 1989). To prevent that patients with dementia become frightened and anxious, frantic and surprising movements and touches should be avoided (DeVos 1989).

► **Important** Further to social touch, contact activities, such as hand games and social dancing, lead to less challenging behavior, increased well-being, and more social interaction between older adults and caregivers (Guzmán-García et al. 2013).

Furthermore, one study showed that patients in institutionalized geriatric care ate **more calories and protein** when they were touched on the arm in addition to being given verbal prompting (Eaton et al. 1986; Lange-Alberts and Shott 1994). In the corresponding experiment, institutionalized older adults with organic brain syndrome were observed during independent food intake in the dining room. The participants were lightly touched on the arm five times during the 1-h meal period and were additionally verbally prompted to eat. Each participant was observed for 3 weeks, and food intake was measured. During the first and third weeks, meals occurred as usual (comparison periods). During the second week, the touch intervention was implemented at breakfast and lunch. The participants in the experimental group consumed significantly more calories and protein during the intervention and the following week than during the first week, as well as compared to the participants in the control group during all 3 weeks (Eaton et al. 1986). This study provides further evidence that brief touch can improve compliance and influence behavior (cf. Sect. 5.2.4). Indeed, in the case of patients' food intake, there are far-reaching consequences. Specifically, if brief touches can improve the absorption of nutrients, the use of artificial feeding methods can possibly be avoided or at least delayed. In addition, brief touches have a similar effect as other social touches, as they also help **reduce social isolation and feelings of being** redundant. These effects, in turn, have a beneficial influence on food intake, as positive emotions have been shown to improve food intake in geriatric patients (Paquet et al. 2003).

▶ **Important** Brief social touches during meals, in addition to verbal encouragement, improve food intake in geriatric patients.

Overall, it is likely that physical contact alone is not responsible for the effects on cognitively impaired older adults (Gallace and Spence 2010). When someone touches another person, this is usually accompanied by other changes in interpersonal contact (e.g., facial expression and tone of voice). One study examined the influence of touch, eye contact, and voice both separately and in combination. The authors found that combining all three forms of communication resulted in more frequent affective and verbal responses in participants (cognitively impaired older adults) than just a single form of communication or a combination of two communication forms (Kramer and Gibson 1991). Furthermore, communication through multiple sensory channels by the caregivers also **increased interaction between the nursing home residents**.

5.5.2.5 Conclusion

It seems almost trivial to point out that touch can be soothing, comforting, or encouraging. Furthermore, each person has an idea of how they would like to be touched in an emotionally stressful situation. However, finding the proper form of touch and overcoming inhibitions can be challenging in healthcare work. Social touching requires a positive relationship, or at least sympathy, between individuals. Nurses who care for a patient over several weeks or even months and years are in a unique position to build a relationship with that patient (and their relatives). Through open-minded attention and social touch gestures that extend beyond physical care, nurses can contribute to the patient's psychological well-being. It is essential for nurses working in the field of geriatric and long-term care to realize that many older adults experience social and emotional deprivation. Importantly, a persistent lack of social feedback and physical contact (at any age) can lead to a decrease in overall life satisfaction and self-esteem. Social touch can build trust and convey affection more quickly and intensely than speech and facial expressions. Caregivers can, thus, help reduce the social isolation of the elderly and seriously ill through the appropriate use of social touch. In addition, social touch helps prevent feelings of depersonalization and dehumanization for both caregivers and patients. However, invariably, nurses should inquire about how each patient feels about touch and reflect on the messages that the touch conveys. In line with the general ethical guidelines of nursing care for working with patients, it is important to avoid provoking feelings of dependency and infantilization (Gleeson and Timmins 2004; Hollinger and Buschmann 1993).

5.5.3 Touch from Close Persons Influences Well-Being, Stress, and Pain

Loving touch (e.g., hugs, hand-holding, and cuddling) between close people is much more than a nonverbal gesture of affection. A growing number of studies have reported that physical closeness is a relevant factor in social support. Positive social interactions and physical contact function as **buffers against stress, reduce pain, improve well-being, and may even protect against illness**. For example, one study investigated the relationship between the frequency of hugs and the susceptibility to colds (Cohen et al. 2015). For this purpose, 404 healthy participants aged 18–55 years were asked on 14 consecutive evenings whether they had experienced a hug or a stressful argument that day. Additionally, perceived social support was assessed. On average, the participants reported being hugged on 67% of the days and experiencing tense situations/conflicts on 7% of the days. At the end of the 14 days, the participants stayed in an isolation room (quarantine) for 1 week, where they were infected with a cold virus and their symptom development was monitored. The results showed that those who experienced more frequent social arguments and fewer hugs had a higher risk of infection (see Fig. 5.4). In contrast, for participants who reported having many hugs, the risk of infection was significantly lower (approximately 20% lower), regardless of the frequency of conflict. Interestingly, the number of hugs did not influence the infection risk in individuals who reported no conflicts. These results suggest that hugging, **as a form of positive social interaction, helps to dampen stress**. Accordingly, physical contact can reduce the negative effects of stress (e.g., on the immune system).

It has yet to be clarified to what extent hugs and social support affect healing processes after an illness has already occurred. However, studies on massage and therapeutic touch suggest positive effects of touch on healing (see Chaps. 6 and 8).

It is well known that various aspects of personal relationships (social support, integration, and conflict) are related to the levels of inflammation in the body. Relationship conflicts and a lack of social support are associated with inflammation-enhancing mechanisms (Kiecolt-Glaser et al. 2010). In contrast, a comprehensive meta-analysis found significantly lower levels of inflammation (fewer cytokines such as C-reactive protein and IL-6 in the blood) in individuals with good social support (Uchino et al. 2018). Additionally, a recent longitudinal study suggested that the frequency of physical contact may influence this association

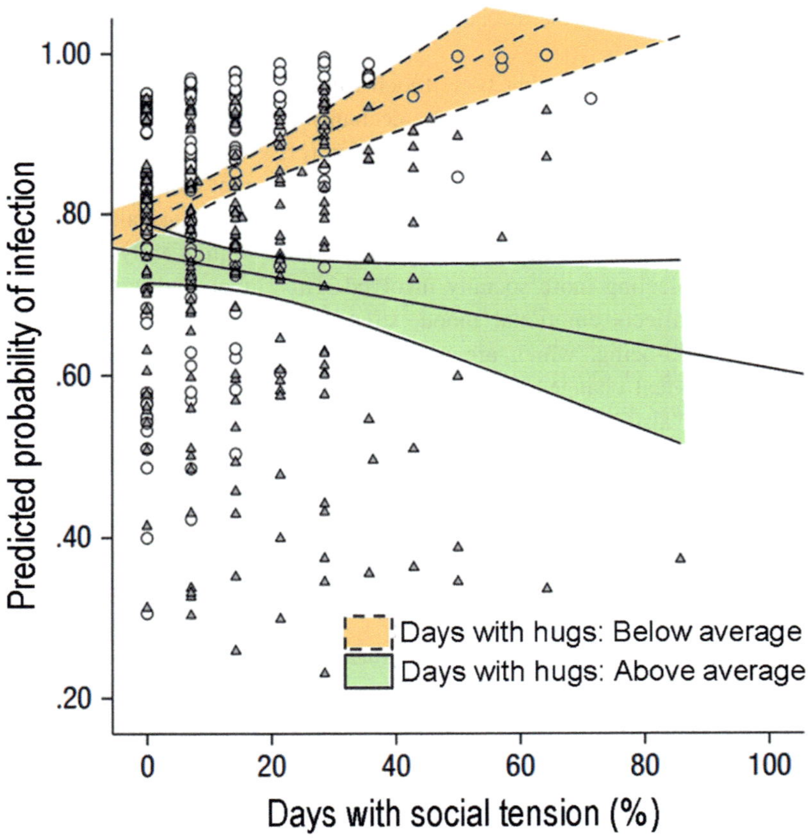

Fig. 5.4 Association between hugs, psychosocial stress, and colds. Individuals who reported having an above-average number of hugs (green) had a *lower* risk of infection, regardless of the number of conflicts reported (days with social tension or arguments). In contrast, individuals who reported having a below-average number of hugs (orange) had an higher risk of infection that *increased* further with number of days with social tension. (Fig. from Cohen et al. 2015)

between inflammation and social support for years into the future (Thomas and Kim 2020). Specifically, the authors examined the **inflammation levels** (C-reactive proteins in the blood; CRP) and the frequency of physical contact in 1124 individuals (age 60+). At the first measurement time point, the mean frequency of physical contact was approximately one time per month, and elevated CRP levels were identified in 20% of the participants. At the second measurement, 5 years later, participants reported experiencing affectionate physical contact only one to two times *per year* on average, and elevated CRP levels were identified in 28% of participants. Interestingly, statistical analyses revealed a relationship between touch frequency at the first measurement time point and CRP levels 5 years later. In contrast, there was no association between touch frequency at the second measurement time point and inflammation levels. The authors concluded that more frequent affectionate physical contact might reduce the likelihood of subsequent elevated inflammation levels. Future studies must examine whether these results can be replicated and the mechanisms that underpin them.

It is safe to assume that body touch triggers physiological and psychological mechanisms that are intertwined in a complex interaction (cf. Fig. 5.5) (Jakubiak and Feeney 2017; Kiecolt-Glaser et al. 2010). Pleasant social touching initiates relationship-promoting processes that lead to the person feeling more socially involved. This positively affects emotional mood, stress, and general well-being, which are associated with neurobiological changes. Furthermore, pleasant touch can also directly lead to biochemical changes (cortisol, oxytocin, and dopamine; see in-depth, Sect. 2.4) that influence stress, emotions, and general health. Less stress and more positive emotions, in turn, contribute to more harmonious relationships, increasing the frequency of pleasant social touches.

Experimental studies have examined the effects of affectionate physical contact on cardiovascular reactivity to stress, the release of cortisol, and the perception of pain.

In order to investigate **cardiovascular reactivity to stress**, couples living together (who were healthy and had normal blood pressure) were studied. They were asked to maintain comfortable physical contact on a sofa for 10 min while talking about a shared pleasurable experience and watching a short romantic video (Grewen et al. 2003). Afterward, the couples were asked to hug each other for 20 s while standing. Participants in the control group sat alone on a sofa for 10 min and then had to stand for 20 s. This was followed by a stress-inducing task that all the participants had to complete alone; specifically, all the participants had to give a 3-min free speech, which was video-recorded. The evaluation showed that the people in the physical contact group showed significantly lower stress reactions during the free speech. Correspondingly, their blood pressure and heart rate rose less than in the control group without physical contact.

A similar study showed that in men and women, **cortisol levels** during a stress-inducing task were influenced by the preceding pleasant physical contact (Ditzen et al. 2019). In this study, the participating couples spent 10 min in a room on a sofa without a specific task. During this period, the couples' level of intimacy (e.g., hand-holding, caressing, kissing, and hugging) was assessed. After the stress tasks, it was found that women who had exchanged more affectionate physical contact with their partner showed significantly lower cortisol levels. In addition, men and women with higher levels of intimacy showed faster recovery of cortisol levels to baseline levels compared to those with little affectionate contact. Additionally, physical contact before a stressful task had a larger positive effect on cortisol response and heart rate than verbal social support from the partner (Ditzen et al. 2007).

The relationship between touch and stress responses can be observed as early as infancy. To investigate this, a **still-face experiment** ("motionless face") was conducted with 53 infants and their mothers (Feldman et al. 2010). The mother showing a motionless face is a stressful situation for the infant. During the experiment, the respective infant sat in a sitting bowl on a table, and the mother sat in front of her infant and played with them. After 3 min of play, the 2-min still-face

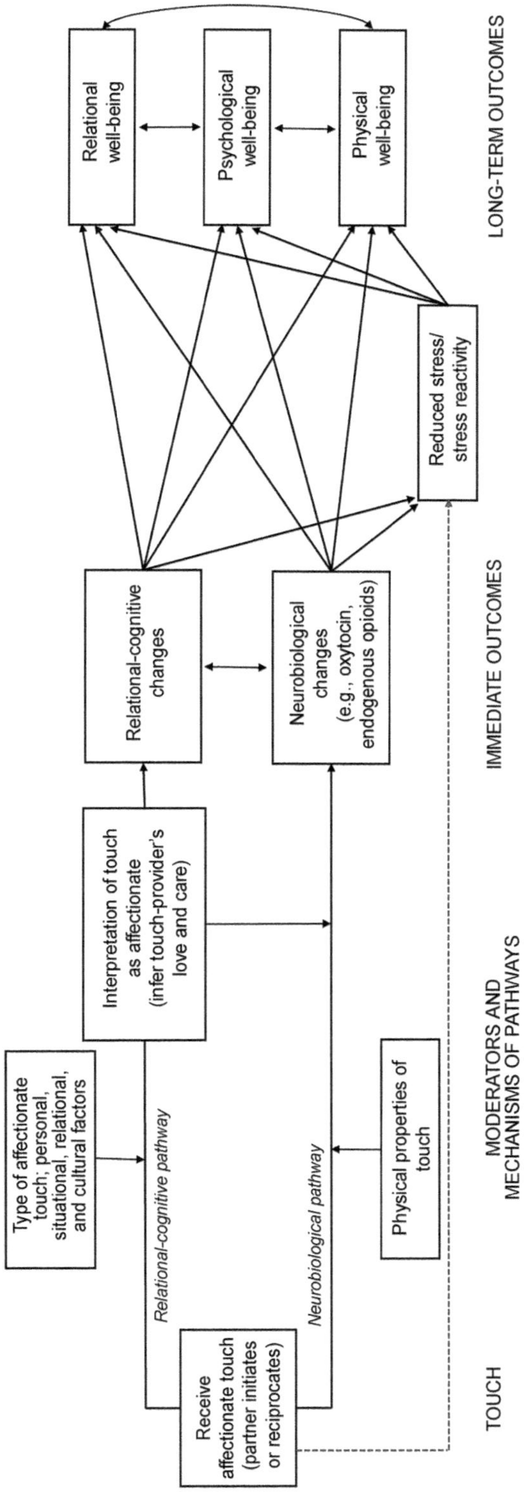

Fig. 5.5 Touch promotes well-being. Theoretical path-model of the relationship between pleasant social touch and social, psychological, and physical well-being. (Fig. from Jakubiak and Feeney 2017)

phase began. During these 2 min, the mother was asked to keep her face motionless and expressionless and not look at her child. The mothers in the experimental group were allowed to touch their children during this time, while the mothers in the control group were not. The evaluation of cortisol levels showed that the children in the experimental group showed a smaller increase in cortisol levels, which quickly returned to baseline levels at the end of the still-face phase. In contrast, in the no-touch control group, the children's cortisol levels continued to rise even after the end of the still-face phase. Some authors hypothesize that early social experiences may help shape the effects of social support on stress responses in adulthood (Hostinar et al. 2014).

Furthermore, there is evidence that individuals who are hugged more frequently in everyday life develop persistently higher levels of **oxytocin** (Light et al. 2005). In both men and women, more positive interactions are associated with higher levels of oxytocin (Gouin et al. 2010). Importantly, high oxytocin levels may have protective effects on the cardiovascular system, lower blood pressure, and buffer against stress (Smith et al. 2013; Grewen and Light 2011). In addition, there is evidence that wounds heal more quickly in individuals with high oxytocin levels than in those with moderate or low oxytocin levels (Gouin et al. 2010).

► **Important** Loving, supportive partnerships, as well as hugs, contribute to better cardiovascular health by dampening individuals' stress responses (Grewen et al. 2003; Robles and Kiecolt-Glaser 2003).

For touch/social support to positively affect stress and cardiovascular outcomes, it must be perceived as supportive rather than evaluative (Kamarck et al. 1990; Edens et al. 1992; Christian and Stoney 2006). The interpretation of touch is influenced by both the behavior of the touching person and the apprehensions, experiences, or self-doubt of the stressed person who is being touched. Results from studies examining whether touch during stressful situations increases or reduces stress are correspondingly varied and contradictory. In studies in which performance tests must be mastered, greater increases in blood pressure and heart rate are often measured when friends or partners are present compared to without them (Christian and Stoney 2006; Allen et al. 2002).

► **Important** Only support (and the accompanying touch) that is perceived as sympathetic has a stress-reducing effect. Conversely, judgmental or evaluative attention ("Can't you do that?" or "I expected more from you!") can intensify stress reactions.

Social support can also have a **pain-reducing** effect. Intuitively, close people hold hands or hug each other in anxious and painful situations. This behavior is particularly pronounced in parents toward their children but persists into old age. For example, in one study, newborns held by a parent during a neonatal heel prick test showed similar or less pain than when given opioids or oral sugar (Axelin et al. 2009). In contrast, an oral water splash (control group) during the heel prick test resulted in significantly greater pain responses than physical contact, opioids, or sugar. In addition, neonates showed fewer adverse side effects (such as a drop in oxygen saturation/heart rate) after opioid administration or body contact than after sugar or water administration. The authors concluded that parental holding and sugar administration were the preferred interventions during very brief, painful procedures in which opioid administration was not absolutely necessary.

In other experimental studies, physical contact has been shown to have a more substantial pain-reducing effect than the mere presence of a person (Field et al. 1997). Indeed, the **empathy and sympathy of** the touching person influence the extent of the pain-reducing effect (Goldstein et al. 2016). For example, adolescents with cancer experienced less pain caused by treatment procedures when they felt safe, less tense, and more distracted (Weekes et al. 1993). To achieve this state, the adolescents preferred to hold their mother's hand or the hand of a nurse they trusted. The relationship and trust with the touching person are crucial for the pain-reducing effects of touch during an acute pain event. Hand-holding by strangers during painful procedures has been found to have a lower pain-reducing effect (Coan et al. 2006), and it may even lead to opposite effects, such as higher pain sensations (Floyd et al. 2018; Yanes et al. 2018). These results contrast with the pain-reducing effects of therapeutic touch in the form of massage (cf. Chap. 8) which is also performed by strangers. Different psychological and physiological mechanisms likely underlie the two processes. Current studies indicate that the anxiety-inhibiting and pain-relieving effects of hand-holding by close people are associated with an alinement of the heartbeat (Goldstein et al. 2017) and the brain activity of those involved (Goldstein et al. 2018). In these situations, the magnitude of empathy correlates with the intensity of cortical coupling and the strength of the pain-relieving effect.

5.5.4 Pets, Animal-Assisted Interventions, and Social Robotics

5.5.4.1 Health-Promoting Effects of Pets

Many recent studies have addressed whether caring for a pet has positive health effects for owners. Initially, the studies yielded conflicting results. However, through extensive reviews, meta-analyses, and detailed investigations, the mechanisms of action in the relationship between pet ownership and health have been extracted (Beetz et al. 2012; Barker and Wolen 2008). These mechanisms of action include:

- The release of oxytocin when petting an animal.
- Changes in stress-induced cardiovascular responses.

The following section addresses the question of whether pets have similar protective effects on health as human social support. In principle, any **interaction with an animal** can be understood as **a form of social behavior.** Depending on the type of animal, this can result in reciprocal and sometimes very long-lasting relationships that, for some individuals, achieve similar emotional significance as interpersonal relationships. In addition, pets can function as social catalysts, serving, for example, as **"icebreakers" to establish contact with other people.** Some surveys suggest that pet owners report less loneliness, better well-being, and even better overall health than those without a pet (McConnell et al. 2011; Headey 1999; Headey et al. 2002). One study that attracted particular attention showed that pet owners with **coronary heart disease** had a better chance of survival (1 year after myocardial infarction or angina pectoris) than individuals without pets (Friedmann et al. 1980). Pet owners even had a higher probability of survival when controlling for their age and severity of disease. Since then, attempts have been made to understand the underlying mechanisms of the effect of pet ownership on health. It is now known that the "pet effect" cannot be explained by physical activity. Studies of the frequency, duration, and intensity of physical activity have failed to find a systematic difference between individuals with and without pets. Indeed, people with medium-to-large-sized dogs who are very committed to their pet's welfare appear to exercise more frequently and regularly than owners of small dogs (Brown and Rhodes 2006; Schofield et al. 2005). Furthermore, the observed health effects are not limited to individuals with dogs but have also been found among owners of other pets (Friedmann et al. 1980).

Furthermore, individuals with pets do not generally show better cardiovascular health, BMI, blood pressure, or heart rate values than those without pets (Friedmann et al. 1980; Parslow and Jorm 2003; Moody et al. 1996). However, there is evidence that pets may improve **cardiovascular reactivity to stress.**

Two studies are presented here as examples of this effect of pets. In the first study, 240 heterosexual couples were examined for their cardiovascular reactivity (increase in blood pressure and heart rate) during stress (Allen et al. 2002). Half of the couples owned a dog or cat, whereas the other half did not own a pet. All the participants were healthy, had normal blood pressure, and were not taking blood pressure or heart medications. Additionally, there were no differences in age, BMI, income, education, or whether their children still lived at home between the couples with and without pets. The participants were assigned to one of four experimental conditions of social support:

(a) Alone.
(b) In the presence of a close friend of the same sex *or* the pet.
(c) In the presence of the life partner.
(d) In the presence of the friend/pet *and* the life partner.

The experiment consisted of two stress tests: an arithmetic task (counting backward out loud in threes from a four-digit number) and a cold stimulus (holding one hand in 2 °C [35.6 °F] cold water for 2 min). Compared to those without pets, participants with pets showed significantly lower heart rates and blood pressures during the rest period, as well as lower increases in heart rate and blood pressure during the stress tests. In addition, pet owners showed faster recovery (time to return to baseline levels) after the stressful stimuli. Of the four social support conditions, participants showed the least stress reactivity when in the company of their pets. In fact, stress reactivity in the presence of the pet was even lower than when the individuals were alone. Moreover, the presence of the pet in addition to the partner resulted in lower cardiovascular reactivity than the presence of the partner alone. The authors concluded that participants felt pressured to perform by their partners and close friends. A crucial factor for the social support effect is that the **support** is **nonjudgmental** (cf. Sect. 5.5.3), and this condition is apparently better fulfilled by (domestic) animals than by humans.

▶ **Important** For a positive effect of social support to occur, the support must not be judgmental. In this regard, pets seem to outclass humans.

The authors conducted another experiment to determine whether the animal's presence causes the effect or whether individuals who acquire an animal systematically differ from others in their stress reactivity (Allen et al. 2001). The study involved 48 people with hypertension who were interested in getting a pet. The participants were randomly assigned to two groups: (a) an experimental group with a pet plus an antihypertensive drug (Lisinopril), and (b) a control group with Lisinopril only. Before the study began, the participants in the two groups did not differ in their mean heart rate and blood pressure, either at rest or under stress (during math and language tests). The participants in the experimental group bought a dog or cat when they began taking the medication, and after 6 months, the participants were examined again. In both groups, Lisinopril use reduced blood pressure at rest by ≈35/20 mmHg. However, a significant difference was seen in stress reactivity, as the increase in heart rate and blood pressure under stress was significantly lower in the experimental group with the pet present than in the control group only taking Lisinopril. The authors interpreted the results as evidence that the pet increased social support in the participants' lives.

These results may be moderated by the **quality of the relationship with the animal** as well as the **oxytocin release when petting an animal** (cf. Sect. 2.4) (Beetz et al. 2012). For example, studies that exposed participants to stress tests while an unfamiliar animal was present showed no altered cardiovascular response to stress (Straatman et al. 1997; Kingwell et al. 2001). Furthermore, it has been shown that more oxytocin is released when petting one's own dog than when petting a stranger's dog (Odendaal 2000).

Other positive physiological changes associated with petting an animal include an increase in the release of beta-endorphin and dopamine and a decrease in cortisol levels (Odendaal and Meintjes 2003). In line with this, some observational studies have reported **mood-elevating effects and increased well-being** in relation to pets (McConnell et al. 2011; Barker and Wolen 2008). Indeed, especially in the case of social rejection, interaction with a pet can serve as a buffer against a negative mood (McConnell et al. 2011).

Nevertheless, social contact with pets cannot replace social interaction with people. The positive effects that can be achieved through the companionship of animals must be understood as a supplement to rather than a substitute for interpersonal relationships (McConnell et al. 2011; Barker and Wolen 2008). For ethical and logistical reasons, appropriate comparative studies do not exist in which participants live completely isolated from other humans for extended periods of time. However, a study with individuals living alone versus in partnerships and with and without pets suggested that pets could attenuate short-term negative moods and reduce feelings of loneliness (Turner et al. 2003). However, pets did not affect the frequency of positive moods. The frequency of positive moods was higher in individuals in partnerships (with or without a pet cat) than in individuals living alone.

▶ **Important** The American Heart Association rates pet ownership as a possible protective factor against cardiovascular disease (Levine et al. 2013). However, more randomized controlled trials are needed to understand the underlying mechanisms of the relationship between pet ownership and health outcomes and to determine the magnitude of the effect. Future studies must also control for risk factors (including smoking and obesity), comorbidities, preventive measures, and psychosocial and socioeconomic factors.

Note

It is not advisable to acquire an animal only for health benefits. In order for the relationship between animals and humans to be pleasant and beneficial for both beings, many conditions must be met. First and foremost, time and space must be available for the animal to ensure that it is kept in a manner appropriate to its species. Lack of time and resources can cause additional stress for the animal and owner, which can ultimately be detrimental to their health. In addition, responsibility for an animal can lead to the postponement or cancellation of hospitalizations and surgeries because care for the animal cannot be provided.

5.5.4.2 Animal-Assisted Interventions

Animal-assisted interventions refer to all activities with animals that do not belong to the patients or clients. For example, this can include interaction with animals as a therapeutic tool and visiting animals in institutions.

As described in the previous section, some effects of animals on health (e.g., the strength of oxytocin release during petting and the reduction of the stress response) depend on the quality of the relationship between the animals and humans. However, the presence of and interaction with unfamiliar animals can also produce surprising effects.

▶ **Important** Animal-assisted interventions can serve as a social catalyst, reduce feelings of loneliness, and positively impact emotional mood.

The biggest difference between animal-assisted interventions and other occupational or psychological approaches is the direct physical contact with a living being that can be touched and that responds to the touch (Bernstein et al. 2000). In this respect, every interaction with an animal is a form of social contact. Moreover, in contrast to many people, animals usually show what they like and do not like in a direct and unfiltered manner. Accordingly, it should come as no surprise that repeated contact with therapy animals can, among other things, **improve social competence** in prison inmates (Fournier et al. 2007). In addition, the release of oxytocin (mentioned above) when petting animals has a stress-reducing and beneficial effect on social compatibility (cf. Sect. 2.4).

However, one of the most frequently demonstrated effects of the presence of an animal is an **increase in social interaction between people**. For this reason, animals are also referred to as social catalysts. This effect can be used in a supportive way, such as in therapy for children with developmental or psychiatric disorders (Beetz et al. 2012; Barker and Wolen 2008). One study indicated that **children with autism** used more language and interacted more socially in the presence of different animals and during therapeutic riding (Sams et al. 2006). Children with autism have also been reported to show less inattention, distractibility, and reduced physical inactivity in such contexts (Bass et al. 2009). In another previous work, **children and adolescents with psychiatric disorders** who participated in an animal-assisted intervention with a dog in addition to standard inpatient therapy showed significant positive effects in terms of vitality, emotional balance, social extraversion, and attention (Basler Befindlichkeitsskala; well-being questionnaire). Additionally, in a control group without animal-assisted intervention, such changes did not occur during the same period (Prothmann et al. 2006).

In another study, **adult inpatients with psychiatric disorders** received 4 weeks of additional animal-assisted intervention (Marr et al. 2000). During this time, their social behavior was assessed daily by an independent observer. Compared to a randomized control group, the patients with animal contact showed significantly more interaction with other patients, showed more frequent smiles and signs of joy, were more sociable and helpful, and were more active and outgoing.

Similar effects have been shown for institutionalized **older adults with psychiatric disorders (including schizophrenia)**. The older adults received animal visitation once per week for 1 year, and positive effects on social behavior and even on coping with activities of daily living (including personal hygiene) were observed both in the short and long terms (Haughie et al. 1992; Barak et al. 2001). Furthermore, the presence of a dog leads to more frequent and longer verbal exchanges between residents of long-term care facilities (Bernstein et al. 2000; Fick 1993), with studies indicating positive effects compared to baseline levels as well as compared to the respective comparison groups.

Additionally, for **geriatric patients with cognitive impairments (dementia)**, positive effects of animal-assisted interventions have been reported. In one study, geriatric dementia patients living in a nursing home had regular contact with a therapy dog for 12 weeks (Walsh et al. 1995). In the presence of the dog, reduced heart rates and a reduction of noise in the ward were observed, and these changes did not occur in the control group. Similarly, other studies have reported significant reductions in agitated behavior (physical and psychological agitation) (Richeson 2003), less need for restraints to prevent self-endangering wandering, and better time orientation of residents (Katsinas 2000). All the studies on animal-assisted interventions have also shown increased social interactions between the residents (Kongable et al. 1989; Richeson 2003).

In addition, some studies have found **positive effects on the mood** of patients who have contact with a therapy animal (Nathans-Barel et al. 2005; Prothmann et al. 2006). However, the long-term outcomes that are associated with this positive mood effect and whether animal-assisted interventions can counteract depression are inconclusive. Nevertheless, study participants in long-term care have reported feeling less lonely when they have regular contact with therapy animals (Banks and Banks 2002, 2005). In this regard, personal time with the animal appears to produce larger effects than animal-assisted group interventions. This is likely due to the greater intensity of contact with the animal (cf. oxytocin release; previous section). However, findings suggest that the positive effects of animal-assisted interventions are not merely due to intensified interpersonal contact but that contact with the animal itself produces positive effects (Beetz et al. 2012). Indeed, studies in which participants were required to care for an animal for several weeks have produced similar results. For example, older adults who cared for a canary showed fewer depressive symptoms and an increase in perceived quality of life after 3 months (Colombo et al. 2006). It can be assumed that regular and prolonged contact with the same animal promotes relationship-building between the human and the animal. These relationships resemble those of pet owners and are also less stressful for the therapy animal. Taking responsibility for an animal can help **structure daily routines** and create a **sense of being needed**.

In the present chapter, care was taken to cite only controlled experimental studies to ensure the reliability of the findings. Studies published on this topic vary greatly in their methodological quality. A large proportion of the publications are merely observational studies without control groups, descriptions of individual cases, or very small samples.

> *Important* **Note!** In general, any animal-assisted therapy must consider both human and animal welfare. The individuals providing animal-assisted interventions require appropriate training to ensure the quality and safety of the intervention, as well as the health and appropriate husbandry of the respective animal species. Various institutions offer appropriate advanced training to become a specialist in animal-assisted therapy.

5.5.4.3 Social Robotics

A recent study investigated the effects of petting a robot in the form of a baby seal ("Paro") on pain perception (heat pain) and oxytocin levels (Geva et al. 2020). The robot responds to petting by moving its tail and winking, and it seeks eye contact and makes sounds like a baby seal. The authors reported that the participants (healthy young adults) who stroked and talked to the robot rated a heat stimulus as less painful than those without the robot (control group). The individuals who played with the seal also showed an unexpected drop in oxytocin levels, whereas in the control group, the oxytocin levels remained stable during the experiment. This effect is unusual because existing research has associated an *increase in* oxytocin with petting animals and social contact (see earlier in this chapter). The observed pain-reducing effects may be due to the **distracting effect of the robot.**

Consistent with this finding, a recent review article reported that children who played with a humanoid or animal-like robot were distracted from medical treatment, showed **less stress and pain**, appeared more relaxed, smiled more, and communicated more (Moerman et al. 2019). The children were usually accompanied by their parents who also interacted with the robot. However, the authors concluded that the observed distraction effects might be short-lived (e.g., during a vaccination), and parental support may be needed for the child to continue playing (Beran et al. 2015). Similar results were obtained in a study of pain-reducing and anxiety-reducing effects from an animal robot; specifically, the effects were largest when parents and children played together with the robot (i.e., when additional interpersonal social support was present) (Okita 2013).

> **Important** Social robots can create distraction effects, thus dampening short-term pain and stress.

One patient group for which the therapeutic use of social robots is increasingly being tested is **children with autism spectrum disorders (ASD)**. The assumption is that social robots:

- Are perceived as less intimidating than humans.
- Are more predictable than animals.
- But at the same time, generate more social engagement than other toys or tablet computers (Krichmar and Chou 2018).

The goal is to use robots to improve these children's social and communication skills. Systematic reviews of studies over the last 15 years indicate that children with ASD show less social anxiety toward social robots and more attentive and responsive behavior than toward humans (Sartorato et al. 2017; Pennisi et al. 2016). In addition, during robot interaction, repetitive and stereotypic behaviors decrease and verbal expressions increase. Furthermore, after the robot-assisted interventions, children with ASD tend to show less negative emotions, anxiety, and withdrawal behaviors (Robinson et al. 2019). Social behaviors toward humans also improve after several weeks of robot interventions, as demonstrated by more frequent eye contact, more verbal expressions, and improved recognition of facial expressions and gestures. Compared to similarly intensive training with human therapists, the robotic interventions do not seem to differ in their effects. Indeed, current results suggest that it is primarily the intensity and focus of the exercises that determine success.

Another possible use of robotic systems is **sensory integration therapy (SIT) for children with neurodevelopmental disorders**. Unlike social robots that focus on eye contact, facial expressions, and attention, these systems are designed to elicit and encourage children's tactile interactions with the robot. Currently, several models are being evaluated (e.g., KASPAR, ROBALL, and CARBO) (Krichmar and Chou 2018). These robotic systems register touch, light up in different colors, move, and make sounds. "Carbo," for example, can recognize the direction and speed with which it is stroked, which allows touch games to be implemented. Specifically, stroking movements must be performed in the specified direction and speed to color the hemisphere-shaped robot the target color. In an exploratory study without a control group, children with attention deficit hyperactivity disorder (ADHD), ASD, anxiety, and oppositional defiant disorder showed high acceptance and willingness to participate. However, comparative studies with conventional therapy are needed to assess the effectiveness of robot-assisted SIT.

▶ **Important** Interactions with robots can strengthen social and communication skills in children with ASD.

As an alternative to animal-assisted interventions, social robots have also been tested **in nursing homes and homes for the elderly.** These technical applications generate much fascination among the residents. However, there are also concerns that their use may further reduce actual interpersonal contact and touch in the context of care (Winkelmann 2019). Due to the current nursing shortage, it is to be feared that such a reduction would affect those patients the most who are already affected by a lack of social contact.

Principally, in any application of technical or social substitutes, it must be considered that humans have basic psychosocial needs and can survive on their own only in exceptional situations. In situations of social deprivation, humans are capable of amazing flexibility. For example, to ensure physical and psychological survival, humans can form attachments with animals and even virtual figures. However, the minimum requirement is that basic psychosocial needs such as security, belonging, empathy, and emotional reciprocity are met. When more of these needs are met, more stable attachments can be formed. Accordingly, findings on the emotionally uplifting effects of pets (cf. earlier in this chapter) show that interpersonal contact has a more reliable mood-stabilizing effect than animal contact, and social robots would likely satisfy fewer needs than pets. Thus far, the extent to which human physical contact needs can be met by social robots has not been researched. In the opinion of the authors of this book, the use of technology to satisfy social and physical contact needs is unethical and psychologically, socially, and biologically unacceptable unless it is **temporary and complementary to real interpersonal relationships**.

Studies conducted to date in nursing homes and homes for older adults have predominantly investigated how patients with dementia respond to the robot seal "Paro". A systematic review of studies conducted in recent years suggests at least three positive effects (Hung et al. 2019):

- Reduction of negative emotions and behaviors.
- Triggering of positive mood expressions.
- Increase in social interaction with other people.

Consequently, the effects are similar to those elicited by animal-assisted intervention (Kramer et al. 2009). Consequently, social robots could substitute animal-assisted interventions in facilities in which real animals are not allowed. However, current barriers to their use include the high initial costs, additional required supervision, hygiene concerns, and fears regarding the stigmatization (infantilization) of older adults (Hung et al. 2019).

5.5.4.4 Methodological Shortcomings of Social Robotics Studies

Despite the rapidly increasing number of studies in social robotics, the vast majority are of low methodological quality due to small sample sizes and the lack of a control group. Usually, additional people are present during the robotic intervention to supervise the technology (Moerman et al. 2019) or instruct the intervention (Kachouie et al. 2014), which increases the likelihood that the effects found are due to **experimenter and Hawthorne effects**. Experimenter effects refer to the fact that the expectations and behavior of the experimenters influence the behavior of the participants. The Hawthorne effect means that participants change their natural behavior because they are given attention and know they are under observation. In addition, the presence of other people obscures whether being alone with a robot would be perceived as creepy. For example, in a field study in which "Paro" was used in a child and adolescent psychiatric ward, some children found the robot unpleasant and scary (Nakadoi 2015). Therefore, the authors recommend that special precautions be taken when using robots in psychiatric settings.

Only a few long-term studies exist, and these were conducted without a control group. The long-term studies suggest that the positive changes triggered by "Paro" extend beyond novelty effects (Wada et al. 2005; Sabanovic et al. 2013). However, the lack of control groups means that it is not possible to distinguish whether the effects were triggered by the robot or by other changes in participants' daily lives associated with the study (e.g., weekly group sessions and regular interviews).

> ▶ **Important** Similar to animal-assisted interventions, social robots in nursing homes and homes for older adults can serve as a welcome change in everyday life and an icebreaker for conversations. These systems can help increase social interaction and have a mood-lifting effect.

5.5.4.5 Haptic Telecommunications

Approaches in which **technology-mediated social touch** is used **to augment telecommunications** are promising. These approaches attempt to supplement telephone or video-based conversations with another sensory channel. Ideally, a friend or family member should be connected as part of this communication. Correspondingly, exploratory research suggests that techno-mediated emotional touch performed by strangers is perceived as unusual or invasive (Wang and Quek 2010). Instead, participants prefer to use haptic communication with close individuals (Suhonen et al. 2012), which indicates that the relationship between the sender and receiver in the communication and the associated feeling of security also play important roles in this type of touch (cf. Sect. 5.1).

Moreover, a study using a pillow in the shape of a human torso showed surprising effects on participants' stress levels. Participants in the study (women, mean age 63) had a standardized conversation over the phone for 15 min with a stranger who knew nothing about the study. The participants were seated in a comfortable chair and used the speakerphone function. During the conversation, the participants in the experimental group hugged the cushion (Sumioka et al. 2013). As a result, the cortisol levels (stress hormone) of the people in the experimental group decreased significantly during the phone call. However, in the control group, no difference was found in cortisol levels before and after the telephone call. Therefore, it would be interesting to investigate what effects such a pillow would have during communication with close individuals and whether such a pillow would be comparable to an approach using weighted/sand blankets (cf. Sect. 8.3.9).

Many tele-touch applications target couples in long-distance relationships to **simulate a sense of physical proximity**. Such communication elements can be PC-linked or Bluetooth-controlled. The use of these applications during phone calls or video-based conversations helps give the technical "touches" social/emotional meaning. The tactile stimulators create vibration, pressure, or heat on the palm, arm, or torso (Kontaris et al. 2012; Gooch and Watts 2010; Sallnäs 2010). Initial results from small samples suggest that this can increase the sense of social presence.

Overall, while many technical approaches to tele-touch exist, few of the prototypes have been evaluated with experimental studies (Huisman 2017; Haans and IJsselsteijn 2006; Wang and Quek 2010). Consequently, it is unknown whether such applications can counteract loneliness and social isolation. Furthermore, in the medical and nursing contexts, no studies have been conducted so far regarding tele-touch applications.

5.6 Summary

- How a touch is evaluated depends on the person's expectations, the situation, which part of the body is touched, and the relationship with the touching person.
- Moods and intentions influence how touch is performed (e.g., rough, gentle, quick, short, or slow stroking), even unconsciously.
- Even a brief touch can reveal the intention and mood of the person performing the touch within seconds.
- Depending on how a touch is evaluated/perceived, it can increase or decrease the arousal levels (stress) of the touched person.
- The strength of the anxiety- and stress-reducing effects of touch depends on the emotional connection and empathy of the person touching.
- Fleeting touches can influence attitudes, moods, and behavior.
- Physical contact is the fastest and most straightforward way to convey love and affection, strengthen relationships, and show sympathy and comfort.
- Social support, hugs, and touch can protect the cardiovascular system, reduce stress, reduce inflammation levels in the blood, and positively affect the immune system.
- For positive effects on stress and the cardiovascular system, it is crucial that the support/touch be perceived as supportive and not as evaluative.
- Physical contact with pets leads to the release of oxytocin.
- Pets may be perceived as social support and reduce cardiovascular reactivity during stress.
- Pets and therapy animals act as social catalysts (i.e., they promote interaction between people).
- Animal-assisted interventions have a mood-lifting effect.

References

Allen K, Shykoff BE, Izzo JL. Pet ownership, but not ACE inhibitor therapy, blunts home blood pressure responses to mental stress. Hypertension. 2001;38(4):815–20. https://doi.org/10.1161/hyp.38.4.815.

Allen K, Blascovich J, Mendes WB. Cardiovascular reactivity and the presence of pets, friends, and spouses: the truth about cats and dogs. Psychosom Med. 2002;64(5):727.

Andersen PA, Guerrero LK. Haptic behavior in social interaction. In: Grunwald M, editor. Human haptic perception: basics and applications. Basel: Birkhäuser; 2008. p. 155–63.

App B, McIntosh DN, Reed CL, Hertenstein MJ. Nonverbal channel use in communication of emotion: how may depend on why. Emotion. 2011;11(3):603–17. https://doi.org/10.1037/a0023164.

Avorn J, Langer E. Induced disability in nursing home patients: a controlled trial. J Am Geriatr Soc. 1982;30(6):397–400. https://doi.org/10.1111/j.1532-5415.1982.tb02839.x.

Axelin A, Salanterä S, Kirjavainen J, Lehtonen L. Oral glucose and parental holding preferable to opioid in pain management in preterm infants. Clin J Pain. 2009;25(2):138–45. https://doi.org/10.1097/AJP.0b013e318181ad81.

Banks MR, Banks WA. The effects of animal-assisted therapy on loneliness in an elderly population in long-term care facilities. J Gerontol A Biol Sci Med Sci. 2002;57(7):M428–32. https://doi.org/10.1093/gerona/57.7.M428.

Banks MR, Banks WA. The effects of group and individual animal-assisted therapy on loneliness in residents of long-term care facilities. Anthrozoös. 2005;18(4):396–408. https://doi.org/10.2752/089279305785593983.

Barak Y, Savorai O, Mavashev S, Beni A. Animal-assisted therapy for elderly schizophrenic

patients: a one-year controlled trial. Am J Geriatr Psychiatry. 2001;9(4):439–42. https://doi.org/10.1097/00019442-200111000-00013.
Barker SB, Wolen AR. The benefits of human-companion animal interaction: a review. J Vet Med Educ. 2008;35(4):487–95. https://doi.org/10.3138/jvme.35.4.487.
Barnett K. A survey of the current utilization of touch by health team personnel with hospitalized patients. Int J Nurs Stud. 1972;9(4):195–209. https://doi.org/10.1016/0020-7489(72)90033-8.
Bartol MA. Dialogue with dementia: nonverbal communication in patients with Alzheimer's disease. J Gerontol Nurs. 1979;5(4):21–31. https://doi.org/10.3928/0098-9134-19790701-06.
Bass MM, Duchowny CA, Llabre MM. The effect of therapeutic horseback riding on social functioning in children with autism. J Autism Dev Disord. 2009;39(9):1261–7. https://doi.org/10.1007/s10803-009-0734-3.
Beetz A, Uvnäs-Moberg K, Julius H, Kotrschal K. Psychosocial and psychophysiological effects of human-animal interactions: the possible role of oxytocin. Front Psychol. 2012;3:234. https://doi.org/10.3389/fpsyg.2012.00234.
Benedetti F. Placebo and the new physiology of the doctor-patient relationship. Physiol Rev. 2013;93(3):1207–46. https://doi.org/10.1152/physrev.00043.2012.
Beran TN, Ramirez-Serrano A, Vanderkooi OG, Kuhn S. Humanoid robotics in health care: an exploration of children's and parents' emotional reactions. J Health Psychol. 2015;20(7):984–9. https://doi.org/10.1177/1359105313504794.
Bernstein PL, Friedmann E, Malaspina A. Animal-assisted therapy enhances resident social interaction and initiation in long-term care facilities. Anthrozoös. 2000;13(4):213–24. https://doi.org/10.2752/089279300786999743.
Breidert M, Hofbauer K. Placebo: Missverständnisse und Vorurteile. Osteopathische Medizin. 2010;11(3):14–8. https://doi.org/10.1016/j.ostmed.2010.03.001.
Brockner J, Pressman B, Cabitt J, Moran P. Nonverbal intimacy, sex, and compliance: a field study. J Nonverbal Behav. 1982;6(4):253–8. https://doi.org/10.1007/bf00987192.
Brown SG, Rhodes RE. Relationships among dog ownership and leisure-time walking in Western Canadian adults. Am J Prev Med. 2006;30(2):131–6. https://doi.org/10.1016/j.amepre.2005.10.007.
Bush E. The use of human touch to improve the Wellbeing of older adults: a holistic nursing intervention. J Holist Nurs. 2001;19(3):256–70.
Carney DR, Cuddy AJC, Yap AJ. Power posing: brief nonverbal displays affect neuroendocrine levels and risk tolerance. Psychol Sci. 2010;21(10):1363–8.
Chae Y, Olausson H. The role of touch in acupuncture treatment. Acupunct Med. 2017;35(2):148–52. https://doi.org/10.1136/acupmed-2016-011178.
Chae Y, Lee Y-S, Enck P. How placebo needles differ from placebo pills? Front Psych. 2018;9:243.
Cho KS, Snyder M. Use of hand massage with presence to increase relaxation in Korean: American elderly. J Nurs Acad Soc. 1996;26(3):623. https://doi.org/10.4040/jnas.1996.26.3.623.
Christian LM, Stoney CM. Social support versus social evaluation: unique effects on vascular and myocardial response patterns. Psychosom Med. 2006;68(6):914–21. https://doi.org/10.1097/01.psy.0000244023.20755.cf.
Coan JA, Schaefer HS, Davidson RJ. Lending a hand: social regulation of the neural response to threat. Psychol Sci. 2006;17(12):1032–9. https://doi.org/10.1111/j.1467-9280.2006.01832.x.
Cocksedge S, George B, Renwick S, Chew-Graham CA. Touch in primary care consultations: qualitative investigation of doctors' and patients' perceptions. Br J Gen Pract. 2013;63(609):e283–90. https://doi.org/10.3399/bjgp13X665251.
Cohen S, Janicki-Deverts D, Turner RB, Doyle WJ. Does hugging provide stress-buffering social support? A study of susceptibility to upper respiratory infection and illness. Psychol Sci. 2015;26(2):135–47. https://doi.org/10.1177/0956797614559284.
Colombo G, Buono MD, Smania K, Raviola R, de Leo D. Pet therapy and institutionalized elderly: a study on 144 cognitively unimpaired subjects. Arch Gerontol Geriatr. 2006;42(2):207–16. https://doi.org/10.1016/j.archger.2005.06.011.
Converso D, Loera B, Viotti S, Martini M. Do positive relations with patients play a protective role for healthcare employees? Effects of patients' gratitude and support on nurses' burnout. Front Psychol. 2015;6:470. https://doi.org/10.3389/fpsyg.2015.00470.
Crane J, Crane FG. Optimal nonverbal communications strategies physicians should engage in to promote positive clinical outcomes. Health Mark Q. 2010;27(3):262–74. https://doi.org/10.1080/07359683.2010.495300.
Crusco AH, Wetzel CG. The Midas touch: the effects of interpersonal touch on restaurant tipping. Pers Soc Psychol Bull. 1984;10(4):512–7.
Curtis R, Groarke AM, Coughlan R, Gsel A. The influence of disease severity, perceived stress, social support and coping in patients with chronic illness: a 1 year follow up. Psychol Health Med. 2004;9(4):456–75. https://doi.org/10.1080/1354850042000267058.
Davidzar R, Giger JN. When touch is not the best approach. J Clin Nurs. 1997;6(3):203–6. https://doi.org/10.1111/j.1365-2702.1997.tb00305.x.
Davin L, Thistlethwaite J, Bartle E, Russell K. Touch in health professional practice: a review. Clin Teach. 2019;16(6):559–64. https://doi.org/10.1111/tct.13089.
DeVos J. The patient with brain dysfunction. In: Manual of psychosocial nursing interventions; 1989. p. 65–88.
Ditzen B, Neumann ID, Bodenmann G, von Dawans B, Turner RA, Ehlert U, Heinrichs M. Effects of different kinds of couple interaction on cortisol and heart rate responses to stress in women. Psychoneuroendocrinology. 2007;32(5):565–74. https://doi.org/10.1016/j.psyneuen.2007.03.011.

Ditzen B, Germann J, Meuwly N, Bradbury TN, Bodenmann G, Heinrichs M. Intimacy as related to cortisol reactivity and recovery in couples undergoing psychosocial stress. Psychosom Med. 2019;81(1):16–25. https://doi.org/10.1097/PSY.0000000000000633.
Dolinski D. Touch, compliance, and homophobia. J Nonverbal Behav. 2010;34(3):179–92. https://doi.org/10.1007/s10919-010-0090-1.
Drescher VM, Gantt WH, Whitehead WE. Heart rate response to touch. Psychosom Med. 1980;42(6):559–65. https://doi.org/10.1097/00006842-198011000-00004.
Drescher VM, Whitehead WE, Morrill-Corbin ED, Cataldo MF. Physiological and subjective reactions to being touched. Psychophysiology. 1985;22(1):96–100. https://doi.org/10.1111/j.1469-8986.1985.tb01565.x.
Dyer I. Preventing the ITU syndrome or how not to torture an ITU patient! Part 2. Intensive Crit Care Nurs. 1995a;11(4):223–32. https://doi.org/10.1016/S0964-3397(95)80618-0.
Dyer I. Preventing the ITU syndrome or how not to torture an ITU patient! Part I. Intensive Crit Care Nurs. 1995b;11(3):130–9. https://doi.org/10.1016/S0964-3397(95)80618-0.
Eaker ED, Pinsky J, Castelli WP. Myocardial infarction and coronary death among women: psychosocial predictors from a 20-year follow-up of women in the Framingham study. Am J Epidemiol. 1992;135(8):854–64. https://doi.org/10.1093/oxfordjournals.aje.a116381.
Eaton M, Mitchell-Bonair IL, Friedmann E. The effect of touch on nutritional intake of chronic organic brain syndrome patients. J Gerontol. 1986;41(5):611–6. https://doi.org/10.1093/geronj/41.5.611.
Edens JL, Larkin KT, Abel JL. The effect of social support and physical touch on cardiovascular reactions to mental stress. J Psychosom Res. 1992;36(4):371–81. https://doi.org/10.1016/0022-3999(92)90073-b.
Ekman P. Facial expression and emotion. Am Psychol. 1993;48(4):384–92. https://doi.org/10.1037/0003-066x.48.4.384.
Ellis RB. Defining communication. In: Ellis RB, Gates RJ, Kenworthy N, editors. Interpersonal communication in nursing: theory and practice. London: Churchill Livingstone; 1995. p. 5–7.
Erceau D, Guéguen N. Tactile contact and evaluation of the toucher. J Soc Psychol. 2007;147(4):441–4. https://doi.org/10.3200/socp.147.4.441-444.
Faulkner M. The onset and alleviation of learned helplessness in older hospitalized people. Aging Ment Health. 2001;5(4):379–86. https://doi.org/10.1080/13607860120080341.
Feldman R, Singer M, Zagoory O. Touch attenuates infants' physiological reactivity to stress. Dev Sci. 2010;13(2):271–8. https://doi.org/10.1111/j.1467-7687.2009.00890.x.
Fick KM. The influence of an animal on social interactions of nursing home residents in a group setting. Am J Occup Ther. 1993;47(6):529–34. https://doi.org/10.5014/ajot.47.6.529.
Field T, Hernandez-Reif M, Taylor S, Quintino O, Burman I. Labor pain is reduced by massage therapy. J Psychosom Obstet Gynaecol. 1997;18(4):286–91. https://doi.org/10.3109/01674829709080701.
Fine L, Rajput V. The smile is stronger than the handshake. MedEdPublish. 2020;9(1):1–5. https://doi.org/10.15694/mep.2020.000068.1.
Fisher JD, Rytting M, Heslin R. Hands touching hands: affective and evaluative effects of an interpersonal touch. Sociometry. 1976;39(4):416. https://doi.org/10.2307/3033506.
Flegal KM, Kit BK, Orpana H, Graubard BI. Association of all-cause mortality with overweight and obesity using standard body mass index categories: a systematic review and meta-analysis. JAMA. 2013;309(1):71–82. https://doi.org/10.1001/jama.2012.113905.
Floyd K, Ray CD, van Raalte LJ, Stein JB, Generous MA. Interpersonal touch buffers pain sensitivity in romantic relationships but heightens sensitivity between strangers and friends. Res Psychol Behav Sci. 2018;6(1):27–34. https://doi.org/10.12691/rpbs-6-1-4.
Fournier AK, Geller ES, Fortney EV. Human-animal interaction in a prison setting: impact on criminal behavior, treatment Progress, and social skills. Behav Soc Iss. 2007;16(1):89–105. https://doi.org/10.5210/bsi.v16i1.385.
Friedman R, Elliot AJ. The effect of arm crossing on persistence and performance. Eur J Soc Psychol. 2008;38(3):449–61. https://doi.org/10.1002/ejsp.444.
Friedmann E, Katcher AH, Lynch JJ, Thomas SA. Animal companions and one-year survival of patients after discharge from a coronary care unit. Public Health Rep. 1980;95(4):307–12.
Gallace A, Spence C. The science of interpersonal touch: an overview. Neurosci Biobehav Rev. 2010;34(2):246–59. https://doi.org/10.1016/j.neubiorev.2008.10.004.
Geva N, Uzefovsky F, Levy-Tzedek S. Touching the social robot PARO reduces pain perception and salivary oxytocin levels. Sci Rep. 2020;10(1):9814. https://doi.org/10.1038/s41598-020-66982-y.
Gleeson M, Timmins F. Touch: a fundamental aspect of communication with older people experiencing dementia. Nurs Older People. 2004;16(2):18–21. https://doi.org/10.7748/nop2004.04.16.2.18.c2302.
Goldstein P, Shamay-Tsoory SG, Yellinek S, Weissman-Fogel I. Empathy predicts an experimental pain reduction during touch. J Pain. 2016;17(10):1049–57. https://doi.org/10.1016/j.jpain.2016.06.007.
Goldstein P, Weissman-Fogel I, Shamay-Tsoory SG. The role of touch in regulating inter-partner physiological coupling during empathy for pain. Sci Rep. 2017;7(1):3252. https://doi.org/10.1038/s41598-017-03627-7.
Goldstein P, Weissman-Fogel I, Dumas G, Shamay-Tsoory SG. Brain-to-brain coupling during handholding is associated with pain reduction. Proc Natl

Acad Sci U S A. 2018;115(11):E2528–37. https://doi.org/10.1073/pnas.1703643115.
Gooch D, Watts L. Communicating social presence through thermal hugs. In: In Proc. Ubicomp 2010 SISSE Workshop; 2010. p. 11–9.
Gouin JP, Carter CS, Pournajafi-Nazarloo H, Glaser R, Malarkey WB, Loving TJ, et al. Marital behavior, oxytocin, vasopressin, and wound healing. Psychoneuroendocrinology. 2010;35(7):1082–90. https://doi.org/10.1016/j.psyneuen.2010.01.009.
Greco A, Steca P, Pozzi R, Monzani D, D'Addario M, Villani A, et al. Predicting depression from illness severity in cardiovascular disease patients: self-efficacy beliefs, illness perception, and perceived social support as mediators. Int J Behav Med. 2014;21(2):221–9. https://doi.org/10.1007/s12529-013-9290-5.
Greenbaum PE, Lumley MA, Turner C, Melamed BG. Dentist's reassuring touch: effects on children's behavior. Pediatr Dent. 1993;15(1):20–4. https://www.ncbi.nlm.nih.gov/pubmed/8233987.
Grewen KM, Light KC. Plasma oxytocin is related to lower cardiovascular and sympathetic reactivity to stress. Biol Psychol. 2011;87(3):340–9. https://doi.org/10.1016/j.biopsycho.2011.04.003.
Grewen KM, Anderson BJ, Girdler SS, Light KC. Warm partner contact is related to lower cardiovascular reactivity. Behav Med. 2003;29(3):123–30. https://doi.org/10.1080/08964280309596065.
Groth M, Grandey A. From bad to worse: negative exchange spirals in employee–customer service interactions. Organ Psychol Rev. 2012;2(3):208–33. https://doi.org/10.1177/2041386612441735.
Grunwald M. Homo hapticus. Warum wir ohne Tastsinn nicht leben können. München: Droemer; 2017.
Guéguen N. Nonverbal encouragement of participation in a course: the effect of touching. Soc Psychol Educ. 2004;7(1):89–98. https://doi.org/10.1023/b:spoe.0000010691.30834.14.
Guéguen N, Fischer-lokou J. An evaluation of touch on a large request: a field setting. Psychol Rep. 2002;90(1):267–9. https://doi.org/10.2466/pr0.2002.90.1.267.
Guéguen N, Fischer-lokou J. Tactile contact and spontaneous help: an evaluation in a natural setting. J Soc Psychol. 2003;143(6):785–7. https://doi.org/10.1080/00224540309600431.
Guéguen N, Jacob C. The effect of touch on tipping: an evaluation in a French bar. Int J Hosp Manag. 2005;24(2):295–9. https://doi.org/10.1016/j.ijhm.2004.06.004.
Guéguen N, Meineri S, Charles-Sire V. Improving medication adherence by using practitioner nonverbal techniques: a field experiment on the effect of touch. J Behav Med. 2010;33(6):466–73. https://doi.org/10.1007/s10865-010-9277-5.
Guéguen N, Afifi F, Brault S, Charles-Sire V, Leforestier PM, Morzedec A, Piron E. Failure of tactile contact to increase request compliance: the case of blood donation behavior. J Articles Supp Null Hypothesis. 2011;8(1):1–8.
Guzmán-García A, Hughes JC, James IA, Rochester L. Dancing as a psychosocial intervention in care homes: a systematic review of the literature. Int J Geriatr Psychiatry. 2013;28(9):914–24. https://doi.org/10.1002/gps.3913.
Haans A, Ijsselsteijn W. Mediated social touch: a review of current research and future directions. Virtual Reality. 2006;9(2–3):149–59. https://doi.org/10.1007/s10055-005-0014-2.
Halbesleben JRB, Rathert C. Linking physician burnout and patient outcomes: exploring the dyadic relationship between physicians and patients. Health Care Manage Rev. 2008a;33(1):29–39. https://doi.org/10.1097/01.HMR.0000304493.87898.72.
Halbesleben JRB, Rathert C. The role of continuous quality improvement and psychological safety in predicting work-arounds. Health Care Manage Rev. 2008b;33(2):134–44. https://doi.org/10.1097/01.HMR.0000304505.04932.62.
Hall JA. Touch, status, and gender at professional meetings. J Nonverbal Behav. 1996;20(1):23–44. https://doi.org/10.1007/BF02248713.
Harlow HF. The nature of love. Am Psychol. 1958;13(12):673–85. https://doi.org/10.1037/h0047884.
Hartnett JJ, Bailey KG, Gibson FW. Personal space as influenced by sex and type of movement. J Psychol. 1970;76(2):139–44. https://doi.org/10.1080/00223980.1970.9916831.
Haughie E, Milne D, Elliott V. An evaluation of companion pets with elderly psychiatric patients. Behav Cogn Psychother. 1992;20(4):367–72. https://doi.org/10.1017/s0141347300017511.
Headey B. Health benefits and health cost savings due to pets: preliminary estimates from an Australian National Survey. Soc Indic Res. 1999;47(2):233–43.
Headey B, Grabka M, Kelley J, Reddy P, Tseng YP. Pet ownership is good for your health and saves public expenditure too: Australian and German longitudinal evidence. Aust Soc Monit. 2002;5(4):93–9.
Henley NM. Status and sex: some touching observations. Bull Psychon Soc. 1973;2(2):91–3. https://doi.org/10.3758/bf03327726.
Hill RA, Dunbar RIM. Social network size in humans. Hum Nat. 2003;14(1):53–72. https://doi.org/10.1007/s12110-003-1016-y.
Hollinger LM, Buschmann MBT. Factors influencing the perception of touch by elderly nursing home residents and their health caregivers. Int J Nurs Stud. 1993;30(5):445–61. https://doi.org/10.1016/0020-7489(93)90054-x.
Holt-Lunstad J. The potential public health relevance of social isolation and loneliness: prevalence, epidemiology, and risk factors. Public Policy Aging Rep. 2017;27(4):127–30. https://doi.org/10.1093/ppar/prx030.
Holt-Lunstad J, Smith TB, Layton JB. Social relationships and mortality risk: a meta-analytic review. PLoS Med. 2010;7:e1000316. https://doi.org/10.1371/journal.pmed.1000316.

Holt-Lunstad J, Smith TB, Baker M, Harris T, Stephenson D. Loneliness and social isolation as risk factors for mortality: a meta-analytic review. Perspect Psychol Sci. 2015;10(2):227–37. https://doi.org/10.1177/1745691614568352.

Hornik J. The effect of touch and gaze upon compliance and interest of interviewees. J Soc Psychol. 1987;127(6):681–3.

Hornik J. Tactile stimulation and consumer response. J Consum Res. 1992;19(3):449. https://doi.org/10.1086/209314.

Hostinar CE, Sullivan RM, Gunnar MR. Psychobiological mechanisms underlying the social buffering of the hypothalamic-pituitary-adrenocortical axis: a review of animal models and human studies across development. Psychol Bull. 2014;140(1):256–82. https://doi.org/10.1037/a0032671.

House JS, Landis KR, Umberson D. Social relationships and health. Science. 1988;241(4865):540–5. https://doi.org/10.1126/science.3399889.

Howard DM. The effects of touch in the geriatric population. Phys Occup Therapy Geriatr. 1988;6(2):35–50. https://doi.org/10.1080/j148v06n02_05.

Howe LC, Leibowitz KA, Crum AJ. When Your Doctor "Gets It" and "Gets You": the critical role of competence and warmth in the patient-provider interaction. Front Psych. 2019;10:475. https://doi.org/10.3389/fpsyt.2019.00475.

Hubble MA, Noble FC, Robinson SE. The effect of counselor touch in an initial counseling session. J Couns Psychol. 1981;28(6):533–5. https://doi.org/10.1037/0022-0167.28.6.533.

Huisman G. Social touch technology: a survey of haptic technology for social touch. IEEE Trans Haptics. 2017;10(3):391–408. https://doi.org/10.1109/toh.2017.2650221.

Hung L, Liu C, Woldum E, Au-Yeung A, Berndt A, Wallsworth C, et al. The benefits of and barriers to using a social robot PARO in care settings: a scoping review. BMC Geriatr. 2019;19(1):232. https://doi.org/10.1186/s12877-019-1244-6.

ICN. Nursing Definitions. International Council of Nurses. 2002. https://www.icn.ch/nursing-policy/nursing-definitions. Accessed 12 Apr 2021.

Ilkilic I, Takim A. Kultur und Gesundheit. Das Informations- und Beratungsangebot zur verbesserten Versorgung von Muslimen im deutschen Gesundheitswesen. Konfliktfelder in der Praxis. Institut für Geschichte, Theorie und Ethik der Medizin der Johannes Gutenberg-Universität Mainz. 2007. http://www.kultur-gesundheit.de/konfliktfelder_in_der_praxis/religioese_grundpflichten/schamgefuehl_und_intimsphaere.php. Accessed 12 Apr 2021.

Jakubiak BK, Feeney BC. Affectionate touch to promote relational, psychological, and physical well-being in adulthood: a theoretical model and review of the research. Pers Soc Psychol Rev. 2017;21(3):228–52. https://doi.org/10.1177/1088868316650307.

Kachouie R, Sedighadeli S, Khosla R, Chu M-T. Socially assistive robots in elderly care: a mixed-method systematic literature review. Int J Human Comput Interact. 2014;30(5):369–93. https://doi.org/10.1080/10447318.2013.873278.

Kamarck TW, Manuck SB, Jennings JR. Social support reduces cardiovascular reactivity to psychological challenge: a laboratory model. Psychosom Med. 1990;52(1):42–58. https://doi.org/10.1097/00006842-199001000-00004.

Kaptchuk TJ, Stason WB, Davis RB, Legedza ART, Schnyer RN, Kerr CE, et al. Sham device v inert pill: randomised controlled trial of two placebo treatments. BMJ. 2006;332(7538):391–7. https://doi.org/10.1136/bmj.38726.603310.55.

Kaptchuk TJ, Kelley JM, Conboy LA, Davis RB, Kerr CE, Jacobson EE, et al. Components of placebo effect: randomised controlled trial in patients with irritable bowel syndrome. BMJ. 2008;336(7651):999–1003. https://doi.org/10.1136/bmj.39524.439618.25.

Katsinas RP. The use and implications of a canine companion in a therapeutic day program for nursing home residents with dementia. Act Adapt Aging. 2000;25(1):13–30. https://ci.nii.ac.jp/naid/10024163120/.

Kelley K, Byrne D. Attraction and altruism: with a little help from my friends. J Res Pers. 1976;10(1):59–68. https://doi.org/10.1016/0092-6566(76)90082-9.

Kelly M, Tink W, Nixon L. Keeping the human touch in medical practice. Acad Med. 2014;89(10):1314. https://doi.org/10.1097/ACM.0000000000000454.

Kerr CE, Shaw JR, Conboy LA, Kelley JM, Jacobson E, Kaptchuk TJ. Placebo acupuncture as a form of ritual touch healing: a neurophenomenological model. Conscious Cogn. 2011;20(3):784–91. https://doi.org/10.1016/j.concog.2010.12.009.

Kiecolt-Glaser JK, Gouin J-P, Hantsoo L. Close relationships, inflammation, and health. Neurosci Biobehav Rev. 2010;35(1):33–8. https://doi.org/10.1016/j.neubiorev.2009.09.003.

Kim EJ, Buschmann MT. The effect of expressive physical touch on patients with dementia. Int J Nurs Stud. 1999;36(3):235–43. https://doi.org/10.1016/s0020-7489(99)00019-x.

Kingwell BA, Lomdahl A, Anderson WP. Presence of a pet dog and human cardiovascular responses to mild mental stress. Clin Auton Res. 2001;11(5):313–7. https://doi.org/10.1007/bf02332977.

Kirsch LP, Krahé C, Blom N, Crucianelli L, Moro V, Jenkinson PM, Fotopoulou A. Reading the mind in the touch: neurophysiological specificity in the communication of emotions by touch. Neuropsychologia. 2018;116(Pt A):136–49. https://doi.org/10.1016/j.neuropsychologia.2017.05.024.

Kleinke CL. Compliance to requests made by gazing and touching experimenters in field settings. J Exp Soc Psychol. 1977;13(3):218–23. https://doi.org/10.1016/0022-1031(77)90044-0.

Kohler J, Borchers F, Endres M, Weiss B, Spies C, Emmrich JV. Cognitive deficits following intensive care. Deutsches Arzteblatt Int. 2019;116(38):627–34. https://doi.org/10.3238/arztebl.2019.0627.

Kongable LG, Buckwalter KC, Stolley JM. The effects of pet therapy on the social behavior of institutionalized Alzheimer's clients. Arch Psychiatr Nurs. 1989;3(4):191–8.

Kontaris D, Harrison D, Patsoule EE, Zhuang S, Slade A. Feelybean: communicating touch over distance. Extended abstracts on human factors in computing systems. In: CHI'12 Extended Abstracts on human factors in computing systems; 2012. p. 1273–8.

Kramer BJ, Gibson JW. The cognitively impaired elderly's response to touch: a naturalistic study. J Gerontol Soc Work. 1991;18(2):175–93.

Kramer A, Heidecke C-D. Kampf gegen Krankenhauskeime: Der Patient gehört mit ins Boot. kma Klinik Management aktuell. 2016;21(11):94–6. https://doi.org/10.1055/s-0036-1594319.

Kramer SC, Friedmann E, Bernstein PL. Comparison of the effect of human interaction, animal-assisted therapy, and AIBO-assisted therapy on long-term care residents with dementia. Anthrozoös. 2009;22(1):43–57. https://doi.org/10.2752/175303708x390464.

Krichmar JL, Chou TS. A tactile robot for developmental disorder therapy. In: Proceedings of the technology, mind, and society conference. technology, mind & society, an interdisciplinary conference: April 2018, Washington, DC. New York, NY: The Association for Computing Machinery (ICPS); 2018.

Lange-Alberts ME, Shott S. Nutritional intake. Use of touch and verbal cuing. J Gerontol Nurs. 1994;20(2):36–40. https://doi.org/10.3928/0098-9134-19940201-08.

Langewitz W. Placebo—Nocebo. In: Köhle K, Herzog W, Joraschky P, Kruse J, Langewitz W, Söllner W, editors. Uexküll Psychosomatische Medizin. Theoretische Modelle und klinische Praxis. 8th ed. München: Elsevier; 2017. p. 475–81.

Langland RM, Panicucci CL. Effects of touch on communication with elderly confused clients. J Gerontol Nurs. 1982;8(3):152–5. https://doi.org/10.3928/0098-9134-19820301-09.

Larsen RJ, Kasimatis M, Frey K. Facilitating the furrowed brow: an unobtrusive test of the facial feedback hypothesis applied to unpleasant affect. Cognit Emot. 1992;6(5):321–38. https://doi.org/10.1080/02699939208409689.

Levine GN, Allen K, Braun LT, Christian HE, Friedmann E, Taubert KA, et al. Pet ownership and cardiovascular risk: a scientific statement from the American Heart Association. Circulation. 2013;127(23):2353–63. https://doi.org/10.1161/CIR.0b013e31829201e1.

Lewis RJ, Derlega VJ, Shankar A, Cochard E, Finkel L. Nonverbal correlates confederates' touch: confounds in touch research. J Soc Behav Pers. 1997;12(3):821–30.

Light KC, Grewen KM, Amico JA. More frequent partner hugs and higher oxytocin levels are linked to lower blood pressure and heart rate in premenopausal women. Biol Psychol. 2005;69(1):5–21. https://doi.org/10.1016/j.biopsycho.2004.11.002.

Lynch JJ, Thomas SA, Mills ME, Malinow K, Katcher AH. The effects of human contact on cardiac arrhythmia in coronary care patients. J Nerv Ment Dis. 1974;158(2):88–99. https://doi.org/10.1097/00005053-197402000-00002.

Makoul G, Zick A, Green M. An evidence-based perspective on greetings in medical encounters. Arch Intern Med. 2007;167(11):1172–6. https://doi.org/10.1001/archinte.167.11.1172.

Mallett J. Communication between nurses and post-anaesthetic patients. Intensive Care Nurs. 1990;6(1):45–53. https://doi.org/10.1016/0266-612x(90)90009-v.

Marr CA, French L, Thompson D, Drum L, Greening G, Mormon J, et al. Animal-assisted therapy in psychiatric rehabilitation. Anthrozoös. 2000;13(1):43–7. https://doi.org/10.2752/089279300786999950.

Marx MS, Werner P, Cohen-Mansfield J. Agitation and touch in the nursing home. Psychol Rep. 1989;64(3 Pt 2):1019–26. https://doi.org/10.2466/pr0.1989.64.3c.1019.

McCann K, McKenna HP. An examination of touch between nurses and elderly patients in a continuing care setting in Northern Ireland. J Adv Nurs. 1993;18(5):838–46. https://doi.org/10.1046/j.1365-2648.1993.18050838.x.

McConnell AR, Brown CM, Shoda TM, Martin CM, Stayton LE. Friends with benefits: on the positive consequences of pet ownership. J Pers Soc Psychol. 2011;101(6):1239–52. https://doi.org/10.1037/e683152011-002.

McCorkle R. Effects of touch on seriously ill patients. Nurs Res. 1974;23(2):125–31. https://doi.org/10.1097/00006199-197403000-00007.

Michalak J, Mischnat J, Teismann T. Sitting posture makes a difference-embodiment effects on depressive memory bias. Clin Psychol Psychother. 2014;21(6):519–24. https://doi.org/10.1002/cpp.1890.

Moerman CJ, van der Heide L, Heerink M. Social robots to support children's well-being under medical treatment: a systematic state-of-the-art review. J Child Health Care. 2019;23(4):596–612. https://doi.org/10.1177/1367493518803031.

Montagu A. Touching. The human significance of the skin. 2nd ed. New York: Harper & Row; 1978.

Moody WJ, Fenwick DC, Blackshaw JK. Pitfalls of studies designed to test the effect pets have on the cardiovascular parameters of their owners in the home situation: a pilot study. Appl Anim Behav Sci. 1996;47(1–2):127–36. https://doi.org/10.1016/0168-1591(95)01016-5.

Moore JR, Gilbert DA. Elderly residents: perceptions of nurses' comforting touch. J Gerontol Nurs. 1995;21(1):6–13. https://doi.org/10.3928/0098-9134-19950101-04.

Mujallad A, Taylor EJ. Modesty among Muslim women: implications for nursing care. Medsurg Nurs. 2016;25(3):169–72.

Nakadoi Y. Usefulness of animal type robot in the treatment in child and adolescent psychiatric ward. Eur Child Adolesc Psychiatry. 2015;1(24):281.

Nannberg JC, Hansen CH. Post-compliance touch: an incentive for task performance. J Soc Psychol. 1994;134(3):301–7. https://doi.org/10.1080/00224545.1994.9711734.

Nathans-Barel I, Feldman P, Berger B, Modai I, Silver H. Animal-assisted therapy ameliorates anhedonia in schizophrenia patients. A controlled pilot study. Psychother Psychosom. 2005;74(1):31–5. https://doi.org/10.1159/000082024.

Nilsen WJ, Vrana SR. Some touching situations: the relationship between gender and contextual variables in cardiovascular responses to human touch. Ann Behav Med. 1998;20(4):270–6. https://doi.org/10.1007/BF02886376.

Odendaal JSJ. Animal-assisted therapy—magic or medicine? J Psychosom Res. 2000;49(4):275–80. https://doi.org/10.1016/s0022-3999(00)00183-5.

Odendaal JSJ, Meintjes RA. Neurophysiological correlates of affiliative behaviour between humans and dogs. Vet J. 2003;165(3):296–301. https://doi.org/10.1016/s1090-0233(02)00237-x.

Okita SY. Self-other's perspective taking: the use of therapeutic robot companions as social agents for reducing pain and anxiety in pediatric patients. Cyberpsychol Behav Soc Netw. 2013;16(6):436–41. https://doi.org/10.1089/cyber.2012.0513.

Olshansky B. Placebo and nocebo in cardiovascular health: implications for healthcare, research, and the doctor-patient relationship. J Am Coll Cardiol. 2007;49(4):415–21. https://doi.org/10.1016/j.jacc.2006.09.036.

Paquet C, DA MK, Kergoat MJ, Ferland G, Dubé L. Direct and indirect effects of everyday emotions on food intake of elderly patients in institutions. J Gerontol A Biol Sci Med Sci. 2003;58(2):153–8. https://doi.org/10.1093/gerona/58.2.M153.

Parslow RA, Jorm AF. Pet ownership and risk factors for cardiovascular disease: another look. Med J Aust. 2003;179(9):466–8. https://doi.org/10.5694/j.1326-5377.2003.tb05649.x.

Patterson ML, Powell JL, Lenihan MG. Touch, compliance, and interpersonal affect. J Nonverbal Behav. 1986;10(1):41–50. https://doi.org/10.1007/bf00987204.

Pedersen DM, Heaston AB. The effects of sex of subject, sex of approaching person, and angle of approach upon personal space. J Psychol. 1972;82(2):277–86. https://doi.org/10.1080/00223980.1972.9923818.

Pennisi P, Tonacci A, Tartarisco G, Billeci L, Ruta L, Gangemi S, Pioggia G. Autism and social robotics: a systematic review. Autism Res. 2016;9(2):165–83. https://doi.org/10.1002/aur.1527.

Pensieri C, Delle Chiaie G, Vincenzi B, Nobile N, Benedictis A, D'aprile M, Alloni R. Doctor-patient communication tricks. Oncological study at Campus bio-Medico University of Rome. LCT. 2018;169(5):e224–30.

Prothmann A, Bienert M, Ettrich C. Dogs in child psychotherapy: effects on state of mind. Anthrozoös. 2006;19(3):265–77. https://doi.org/10.2752/089279306785415583.

Pschyrembel Klinisches Wörterbuch. 268. neu bearbeitete Auflage. Berlin, Boston: De Gruyter; 2020.

Richeson NE. Effects of animal-assisted therapy on agitated behaviors and social interactions of older adults with dementia. Am J Alzheimers Dis Other Demen. 2003;18(6):353–8. https://doi.org/10.1177/153331750301800610.

Riskind JH, Gotay CC. Physical posture: could it have regulatory or feedback effects on motivation and emotion? Motiv Emot. 1982;6(3):273–98. https://doi.org/10.1007/bf00992249.

Roberts KJ. Physician-patient relationships, patient satisfaction, and antiretroviral medication adherence among HIV-infected adults attending a public health clinic. AIDS Patient Care STDS. 2002;16(1):43–50. https://doi.org/10.1089/108729102753429398.

Robinson NL, Cottier TV, Kavanagh DJ. Psychosocial health interventions by social robots: systematic review of randomized controlled trials. J Med Internet Res. 2019;21(5):e13203. https://doi.org/10.2196/13203.

Robles TF, Kiecolt-Glaser JK. The physiology of marriage: pathways to health. Physiol Behav. 2003;79(3):409–16. https://doi.org/10.1016/s0031-9384(03)00160-4.

Rosenberger LA, Ree A, Eisenegger C, Sailer U. Slow touch targeting CT-fibres does not increase prosocial behaviour in economic laboratory tasks. Sci Rep. 2018;8(1):1–14. https://doi.org/10.1038/s41598-018-25601-7.

Roter DL, Frankel RM, Hall JA, Sluyter D. The expression of emotion through nonverbal behavior in medical visits. Mechanisms and outcomes. J Gen Intern Med. 2006;21 Suppl 1(1):28–34. https://doi.org/10.1111/j.1525-1497.2006.00306.x.

Routasalo P. Non-necessary touch in the nursing care of elderly people. J Adv Nurs. 1996;23(5):904–11. https://doi.org/10.1046/j.1365-2648.1996.00947.x.

Routasalo P, Isola A. The right to touch and be touched. Nurs Ethics. 1996;3(2):165–76. https://doi.org/10.1177/096973309600300209.

Routasalo PE, Savikko N, Tilvis RS, Strandberg TE, Pitkälä KH. Social contacts and their relationship to loneliness among aged people—a population-based study. Gerontology. 2006;52(3):181–7. https://doi.org/10.1159/000091828.

Sabanovic S, Bennett CC, Wan-Ling C, Huber L. PARO robot affects diverse interaction modalities in group sensory therapy for older adults with dementia. In: IEEE International Conference on Rehabilitation Robotics (ICORR). Seattle, WA/Piscataway, NJ: Institute of Electrical and Electronics Engineers/IEEE; 2013.

Sallnäs EL. Haptic feedback increases perceived social presence. In: Kappers AML, van Erp JBF, Bergmann Tiest WM, van der Helm FCT, editors. Haptics: generating and perceiving tangible sensations. Berlin, Heidelberg: Springer; 2010. p. 178–85.

Sams MJ, Fortney EV, Willenbring S. Occupational therapy incorporating animals for children with autism: a pilot investigation. Am J Occup Ther. 2006;60(3):268–74. https://doi.org/10.5014/ajot.60.3.268.

Sartorato F, Przybylowski L, Sarko DK. Improving therapeutic outcomes in autism spectrum disorders: enhancing social communication and sensory processing through the use of interactive robots. J Psychiatr Res. 2017;90:1–11. https://doi.org/10.1016/j.jpsychires.2017.02.004.

Savageau J, Ciociolo G, Sullivan IK, Tripathi A. Patient perspectives towards physician handshakes in the primary care setting. In: STFM conference on medical student education, Portland, OR; 2020. https://resourcelibrary.stfm.org/higherlogic/system/downloaddocumentfile.ashx?documentfilekey=9fd80ed5-71e7-a9f1-f48c-cd951d571e79&forcedialog=1. Accessed 12 Apr 2021.

Scheel K. Ethische Aspekte des Berührens. Der Schmerzpatient. 2019;2(02):62–5. https://doi.org/10.1055/a-0823-0744.

Scherer KR, Johnstone T, Klasmeyer G. Vocal expression of emotion. In: Davidson RJ, Goldsmith HH, editors. Handbook of affective sciences. Oxford, New York: Oxford University Press; 2003. p. 433–56.

Schoenhofer SO. Affectional touch in critical care nursing: a descriptive study. Heart Lung. 1989;18:146–54.

Schofield G, Mummery K, Steele R. Dog ownership and human health-related physical activity: an epidemiological study. Health Promot J Austr. 2005;16(1):15–9. https://doi.org/10.1071/he05015.

Schroeder J, Risen JL, Gino F, Norton MI. Handshaking promotes deal-making by signaling cooperative intent. J Pers Soc Psychol. 2019;116(5):743–68. https://doi.org/10.1037/pspi0000157.

Sklansky M, Nadkarni N, Ramirez-Avila L. Banning the handshake from the health care setting. JAMA. 2014;311(24):2477–8. https://doi.org/10.1001/jama.2014.4675.

Smith TW, Uchino BN, MacKenzie J, Hicks AM, Campo RA, Reblin M, et al. Effects of couple interactions and relationship quality on plasma oxytocin and cardiovascular reactivity: empirical findings and methodological considerations. Int J Psychophysiol. 2013;88(3):271–81. https://doi.org/10.1016/j.ijpsycho.2012.04.006.

Sorajjakool S, Carr MF, Nam JJ, Bursey E. World religions for healthcare professionals. 2nd ed. Abingdon, Oxon, New York: Routledge; 2017.

Soussignan R. Duchenne smile, emotional experience, and autonomic reactivity: a test of the facial feedback hypothesis. Emotion. 2002;2(1):52–74. https://doi.org/10.1037/1528-3542.2.1.52.

Spitz RA. The role of ecological factors in emotional development in infancy. Child Dev. 1949;20(3):S. 145. https://doi.org/10.2307/1125870.

Stein N, Sanfilipo M. Depression and the wish to be held. J Clin Psychol. 1985;41(1):3–9. https://doi.org/10.1002/1097-4679(198501)41:1<3::aid-jclp2270410102>3.0.co;2-m.

Stepper S, Strack F. Proprioceptive determinants of emotional and nonemotional feelings. J Pers Soc Psychol. 1993;64(2):211–20. https://doi.org/10.1037/0022-3514.64.2.211.

Steptoe A, Shankar A, Demakakos P, Wardle J. Social isolation, loneliness, and all-cause mortality in older men and women. Proc Natl Acad Sci. 2013;110(15):5797–801. https://doi.org/10.1073/pnas.1219686110.

Steward AL, Lupfer M. Touching as teaching: the effect of touch on Students' perceptions and performance. J Appl Social Pyschol. 1987;17(9):800–9. https://doi.org/10.1111/j.1559-1816.1987.tb00340.x.

Stolze H, editor. KBT Die Konzentrative Bewegungstherapie. Grundlagen und Erfahrungen. Dritte. ergänzte Auflage ed. Berlin, Heidelberg: Springer; 2002.

Storch M, Cantieni B, Hüther G, Tschacher W. Embodiment. Die Wechselwirkung von Körper und Psyche verstehen und nutzen. 3 unveränderte Auflage ed. Bern: Hogrefe; 2017.

Straatman I, Hanson EKS, Endenburg N, Mol JA. The influence of a dog on male students during a stressor. Anthrozoös. 1997;10(4):191–7. https://doi.org/10.2752/089279397787001012.

Strack F, Martin LL, Stepper S. Inhibiting and facilitating conditions of the human smile: a nonobtrusive test of the facial feedback hypothesis. J Pers Soc Psychol. 1988;54(5):768–77. https://doi.org/10.1037/0022-3514.54.5.768.

Suhonen K, Väänänen-Vainio-Mattila K, Mäkelä K. User experiences and expectations of vibrotactile, thermal and squeeze feedback in interpersonal communication. In: The 26th BCS Conference on Human Computer Interaction: BCS Learning & Development; 2012. p. 205–14.

Sumioka H, Nakae A, Kanai R, Ishiguro H. Huggable communication medium decreases cortisol levels. Sci Rep. 2013;3(1):3034. https://doi.org/10.1038/srep03034.

Sussman NM, Rosenfeld HM. Touch, justification, and sex: influences on the aversiveness of spatial violations. J Soc Psychol. 1978;106(2):215–25. https://doi.org/10.1080/00224545.1978.9924173.

Suvilehto JT, Glerean E, Dunbar RIM, Hari R, Nummenmaa L. Topography of social touching depends on emotional bonds between humans. Proc Natl Acad Sci U S A. 2015;112(45):13811–6. https://doi.org/10.1073/pnas.1519231112.

Suvilehto JT, Nummenmaa L, Harada T, Dunbar RIM, Hari R, Turner R, et al. Cross-cultural similarity in relationship-specific social touching. Proc Biol Sci. 2019;286(1901):20190467. https://doi.org/10.1098/rspb.2019.0467.

Takemura K. The effect of interpersonal sentiments on behavioral intention of helping behavior among Japanese students. J Soc Psychol. 1993;133(5):675–81. https://doi.org/10.1080/00224545.1993.9713922.

Thomas PA, Kim S. Lost touch? Implications of Physical Touch for Physical Health. J Gerontol B Psychol Sci Soc Sci. 2020;76:e111.

Turner DC, Rieger G, Gygax L. Spouses and cats and their effects on human mood. Anthrozoös. 2003;16(3):213–28. https://doi.org/10.2752/089279303786992143.
Uchino BN, Trettevik R, de Grey K, Robert G, Cronan S, Hogan J, Baucom BRW. Social support, social integration, and inflammatory cytokines: a meta-analysis. Health Psychol. 2018;37(5):462–71. https://doi.org/10.1037/hea0000594.
Victor C, Scambler S, Bond J, Bowling A. Being alone in later life: loneliness, social isolation and living alone. Rev Clin Gerontol. 2000;10(4):407–17. https://doi.org/10.1017/s0959259800104101.
Wada K, Shibata T, Saito T, Sakamoto K, Tanie K. Psychological and social effects of one year robot assisted activity on elderly people at a health service facility for the aged. In: IEEE International Conference on robotics and automation (ICRA). Barcelona, Spain, 18-22 April, 2005. Piscataway, NJ: IEEE Robotics and Automation Society; 2005.
Walsh PG, Mertin PG, Verlander DF, Pollard CF. The effects of a 'pets as therapy' dog on persons with dementia in a psychiatric ward. Aust Occup Ther J. 1995;42(4):161–6. https://doi.org/10.1111/j.1440-1630.1995.tb01331.x.
Wang R, Quek F. Touch & talk: contextualizing remote touch for affective interaction. In: Proceedings of the 4th International Conference on Tangible and Embedded Interaction 2010, Cambridge, MA, USA, January 24–27, 2010; 2010. p. 13–20.
Watson WH. The meanings of touch: geriatric nursing. J Commun. 1975;25(3):104–12. https://doi.org/10.1111/j.1460-2466.1975.tb00611.x.
Weekes DP, Kagan SH, James K, Seboni N. The phenomenon of hand holding as a coping strategy in adolescents experiencing treatment-related pain. J Pediatr Oncol Nurs. 1993;10(1):19–25. https://doi.org/10.1177/104345429301000105.
Whitcher SJ, Fisher JD. Multidimensional reaction to therapeutic touch in a hospital setting. J Pers Soc Psychol. 1979;37(1):87–96. https://doi.org/10.1037/0022-3514.37.1.87.
Wilda-Kiesel A, Tögel A, Wutzler U. Kommunikative Bewegungstherapie. Brücke zwischen Psychotherapie und Körpertherapie. 1st ed. Bern: Huber; 2011.
Wilhelm FH, Kochar AS, Roth WT, Gross JJ. Social anxiety and response to touch: incongruence between self-evaluative and physiological reactions. Biol Psychol. 2001;58(3):181–202. https://doi.org/10.1016/s0301-0511(01)00113-2.
Wilkes C, Kydd R, Sagar M, Broadbent E. Upright posture improves affect and fatigue in people with depressive symptoms. J Behav Ther Exp Psychiatry. 2017;54:143–9. https://doi.org/10.1016/j.jbtep.2016.07.015.
Williams GP, Kleinke CL. Effects of mutual gaze and touch on attraction, mood, and cardiovascular reactivity. J Res Pers. 1993;27(2):170–83. https://doi.org/10.1006/jrpe.1993.1012.
Willis FN, Briggs LF. Relationship and touch in public settings. J Nonverbal Behav. 1992;16(1):55–63. https://doi.org/10.1007/bf00986879.
Willis FN, Hamm HK. The use of interpersonal touch in securing compliance. J Nonverbal Behav. 1980;5(1):49–55. https://doi.org/10.1007/bf00987054.
Winkelmann C. Untersuchung zum Benefit durch digitale Ausstattung aus Sicht von Mitarbeitenden in Altenpflegeeinrichtungen. Poster. 124. München: Jahreskongress der Deutschen Gesellschaft für Physikalische und Rehabilitative Medizin; 2019.
Wycoff EB, Holley JD. Effects of flight Attendants' touch upon airline Passengers' perceptions of the attendant and the airline. Percept Mot Skills. 1990;71(3):932–4. https://doi.org/10.2466/pms.1990.71.3.932.
Yanes AF, Weil A, Furlan KC, Poon E, Alam M. Effect of stress ball use or hand-holding on anxiety during skin cancer excision: a randomized clinical trial. JAMA Dermatol. 2018;154(9):1045–9. https://doi.org/10.1001/jamadermatol.2018.1783.
Zhou L, Wei H, Zhang H, Li X, Bo C, Wan L, et al. The influence of expectancy level and personal characteristics on placebo effects: psychological underpinnings. Front Psych. 2019;10:20. https://doi.org/10.3389/fpsyt.2019.00020.
Zolnierek KB, Dimatteo MR. Physician communication and patient adherence to treatment: a meta-analysis. Med Care. 2009;47(8):826–34. https://doi.org/10.1097/mlr.0b013e31819a5acc.

Relevance of Touch During Pregnancy and Birth

6

Stephanie Margarete Mueller and Martin Grunwald

Contents

6.1 Effects of Manual Techniques in the Course of Pregnancy

The time of pregnancy as the earliest stage of human development can influence the individual's biological and psychological development into adulthood. From this perspective, good conditions for optimal development are desirable. Human touch and massage have the potential to trigger complex biochemical reactions in people of all ages. These reactions can positively affect the physical and psychological state of an individual (cf. Sect. 2.4). Furthermore, physical stimulation of the maternal body during pregnancy influences both the mother and the fetus.

S. M. Mueller (✉) · M. Grunwald
Haptic Research Lab, Paul-Flechsig-Institute for Brain Research, Leipzig University, Leipzig, Germany
e-mail: s.mueller@medizin.uni-leipzig.de; mgrun@medizin.uni-leipzig.de

S. M. Mueller et al., *Human Touch in Healthcare*, https://doi.org/10.1007/978-3-662-67860-2_6

6.1.1 Background: Consequences of Stress During Pregnancy

Stress, which could be triggered by interpersonal problems, extreme life events, or mental illnesses, is one of the main risk factors for the mother and child during pregnancy (for more details, see the box on the consequences of stress during pregnancy). For this reason, it is important to avoid stress during pregnancy as much as possible. However, since not all stress can be avoided, applying techniques that reduce stress and counteract its physiological consequences is a sensible strategy to employ. Physical activity (e.g., pregnancy yoga) and relaxation techniques (e.g., progressive muscle relaxation, autogenic training, and Feldenkrais) are possible options for stress reduction. Another option is relaxation massages (e.g., effleurage and Swedish massage). Problematically, massages are still often undervalued as simply being "feel-good" treatments, and their positive effects on biochemical, immunological, and hormonal processes are largely underestimated. Some physiotherapists and massage practitioners may refuse massage treatments for pregnant women out of fear of causing miscarriages, referencing alleged contraindications or knowledge taught in training. However, this fear is unfounded if a few key rules are observed (For more information on precautionary measures, see Sect. 6.1.7).

Consequences of Stress, Depression, and Anxiety During Pregnancy on the Fetus and Mother

Pregnancy Complications

Psychosocial stress, anxiety, and depression are among the main risk factors during pregnancy, and they affect both the health of the mother and the maturation and growth of the fetus (Coussons-Read et al. 2007, 2012; Field and Diego 2008; Lundy et al. 1999). The increased release of stress hormones during stress, anxiety, and depression is the leading cause of their negative consequences during pregnancy (Talge et al. 2007). High concentrations of stress hormones (cortisol, catecholamine, and norepinephrine) during pregnancy are likely related to the development of **pre-eclampsia and birth complications** (Glover 2015; Paarlberg et al. 1995). Pregnant women with insufficiently treated depression are also more prone to pregnancy complications (Bonari et al. 2004; Dennis and Dowswell 2013) and cesarean deliveries (Chung et al. 2001; Oberlander et al. 2006). Furthermore, maternal stress negatively affects pregnancy duration and may promote **preterm births** (Ruiz et al. 2003; Dayan et al. 2002; Wadhwa et al. 1998). Finally, stress and mental disorders are associated with increased alcohol, drug, and tobacco use during pregnancy.

Physical Development of the Fetus

In animal models, maternal stress hormones have been shown to delay fetal growth, lead to lower birth and brain weights, and negatively affect the development of the fetus's heart, blood vessels, and endocrine system (Kutzler et al. 2004; Jensen et al. 2002). In this regard, both few high doses of stress hormones and multiple low doses delivered over a long period of time negatively affected fetal development (Newnham and Moss 2001). Analogously, in humans, children of depressed mothers are born with **lower birth weight and smaller head circumferences** than children of healthy mothers (Bonari et al. 2004; Gilles et al. 2018), and they are also more likely to have respiratory distress or feeding difficulties (Oberlander et al. 2006). In addition, high maternal stress hormone concentrations during pregnancy are suspected to cause **vulnerability to chronic diseases** in the offspring (fetal programming) (Lesage et al. 2004). According to this hypothesis, prenatal stress alters fetal physiology in ways that increase the likelihood of cardiovascular, metabolic, and neuroendocrine diseases (such as coronary heart disease or type-2 diabetes) in the adult offspring (Cottrell and Seckl 2009;

Arck and Hecher 2014; Plagemann 2016; Entringer et al. 2008).

Emotional and Cognitive Effects

Diverse studies have shown that the concentrations of maternal biochemical messengers influence the biochemical conditions of the fetus (Lundy et al. 1999): For example, children whose mothers had increased cortisol and norepinephrine levels and low dopamine and serotonin levels are more likely to show depression-like symptoms after birth, as well as comparable neurotransmitter ratios to their mothers (Lundy et al. 1999; Ashman et al. 2002; Field 1998). In addition, depression during pregnancy can cause fetal growth retardation and delayed cognitive, motor, and emotional development in infancy and childhood (Evans et al. 2012; Lundy et al. 1999; Luoma et al. 2001; Field et al. 2009b). Other studies have shown that children whose mothers suffered from psychosocial stress or anxiety disorders during pregnancy are significantly more likely to experience **emotional and cognitive developmental disorders** such as anxiety, ADHD, and delays in language development (Talge et al. 2007; O'Connor et al. 2002; van den Bergh and Marcoen 2004). Prenatal maternal depression is also one of the strongest risk factors for postpartum depression, and postpartum depression itself poses significant risks for delayed development in infancy and toddlerhood (Beck 2001).

▶ **Important** Stress triggered by psychosocial factors (e.g., bullying, problematic relationships with the partner/family, and precarious work situation), dramatic life events (e.g., illness, death), and mental illness (including depression, anxiety disorder, and addiction), increases the likelihood of pregnancy complications, premature birth, and developmental disorders in the fetus and infant. The consequences can continue into the offspring's adulthood.

6.1.2 In Vitro Fertilization

In addition to biological factors, psychological stress can negatively affect the reproductive system of both men and women and reduce fertility (Fogarty 2018). This is also true for the process of artificial insemination. It is well known that many patients undergoing in vitro fertilization (IVF) are under considerable emotional pressure, and the resulting mental and physical tension has been suggested as one possible reason for the high IVF failure rates.

To date, only one group of researchers has investigated whether relaxing massages can increase the success of IVF (Okhowat et al. 2015). In that study, the participating women were not massaged using traditional manual techniques but lay on an andullation table for 30 min immediately before the fertilized eggs were transferred to the uterus. During the andullation treatment, the person lays on a mattress that delivers multidirectional stochastic vibrations (10–80 Hz), and infrared light is used to warm the muscles to increase the relaxation effect of the whole-body vibration. In this study, significantly higher pregnancy rates (58.9% vs. 41.7%) and birth rates (32.0% vs. 20.3%) were reported in the group treated with andullation compared to the control group. However, the reliability of the effect needs to be tested in further studies.

▶ **Important** Relaxation massage, whole body vibration, and infrared therapy immediately before the fertilized eggs are implanted may increase the likelihood of successful IVF pregnancy.

6.1.3 Prevention of Pregnancy Complications

Even when pregnancies proceed without complications and the women are not exposed to any particular stress, relaxation procedures have a positive effect on the development of the fetus and the health of the mother (Fink et al. 2012; Mueller and Grunwald 2019, 2021).

Four studies have explicitly investigated the effects of full-body massage on psychologically and physically healthy pregnant women. In the earliest study, the women received 20-min massage treatments twice per week for 5 weeks (Field et al. 1999), and their outcomes were compared to those of a control group that performed guided progressive muscle relaxation (PMR) twice per week. At the end of the study, the women in the massage group showed the following outcomes:

- Less anxiety.
- Higher dopamine levels.
- Better mood.
- Calmer and deeper sleep.
- Less leg and back pain.
- Lower norepinephrine levels.
- Fewer birth complications.
- A lower preterm birth rate.
- Fewer postnatal complications in the infants.

In the PMR control group, positive effects of the treatment were found only for leg pain, anxiety, and dopamine levels (Field et al. 1999).

Positive effects of relaxation massage on pregnancy-related anxiety, sleep difficulties, and back pain have been confirmed by other studies (Khojasteh et al. 2016; El-Hosary et al. 2016). In addition, significant improvements have been shown for headaches and muscle spasms but not for joint pain (El-Hosary et al. 2016).

Another study compared the cortisol and immunoglobulin A (IgA) levels of women treated with massage (intervention group) and women who received standard medical care (control group). Women in the intervention group received a 70-min massage with aroma oil (2% lavender oil; for precautions on massage during pregnancy, see Sect. 6.1.7) every other week (10 times in total) from 16 weeks to 36 weeks of pregnancy. Immediately following each intervention, **reduced cortisol and increased IgA levels** were measured. In the intervention group, the IgA levels also increased continuously across the 10 measurement time points, suggesting a cumulative positive effect of regular massage on the immune system (Chen et al. 2017).

▶ **Important** Massages during pregnancy strengthen the immune system of pregnant women, improve mood, reduce stress hormones, reduce leg and back pain, and reduce the premature birth rate.

6.1.3.1 What Is the Partner Allowed to Do at Home?

For pregnant women, the partner or another trusted person can perform gentle stroking massages of the head, face, neck, shoulders, back, sacrum, hands, and feet. Relaxation massages in the area of the lower back and foot massages are particularly beneficial. Due to the **increased risk of thrombosis** during pregnancy, vigorous massages of the legs and arms should be avoided as a precaution. For further precautions for massage during pregnancy, see Sect. 6.1.7.

Application Example: Partner Massage
The pregnant woman lies down on one side of her body with her legs slightly bent. The position can be stabilized with pillows behind the back and between the knees and ankles. The head, shoulder, back, hand, and feet are massaged successively. After 10 min, the woman turns to the other side, and the massage is repeated.

Frequency: Once or twice a week between the 16th week and 36th week of pregnancy.

Note! Crucial for the effectiveness of the massage is the application of medium pressure that is perceived as pleasant and not painful. Mutual interaction through communication is essential to avoid pain and ensure pleasant relaxation. The safety precautions for massage during pregnancy should also be observed (Sect. 6.1.7). ◄

6.1.4 Pregnancy-Related Pain

Many pregnant women wish to use physical therapy to relieve lower back and pelvic girdle pain, especially later in pregnancy. In Sect. 6.1.3, study results were reported showing that relaxation massages can reduce pregnancy-related back and leg pain. However, some physical therapists avoid treating pregnant women due to concerns about inducing preterm labor. One of the underlying fears in this context is that the treatment may be too intense or strenuous, which could harm the mother or baby. Pregnancy is always a relative contraindication for manual therapy; as a result, consultations with the treating gynecologist are advisable to determine whether a certain manual treatment is safe during pregnancy. However, intense manual therapy treatments may not be necessary to achieve the desired pain relief. Recent meta-analyses suggest that even gentle massaging treatments can significantly reduce pain in the lower back and pelvic girdle (Liddle and Pennick 2015; Hall et al. 2016; Keifel et al. 2020, among others). In this regard, **massages are more successful than relaxation techniques** (PMR) and **as successful as gymnastic exercises**. It should be emphasized that no manual therapy techniques were used in the cited studies (Hall et al. 2016), despite the fact that the title of the review article suggests that. The studies included in the meta-analysis were based only on gentle osteopathic manipulation techniques and Swedish massage techniques with moderate pressure (without inducing pain). Interestingly, when comparing osteopathic manipulation techniques and placebo ultrasound (i.e., moving the scanning device across the lower back without emitting ultrasound), large pain-reducing effects were found for both of these two techniques. Consistent with the positive effects of relaxation massage on pregnancy-related pain, the findings of the meta-analysis suggest that **mild to moderate touch interventions** are sufficient to reduce headache, back pain, and pelvic girdle pain and to prevent muscle spasms. Accordingly, pregnancy-related discomfort can be alleviated without using intensive manual therapy techniques.

▶ **Important** Relaxation massages are more effective than manual therapy and progressive muscle relaxation, and just as effective as gymnastic exercises in reducing pregnancy-related pain.

6.1.5 Massage for Prenatal Depression

Depression and other affective disorders during pregnancy are risk factors for both adverse maternal health and child development outcomes (cf. Sect. 6.1.1). Long-term studies have demonstrated the association of maternal depressive symptoms and pregnancy complications, premature births, forceps and cesarean deliveries, smaller child head circumference, lower birth weight, postpartum depression, and attachment disorders between the mother and child (Smorti et al. 2019).

Complicating matters, the use of **selective serotonin reuptake inhibitors** (SSRIs; antidepressants) during pregnancy is suspected of negatively affecting fetal development and increasing the likelihood of pregnancy complications (Oberlander et al. 2006; Hendrick et al. 2003a, b; Auerbach et al. 1992; Previti et al. 2014). For this reason, the search for complementary treatments that can be used in support of psychotherapeutic approaches is urgent.

Studies investigating the effects of relaxation massage on clinical depression during pregnancy have confirmed the same effects as those observed in healthy pregnant women. Accordingly, pregnant women with depression treated with massage tend to report **lower depression and anxiety scores** (Field et al. 1996, 2004, 2008, 2012) and less leg and back pain during pregnancy than pregnant women with depression who are not treated with massage. Massage treatments also increase the willingness of pregnant women with depression to regularly attend concurrent psychotherapy sessions and continue them for several weeks (Field et al. 2009a). In one study, the group that received both relaxation massage and psychotherapy showed more extensive reductions in depression, anxiety, and cortisol levels than the control group treated with psychotherapy alone (Field et al. 2009a). The results of another study also confirm the positive effect of massage on reducing the cortisol and norepinephrine levels and increasing the concentration of dopamine and serotonin in pregnant women with depression, which underlines the findings of lower anxiety and depression after massage treatment (Field et al. 2004).

Furthermore, the effects of the massage treatments persist beyond birth in both the mother and the children; in particular, mothers who have received massage during pregnancy tend to show **lower levels of postpartum depression** and **lower postpartum cortisol concentrations** than control mothers (Field et al. 2012). (For effects on fetal development, see Sect. 6.1.6.)

> **Important** The positive effects of massage treatments are often underestimated and need to be optimally utilized. A change in perception is needed so that more people can access the positive physiological and psychological effects of massage (Mueller and Grunwald 2021).

6.1.6 Effects on the Maturation of the Fetus

Massages during pregnancy not only have a positive effect on the well-being, immune system, and pregnancy progress of the expectant mother. Regular relaxation massages can also have a positive effect on the development and growth of the fetus.

Many studies describe the adverse consequences of maternal stress on the development of the fetus. In turn, the relaxing effects of massages can reduce the adverse biological effects of stress (Sect. 6.1.1). The effects of regular massage on fetal development have been studied primarily in pregnant women with depression. However, it can be assumed that the direction of the effects of massage would be similar for other psychosocial stressors. In particular, it has been shown that women with depression who undergo regular treatment with relaxation massages during pregnancy have a **lower incidence of preterm birth** and give birth to **children with higher birth weights** than women in the control groups. Similar positive effects can be achieved through 20-min yoga exercises once or twice per week (Field et al. 2009b, 2012). In addition, the newborns of depressed mothers who received massage treatments during their pregnancy tend to show lower cortisol levels several days after birth and score better on behavioral and neurological assessments than infants of mothers with depression who did not receive massages during pregnancy (Field et al. 2006, 2009b).

> **Important** Massage during pregnancy can reduce the concentration of stress hormones in the mother and fetus. This facilitates the growth and development of the fetus and promotes a longer stay in the womb, as well as improving the mother–child bond. In addition, postnatally, newborns of mothers who have undergone regular massage during pregnancy show better results in neurological and behavioral tests (cf. Fig. 6.1).

6.1.7 Precautions for Massage During Pregnancy

Studies investigating the effects of massage during pregnancy usually exclude women with complicated pregnancies or pre-existing complications (e.g., placenta previa, preterm labor, and blood clotting disorders). Accordingly, there are no scientifically based results to determine whether relaxation massages would alleviate or aggravate complicated pregnancies. Currently, only one study exists (non-randomized, no control group) in which hospitalized women (high-risk pregnancies) were provided with various touch interventions (Schlegel et al. 2016). The women received Swedish massage therapy, reflexology, or Reiki (hands laying on the body), and no adverse side effects were observed in any of the women.

To prevent adverse side effects during outpatient care, practitioners should consult the attending gynecologist to learn about the complications and risk factors of each individual's pregnancy. Since new complications may arise during the course of pregnancy, it is always advisable to keep the dialogue going with the pregnant woman and the attending doctor. Furthermore, which treatments are safe should be decided on a case-by-case basis. In uncomplicated pregnancies, massages are *not* contraindicated over the entire course of pregnancy (Fogarty et al. 2019, 2023).

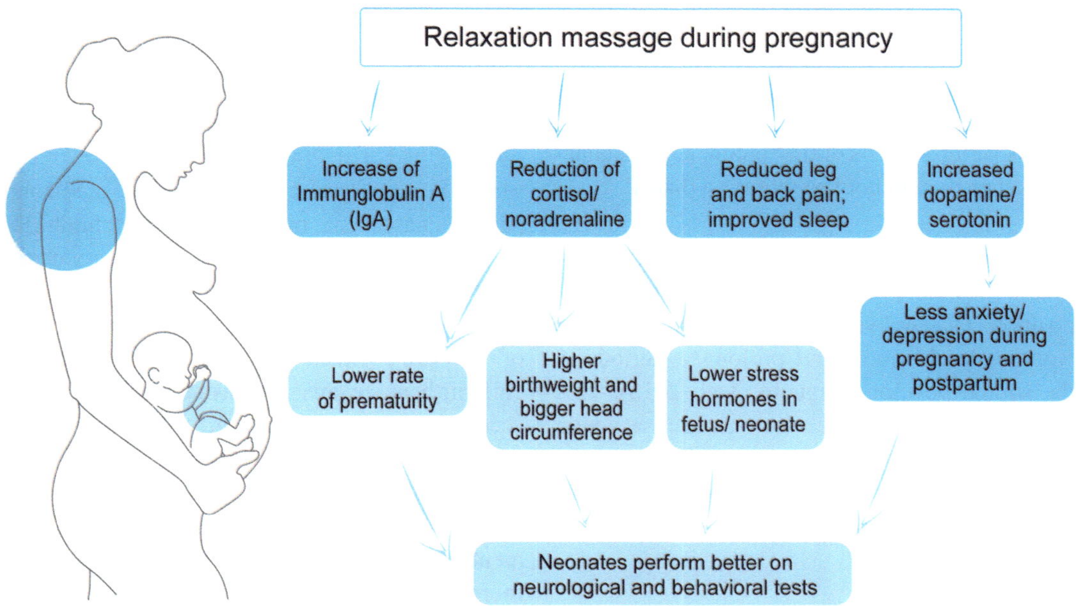

Fig. 6.1 Effects of pregnancy massages. Effects that can be achieved through relaxation massages during pregnancy for the mother (dark blue) and child (light blue). (Fig. adapted from Mueller and Grunwald 2019)

For these women, the determining factor for choosing an intervention is what feels good to the individual and what she finds pleasant and not painful.

However, some fundamental precautions must always be considered:

6.1.7.1 Risk of Thrombosis

Pulmonary embolism secondary to deep vein thrombosis (DVT) is the leading cause of death during pregnancy in industrialized countries (Devis and Knuttinen 2017). The likelihood of developing deep vein thrombosis is increased fivefold during pregnancy (Devis and Knuttinen 2017). Additionally, it can be difficult to diagnose DVT because the symptoms (including leg swelling, leg pain, and back pain) can also occur in healthy pregnant women. Leg massages during pregnancy can be life-threatening if DVT occurs and goes undetected (Sutham et al. 2020). Therefore, no massages should be performed on the arms and especially the legs with pressure into the deep muscles to avoid loosening possible blood clots or causing hematomas. However, superficial lymphatic drainage and gentle, stroking, circular touches are possible to relieve edema (Sutham et al. 2020).

6.1.7.2 Avoid Massage of the Abdomen

During pregnancy, the abdomen should not be massaged, only stroked. This is because heavy pressure can cause the uterus or placenta to rupture, resulting in the termination of pregnancy or even the death of the mother (Ugboma and Akani 2004).

6.1.7.3 Whole-Body Vibration (Andullation)

Whole-body vibration in the form of andullation during pregnancy is usually discouraged by product providers. However, no studies exist showing negative effects of andullation during pregnancy. On the contrary, studies investigating sporting activity during pregnancy have shown protective effects on preterm birth rates, even though many of the sports are associated with considerable body vibrations (including jogging, cycling, handball, volleyball, and tennis) (Misra et al. 1998; Hegaard et al. 2008; Juhl et al. 2008). Furthermore, since the risk of overstraining, injury, and falling during sporting activity is considerably higher than during relaxation-promoting vibration treatment, a general risk due to andullation cannot be assumed. However, systematic studies are not yet available.

▶ **Important** *Note!* Vibration plates, which serve as training and fitness equipment, are also referred to as "whole-body vibration" by some suppliers. However, due to the increased risk of thrombosis during pregnancy, pregnant women should not use vibration plates!

6.1.7.4 Lateral Position

Massages should only be performed in the lateral position. To avoid vena cava syndrome, pregnant women should not spend prolonged periods in the supine position (Higuchi et al. 2015). This also applies to other interventions, such as dental work. In addition, pregnant women should not be massaged in a prone position because many perceive it as uncomfortable, which, thus, hinders relaxation.

6.1.7.5 Acupressure and Reflexology

Some practitioners believe that stimulating specific acupressure points or reflex zones could induce labor during pregnancy. However, to date, no scientific studies have confirmed this belief. A randomized controlled trial found no effect of acupressure on the onset of labor within 97 h after treatment (Torkzahrani et al. 2017). Interestingly, during the birth process, acupressure can have a pain-relieving effect (Smith et al. 2011) (see also Sect. 6.2.1). In studies in which pregnant women received foot reflexology massages, no adverse effects on the course of pregnancy were found (Shobeiri et al. 2017; Mollart 2003).

6.1.7.6 Essential Oils

Highly concentrated essential oils (aromatherapy) should not be used for massages during pregnancy, as some aroma oils are suspected to be labor-inducing and many pregnant women are very sensitive to smell. However, massages with highly diluted essential oils (e.g., 2% lavender oil) have not been found to have any adverse side effects in studies (Chen et al. 2017), so these types of oils could be used for massages, as long as the concentration of the oils is carefully controlled and the expectant mother approves. During the birth process, aromatic oils (inhalation and massage) may be perceived as pain-reducing and relaxing (Dhany et al. 2012).

6.2 Birth

6.2.1 Manual Techniques Such as Acupressure and Effleurage

Many women try to avoid invasive or medicinal pain management methods during childbirth, and, thus, the popularity of complementary methods for pain reduction is high. Although the number of studies devoted to examining the efficacy of non-drug-related pain management during childbirth is steadily increasing, few studies of acceptable methodological quality exist. Nevertheless, those studies with acceptable methodological quality have systematically shown positive effects of non-drug-related pain management on **pain and anxiety reduction** and **increased satisfaction with the birth experience** (Mueller and Grunwald 2021). Specifically, such positive effects have been demonstrated for water birth, cognitive relaxation techniques, and acupuncture, but especially for acupressure and massage techniques (Jones et al. 2012).

In contrast, biofeedback, hypnosis, sterile water injections, aromatherapy (inhalation), and TENS (transcutaneous electrical nerve stimulation; Jones et al. 2012) have only been investigated in studies with poor methodological quality. Studies with inadequate research methods yield results that are unreliable, and consequently, no conclusions can be drawn about their validity or effect sizes.

6.2.1.1 Back, Hand, and Foot Massages

The effects of massage on reducing pain and anxiety during labor have been studied predominantly for the first stage of labor (dilation/active phase). For some women, massages are also pleasant during the transition phase of labor (second stage). For this purpose, the partner or another trusted person can perform **rhythmic stroking movements (effleurage)** with medium pressure on the preferred body regions. Massages of the shoulders, sacral region, hands, and feet are usually perceived as pleasant, and it is also possible to apply effleurage on the abdomen of the expectant mother during labor. Studies report that massage was applied for 20–30 min when contractions occurred (Field et al. 1997; Chang et al. 2002; Karami et al. 2008), and the mothers in the experimental groups reported significantly lower pain levels, less anxiety, and less tension during the first stage of labor than the women in the control groups (standard treatment).

Some findings also suggest that nonpharmacologic approaches may reduce the use of epidural anesthesia and obstetric instruments and reduce the likelihood of cesarean delivery (Chaillet et al. 2014; Smith et al. 2018a). Moreover, massage and cognitive relaxation methods may positively affect the **duration of labor** (Smith et al. 2018b; Chaillet et al. 2014). However, more standardized studies are required to draw firm conclusions regarding these effects.

6.2.1.2 Acupressure

Particularly strong effects on pain reduction during the latent phase (first stage of labor) can be achieved by acupressure. In several studies, one of three acupressure points (SP6, LI4, BL67, see Fig. 6.2) was treated for 30 min during each contraction. Women in the control groups were either touched only gently at acupressure points or given standard treatment. The results of these studies indicate that both gentle touch and acupressure can significantly reduce perceived pain during the first stage of labor (Hjelmstedt et al. 2010; Kashanian and Shahali 2009; Chung et al. 2003). However, in one study, acupressure produced stronger effects than gentle touch, and these effects were measurable both immediately and up to 2 h after the intervention (Hamidzadeh et al. 2012). Additionally, which specific acupressure points were treated did not affect the outcomes (Kim et al. 2002). For example, if the pregnant woman refused SP6 acupressure because the treatment was too uncomfortable, it was possible to stimulate one of the other points (Hjelmstedt et al. 2010). In all of the above studies, a significant shortening of the first stage of labor was also reported in women treated with acupressure.

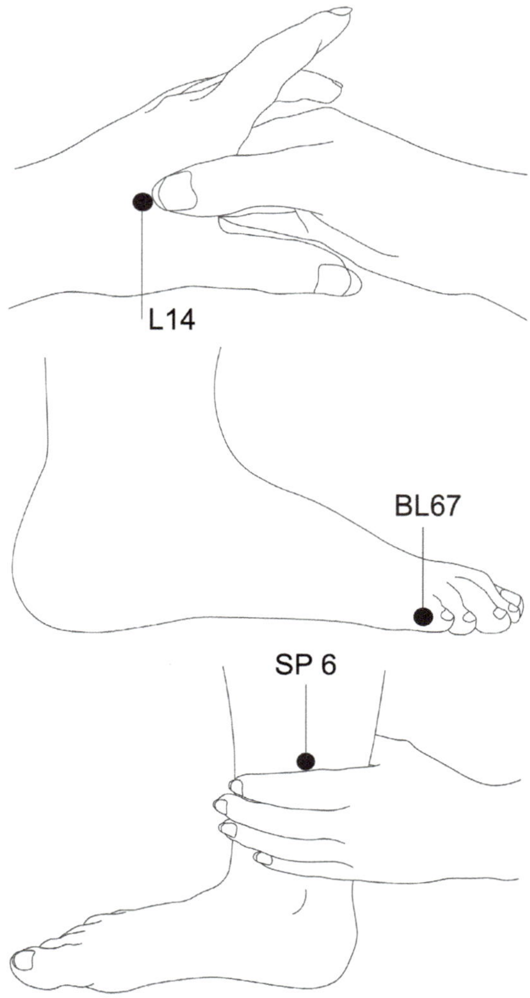

Fig. 6.2 Possible acupressure points for the treatment of labor pain. (Illustration: Anna Zender)

6.2.1.3 Social Support

Some research suggests that the experience and training of the person delivering the interventions are less important than the person's relationship with the expectant mother in terms of keeping the mother calm during labor. For example, studies on social support suggest that **close confidants** can elicit stronger calming effects than strangers in acutely stressful situations (Edens et al. 1992; Lepore et al. 1993). The quality of the relationship also plays a crucial role: if the relationship is predominantly harmonious, this may enhance the effectiveness of a relaxing intervention (Lidderdale and Walsh 1998). (For more details, see Sect. 5.5.)

> **Important** The quality of the relationship between the pregnant woman and the person performing the massage increases its effectiveness.

6.2.2 Perineal Massage

Most women experience pain and discomfort for several days to weeks after a vaginal birth. However, compared to women with an intact perineum, women who have suffered perineal injuries (perineal tear or incision) during childbirth report more severe pain, which can sometimes last 3 months or longer after delivery.

Higher-degree injuries (third or fourth degree perineal tears) are associated with longer healing times and a higher risk of complications and long-lasting impairments (Beckmann and Stock 2013). In addition to pain, fecal incontinence, which may last for years in some women, is the main burdening consequence. In addition, sexual functions can be impaired, or the pain can lead to sexual avoidance behavior.

In light of these issues, birthing techniques that reduce the likelihood of perineal injury are required. For example, the World Health Organization (WHO) discourages the routine performance of perineal incisions (World Health Organization 2018). Restrictions on the use of perineal incisions also reduce the need for surgical sutures and the complications associated with healing (Beckmann and Stock 2013). Moreover, a study of 6041 primiparous women found that a prolonged duration of expulsion (up to 5 h) did not have negative consequences (e.g., risk of suffocation) for the fetus. Consequently, arbitrary shortening of the expulsion phase should be avoided, and the use of instruments (forceps, suction cups) should be restrictive to prevent perineal injuries (Menticoglou et al. 1995).

Additionally, perineal massages can contribute to the prevention of perineal tears. The term perineal massages refers to two different techniques:

(a) Stretching exercises performed by the expectant mothers themselves during the last trimester.
(b) Manual techniques of the midwife or obstetrician during the expulsion phase.

6.2.2.1 Perineal Massage During Pregnancy

Application Example: Perineal Massage
Perineal massage should be performed at least once per week from the 34th week of pregnancy by the pregnant woman or her partner. To do this, the person inserts one or two fingers 3–4 cm (approximately 1 inch) into the vagina, and then, the walls of the vagina are alternately stretched backward (perineal) and sideways for 2 min each. Almond oil is recommended for lubrication. However, other oil- or water-based lubricants may be used. It should be noted that before the perineal massage, the hands should be carefully washed and made warm. Therefore, the treatment is best performed after bathing or showering. ◄

Perineal massage during the last trimester of pregnancy may reduce the likelihood of severe perineal injuries. In this regard, a lower incidence of perineal incisions was reported following the use of perineal massage among first-time mothers who delivered their babies in a clinic. This effect is likely due to several factors:

- Women who have learned perineal massage are likely to be better informed about birth practices, episiotomies, and the benefits of an intact perineum. They may be more willing, even against medical advice, to request a longer second stage of labor and to delay or refuse an episiotomy (Beckmann and Stock 2013).
- Perineal massages improve the elasticity of the perineum and thereby prevent injuries.

Some treatments that are specific to inpatient deliveries (e.g., oxytocin administration to accelerate the expulsion phase, epidural anesthesia, forceps delivery, and routine perineal incisions) increase the likelihood of perineal injuries. One study investigated only home births in order to exclude the possible influencing factors of hospital delivery. This study showed that women who had prenatally performed perineal massages had significantly fewer severe perineal injuries than women who did not use perineal massage during the last trimester (Davidson et al. 2000).

> **Important** Perineal massage during pregnancy can reduce the risk of injury (perineal incisions and tears) during childbirth (through increased elasticity of the perineum).

6.2.2.2 Perineal Massage During the Birth Process

During the birth process, some techniques may help prevent perineal injuries. However, the studies that exist to date are mostly of poor methodological quality, making conclusions about the effect sizes difficult. Nevertheless, preliminary evidence suggests that the application of warm compresses during the second stage of labor and perineal-protective manual techniques reduce the likelihood of third and fourth degree tears (Aasheim et al. 2017). For this reason, the WHO recommends the use of warm compresses as well as manual techniques (including perineal massage) to protect the perineum during the expulsion phase (World Health Organization 2018).

6.2.3 Cesarean Section and Vaginal Birth

Critical birth situations, such as a placenta previa or other factors that endanger the health of mother and child, can justify the medical decision to use a cesarean section. However, the cesarean section rate has been increasing globally since the 1990s. Countries with the highest rates of cesarean section are Brazil (55.6%), the Dominican Republic (56.4%), Egypt (51.8%), Iran (47.9%), Turkey (47.5%), Italy (38.1%), New Zealand (33.4%), and the United States (32.8%) (Betran et al. 2016). So-called "elective cesarean deliveries," which involve choosing a cesarean section delivery that is not medically motivated, are contributing to the worldwide increase in cesarean births (Betran et al. 2016).

The short-term outcome of cesarean and vaginal births is similar; in each case, the fetus must leave the mother's womb and start its vital functions immediately after birth. However, although these types of births are similar in their initial outcomes, they differ greatly in their potential consequences for the mother and child. Surgically assisted birth, especially elective cesarean delivery, is not physically demanding for the child. The careful removal of the child from the uterus causes only moderate physical sensations in the child. Indeed, if the cesarean section is planned, the fetus does not experience any anticipatory labor contractions. A cesarean delivery takes about 1 h, with the actual operation requiring only 15 min to 30 min from the initial abdominal incision to the cutting of the umbilical cord.

The situation is quite different for a child already positioned in the maternal pelvis and experiencing the eruptive contractions of maternal labor. The contractions of the maternal uterus begin many hours before the completion of labor and are intense physical events for both the mother and the fetus. Provided the fetal head is ideally located in the mother's pelvic region, the rhythmic and powerful contractions of the cervix and uterine wall result in intense haptic stimulation of the fetus's body and face. For the fetus, the continuous and impulsive facial and body stimulations during labor are probably as extraordinary as labor is for the mother. The total duration of labor can be 14 h or even longer for first-time mothers. Due to the contractions, the cervix finally pushes over the top of the fetus' head. In the expulsion phase, which is the last phase of natural birth, the number of contractions increases to six or seven every 15 min. In addition, strong and reflexive contractions of the maternal abdominal muscles occur and create the necessary pressure on the fetus's body to push the head, the shoulders, and the rest of the body through the birth canal. This process requires great physical effort for the mother and the fetus. The fetus' significantly increased heart rate during birth suggests that the large-scale deformation of its body, the successive increase in the expulsive pressure forces, and the partial lack of oxygen elicit a strong physiological reaction in the fetus.

However, as the fetus passes through the birth canal, not only physical stimuli are transmitted to it; but the mother's rich microbiological flora is also passed to the infant (Funkhouser and Bordenstein 2013; Ferretti et al. 2018; Wampach et al. 2018). The maternal bacterial cultures later colonize the oral mucosa and the intestine of the infant. In light of a steadily increasing number of cesarean births, increasing numbers of research projects are investigating whether these microbiological colonizations are beneficial or detrimental to the child's health (Funkhouser and Bordenstein 2013). During cesarean deliveries, the child is predominantly exposed to the mother's skin bacteria (Montoya-Williams et al. 2018). Therefore, scientific studies have discussed the possibility that the higher risk of people born via cesarean section suffering from asthma, diabetes, or autoimmune diseases could be related to the lack of transfer of maternal bacterial flora during birth (Sandall et al. 2018; Cardwell et al. 2008; Sevelsted et al. 2015). Systematic studies are currently investigating the impact of the subsequent transfer of vaginal bacterial flora in cesarean births on the health of children born via cesarean section (Dominguez-Bello et al. 2016).

The biological advantages of vaginal birth are also relevant for the respiratory function of the newborn. During the narrow passage through the birth canal in a vaginal birth, the amniotic fluid is squeezed out of the fetal lungs. In contrast, following a cesarean birth, the pulmonary alveoli may stick together due to the remaining amniotic fluid. The result is the respiratory dysfunction often seen in newborns delivered by cesarean section, which requires intensive medical care (Offermann et al. 2015). Finally, intensive medical care after cesarean section requires the physical separation of the newborn from the mother. In contrast, after vaginal delivery, the newborn's lung and respiratory function can oxygenate the blood immediately after birth through independent breathing.

References

Aasheim V, Nilsen ABV, Reinar LM, Lukasse M. Perineal techniques during the second stage of labour for reducing perineal trauma. Cochrane Database Syst Rev. 2017;6:CD006672. https://doi.org/10.1002/14651858.CD006672.pub3.

Arck PC, Hecher K. Pränatale, geschlechtsspezifische Programmierung und chronische Erkrankungen oder Finis Ab Orígine Pendet. Bundesgesundheitsblatt Gesundheitsforschung Gesundheitsschutz. 2014;57(9):1061–6. https://doi.org/10.1007/s00103-014-2015-3.

Ashman SB, Dawson G, Panagiotides H, Yamada E, Wilkinson CW. Stress hormone levels of children of depressed mothers. Dev Psychopathol. 2002;14(2):333–49.

Auerbach JG, Hans SL, Marcus J, Maeir S. Maternal psychotropic medication and neonatal behavior. Neurotoxicol Teratol. 1992;14(6):399–406.

Beck CT. Predictors of postpartum depression - an update. Nurs Res. 2001;50(5):275–85.

Beckmann MM, Stock OM. Antenatal perineal massage for reducing perineal trauma. Cochrane Database Syst Rev. 2013;4:CD005123. https://doi.org/10.1002/14651858.CD005123.pub3.

Betran AP, Torloni MR, Zhang JJ, Gülmezoglu AM. WHO statement on caesarean section rates. BJOG. 2016;123(5):667–70. https://doi.org/10.1111/1471-0528.13526.

Bonari L, Pinto N, Ahn E, Einarson A, Steiner M, Koren G. Perinatal risks of untreated depression during pregnancy. Can J Psychiatry. 2004;49(11):726–35.

Cardwell CR, Stene LC, Joner G, Cinek O, Svensson J, Goldacre MJ, et al. Caesarean section is associated with an increased risk of childhood-onset type 1 diabetes mellitus: a meta-analysis of observational studies. Diabetologia. 2008;51(5):726–35. https://doi.org/10.1007/s00125-008-0941-z.

Chaillet N, Belaid L, Crochetière C, Roy L, Gagné G-P, Moutquin JM, et al. Nonpharmacologic approaches for pain management during labor compared with usual care: a meta-analysis. Birth. 2014;41(2):122–37. https://doi.org/10.1111/birt.12103.

Chang M-Y, Wang S-Y, Chen C-H. Effects of massage on pain and anxiety during labour: a randomized controlled trial in Taiwan. J Adv Nurs. 2002;38(1):68–73. https://doi.org/10.1046/j.1365-2648.2002.02147.x.

Chen P-J, Chou C-C, Yang L, Tsai Y-L, Chang Y-C, Liaw J-J. Effects of aromatherapy massage on pregnant Women's stress and immune function: a longitudinal, prospective, randomized controlled trial. J Altern Complement Med. 2017;23(10):778–86. https://doi.org/10.1089/acm.2016.0426.

Chung TK, Lau TK, Yip AS, Chiu HF, Lee DT. Antepartum depressive symptomatology is associated with adverse obstetric and neonatal outcomes. Psychosom Med. 2001;63(5):830–4.

Chung U-L, Hung L-C, Kuo S-C, Huang C-L. Effects of LI4 and BL 67 acupressure on labor pain and uterine contractions in the first stage of labor. J Nurs Res. 2003;11(4):251–60. https://doi.org/10.1097/01.jnr.0000347644.35251.c1.

Cottrell EC, Seckl JR. Prenatal stress, glucocorticoids and the programming of adult disease. Front Behavior Neurosci. 2009;3(19):1–9. https://doi.org/10.3389/neuro.08.019.2009.

Coussons-Read ME, Okun ML, Nettles CD. Psychosocial stress increases inflammatory markers and alters cytokine production across pregnancy. Brain Behav Immun. 2007;21(3):343–50. https://doi.org/10.1016/j.bbi.2006.08.006.

Coussons-Read ME, Lobel M, Chris CJ, Kreither Marianne O, Kimberly D, Laura A, et al. The occurrence of preterm delivery is linked to pregnancy-specific distress and elevated inflammatory markers across gestation. Brain Behav Immun. 2012;26(4):650–9. https://doi.org/10.1016/j.bbi.2012.02.009.

Davidson K, Jacoby S, Brown MS. Prenatal perineal massage: preventing lacerations during delivery. J Obstet Gynecol Neonatal Nurs. 2000;29(5):474–9. https://doi.org/10.1111/j.1552-6909.2000.tb02768.x.

Dayan J, Creveuil C, Herlicoviez M, Herbel C, Baranger E, Savoye C, Thouin A. Role of anxiety and depression in the onset of spontaneous preterm labor. Am J Epidemiol. 2002;155(4):293–301.

Dennis C-L, Dowswell T. Interventions (other than pharmacological, psychosocial or psychological) for treating antenatal depression. Cochrane Database Syst Rev. 2013;7:CD006795. https://doi.org/10.1002/14651858.CD006795.pub3.

Devis P, Knuttinen MG. Deep venous thrombosis in pregnancy: incidence, pathogenesis and endovascular management. Cardiovasc Diagn Ther. 2017;7(Suppl 3):S309–19. https://doi.org/10.21037/cdt.2017.10.08.

Dhany AL, Mitchell T, Foy C. Aromatherapy and massage intrapartum service impact on use of analgesia and anesthesia in women in labor: a retrospective case note analysis. J Altern Complement Med. 2012;18(10):932–8. https://doi.org/10.1089/acm.2011.0254.

Dominguez-Bello MG, Jesus-Laboy KM, Shen N, Cox LM, Amir A, Gonzalez A, et al. Partial restoration of the microbiota of cesarean-born infants via vaginal microbial transfer. Nat Med. 2016;22(3):250–3. https://doi.org/10.1038/nm.4039.

Edens JL, Larkin KT, Abel JL. The effect of social support and physical touch on cardiovascular reactions to mental stress. J Psychosom Res. 1992;36(4):371–81.

El-Hosary EA, Soliman HFA, El-Homosy SM. Effect of therapeutic massage on relieving pregnancy discomforts. IOSR. 2016;05(04):57–64. https://doi.org/10.9790/1959-0504025764.

Entringer S, Wüst S, Kumsta R, Layes IM, Nelson EL, Hellhammer DH, Wadhwa PD. Prenatal psychosocial stress exposure is associated with insulin resistance in young adults. Am J Obstet Gynecol. 2008;199(5):498.e1–7. https://doi.org/10.1016/j.ajog.2008.03.006.

Evans J, Melotti R, Heron J, Ramchandani P, Wiles N, Murray L, Stein A. The timing of maternal depressive symptoms and child cognitive development. A longitudinal study. J Child Psychol Psychiatry. 2012;53(6):632–40. https://doi.org/10.1111/j.1469-7610.2011.02513.x.

Ferretti P, Pasolli E, Tett A, Asnicar F, Gorfer V, Fedi S, et al. Mother-to-infant microbial transmission from different body sites shapes the developing infant gut microbiome. Cell Host Microbe. 2018;24(1):133–145.e5. https://doi.org/10.1016/j.chom.2018.06.005.

Field T. Maternal depression effects on infants and early interventions. Prev Med. 1998;27(2):200–3. https://doi.org/10.1006/pmed.1998.0293.

Field T, Diego M. Cortisol: the culprit prenatal stress variable. Int J Neurosci. 2008;118(8):S. 1181. https://doi.org/10.1080/00207450701820944.

Field T, Grizzle N, Scafidi F, Schanberg S. Massage and relaxation therapies' effects on depressed adolescent mothers. Adolescence. 1996;31(124):903–11.

Field T, Hernandez-Reif M, Taylor S, Quintino O, Burman I. Labor pain is reduced by massage therapy. J Psychosom Obstet Gynaecol. 1997;18(4):286–91. https://doi.org/10.3109/01674829709080701.

Field T, Hernandez-Reif M, Hart S, Theakston H, Schanberg S, Kuhn C. Pregnant women benefit from massage therapy. J Psychosom Obstet Gynaecol. 1999;20(1):31–8.

Field T, Diego MA, Hernandez-Reif M, Schanberg S, Kuhn C. Massage therapy effects on depressed pregnant women. J Psychosom Obstet Gynaecol. 2004;25(2):115–22.

Field T, Hernandez-Reif M, Diego M. Newborns of depressed mothers who received moderate versus light pressure massage during pregnancy. Infant Behav Dev. 2006;29(1):54–8. https://doi.org/10.1016/j.infbeh.2005.07.004.

Field T, Figueiredo B, Hernandez-Reif M, Diego M, Deeds O, Ascencio A. Massage therapy reduces pain in pregnant women, alleviates prenatal depression in both parents and improves their relationships. J Bodyw Mov Ther. 2008;12(2):146–50. https://doi.org/10.1016/j.jbmt.2007.06.003.

Field T, Deeds O, Diego M, Hernandez-Reif M, Gauler A, Sullivan S, et al. Benefits of combining massage therapy with group interpersonal psychotherapy in prenatally depressed women. J Bodyw Mov Ther. 2009a;13(4):297–303. https://doi.org/10.1016/j.jbmt.2008.10.002.

Field T, Diego M, Hernandez-Reif M, Deeds O, Figueiredo B. Pregnancy massage reduces prematurity, low birthweight and postpartum depression. Infant Behav Dev. 2009b;32(4):454–60. https://doi.org/10.1016/j.infbeh.2009.07.001.

Field T, Diego M, Hernandez-Reif M, Medina L, Delgado J, Hernandez A. Yoga and massage therapy reduce prenatal depression and prematurity. J Bodyw Mov

Ther. 2012;16(2):204–9. https://doi.org/10.1016/j.jbmt.2011.08.002.

Fink NS, Urech C, Cavelti M, Alder J. Relaxation during pregnancy. What are the benefits for mother, fetus, and the newborn? A systematic review of the literature. J Perinat Neonatal Nurs. 2012;26(4):296–306. https://doi.org/10.1097/JPN.0b013e31823f565b.

Fogarty S. Fertility massage: an unethical practice? Int J Therapeut Massage Bodywork. 2018;11(1):17–20.

Fogarty S, McInerney C, Stuart C, Hay P. The side effects and mother or child related physical harm from massage during pregnancy and the postpartum period: an observational study. Complement Ther Med. 2019;42:89–94. https://doi.org/10.1016/j.ctim.2018.11.002.

Fogarty S, Werner R, James JL. Applying scientific rationale to the current perceptions and explanations of massage and miscarriage in the first trimester. Int J Therapeut Massage Bodywork Res Educ Pract. 2023;16(1):30–43.

Funkhouser LJ, Bordenstein SR. Mom knows best: the universality of maternal microbial transmission. PLoS Biol. 2013;11(8):e1001631. https://doi.org/10.1371/journal.pbio.1001631.

Gilles M, Otto H, Wolf IAC, Scharnholz B, Peus V, Schredl M, et al. Maternal hypothalamus-pituitary-adrenal (HPA) system activity and stress during pregnancy: effects on gestational age and infant's anthropometric measures at birth. Psychoneuroendocrinology. 2018;94:152–61. https://doi.org/10.1016/j.psyneuen.2018.04.022.

Glover V. Prenatal stress and its effects on the fetus and the child. Possible underlying biological mechanisms. Adv Neurobiol. 2015;10:269–83. https://doi.org/10.1007/978-1-4939-1372-5_13.

Hall H, Cramer H, Sundberg T, Ward L, Adams J, Moore C, et al. The effectiveness of complementary manual therapies for pregnancy-related back and pelvic pain: a systematic review with meta-analysis. Medicine. 2016;95(38):e4723. https://doi.org/10.1097/MD.0000000000004723.

Hamidzadeh A, Shahpourian F, Orak RJ, Montazeri AS, Khosravi A. Effects of LI4 acupressure on labor pain in the first stage of labor. J Midwifery Womens Health. 2012;57(2):133–8. https://doi.org/10.1111/j.1542-2011.2011.00138.x.

Hegaard HK, Hedegaard M, Damm P, Ottesen B, Petersson K, Henriksen TB. Leisure time physical activity is associated with a reduced risk of preterm delivery. Am J Obstet Gynecol. 2008;198(2):180.e1–5. https://doi.org/10.1016/j.ajog.2007.08.038.

Hendrick V, Smith LM, Suri R, Hwang S, Haynes D, Altshuler L. Birth outcomes after prenatal exposure to antidepressant medication. Am J Obstet Gynecol. 2003a;188(3):812–5. https://doi.org/10.1067/mob.2003.172.

Hendrick V, Stowe ZN, Altshuler LL, Hwang S, Lee E, Haynes D. Placental passage of antidepressant medications. Am J Psychiatry. 2003b;160(5):993–6. https://doi.org/10.1176/appi.ajp.160.5.993.

Higuchi H, Takagi S, Zhang K, Furui I, Ozaki M. Effect of lateral tilt angle on the volume of the abdominal aorta and inferior vena cava in pregnant and nonpregnant women determined by magnetic resonance imaging. Anesthesiology. 2015;122(2):286–93.

Hjelmstedt A, Shenoy ST, Stener-Victorin E, Lekander M, Bhat M, Balakumaran L, Waldenström U. Acupressure to reduce labor pain: a randomized controlled trial. Acta Obstet Gynecol Scand. 2010;89(11):1453–9. https://doi.org/10.3109/00016349.2010.514323.

Jensen EC, Gallaher BW, Breier BH, Harding JE. The effect of a chronic maternal cortisol infusion on the late-gestation fetal sheep. J Endocrinol. 2002;174(1):27–36.

Jones L, Othman M, Dowswell T, Alfirevic Z, Gates S, Newburn M, et al. Pain management for women in labour: an overview of systematic reviews. Cochrane Database Syst Rev. 2012;3:CD009234. https://doi.org/10.1002/14651858.CD009234.pub2.

Juhl M, Andersen PK, Olsen J, Madsen M, Jørgensen T, Nøhr EA, Andersen AM. Physical exercise during pregnancy and the risk of preterm birth: a study within the Danish National Birth Cohort. Am J Epidemiol. 2008;167(7):859–66. https://doi.org/10.1093/aje/kwm364.

Karami NK, Safarzadeh A, Fathizadeh N. Effect of massage therapy on severity of pain and outcome of labor in Primipara. Iran J Nurs Midwifery Res. 2008;12(1):6–9.

Kashanian M, Shahali S. Effects of acupressure at the Sanyinjiao point (SP6) on the process of active phase of labor in nulliparas women. J Matern Fetal Neonatal Med. 2009;23(7):638–41. https://doi.org/10.1080/14767050903277662.

Keifel F, Beyer L, Winkelmann C. Wirksamkeit klassischer Massagetherapie bei chronischen Rückenschmerzen und Funktionsstörungen im Bewegungssystem. Man Med. 2020;58(6):321–6. https://doi.org/10.1007/s00337-020-00732-z.

Khojasteh F, Rezaee N, Safarzadeh A, Sahlabadi R, Shahrakipoor M. Comparison of the effects of massage therapy and guided imagery on anxiety of nulliparous women during pregnancy. Depression. 2016;8(13):1–7.

Kim YR, Chang SB, Lee MK, Maeng WJ. Effects on labor pain and length of delivery time for Primipara women treated by san-yin-Jian(SP-6) acupressure and hob-Gog(LI-4) acupressure. Korean J Women Health Nurs. 2002;8(2):244–56. https://doi.org/10.4069/kjwhn.2002.8.2.244.

Kutzler MA, Ruane EK, Coksaygan T, Vincent SE, Nathanielsz PW. Effects of three courses of maternally administered dexamethasone at 0.7, 0.75, and 0.8 of gestation on prenatal and postnatal growth in sheep. Pediatrics. 2004;113(2):313–9.

Lepore SJ, Allen KA, Evans GW. Social support lowers cardiovascular reactivity to an acute stressor. Psychosom Med. 1993;55(6):518–24.

Lesage J, Del-Favero F, Leonhardt M, Louvart H, Maccari S, Vieau D, Darnaudery M. Prenatal stress induces

intrauterine growth restriction and programmes glucose intolerance and feeding behaviour disturbances in the aged rat. J Endocrinol. 2004;181(2):291–6.
Lidderdale JM, Walsh JJ. The effects of social support on cardiovascular reactivity and perinatal outcome. Psychol Health. 1998;13(6):1061–70. https://doi.org/10.1080/08870449808407450.
Liddle SD, Pennick V. Interventions for preventing and treating low-back and pelvic pain during pregnancy. Cochrane Database Syst Rev. 2015;2015(9):CD001139.
Lundy BL, Jones NA, Field T, Nearing G, Davalos M, Pietro PA, et al. Prenatal depression effects on neonates. Infant Behav Dev. 1999;22(1):119–29.
Luoma I, Tamminen T, Kaukonen P, Laippala P, Puura K, Salmelin R, Almqvist F. Longitudinal study of maternal depressive symptoms and child well-being. J Am Acad Child Adolesc Psychiatry. 2001;40(12):1367–74. https://doi.org/10.1097/00004583-200112000-00006.
Menticoglou SM, Manning F, Harman C, Morrison I. Perinatal outcome in relation to second-stage duration. Am J Obstet Gynecol. 1995;173(3):906–12. https://doi.org/10.1016/0002-9378(95)90364-x.
Misra DP, Strobino DM, Stashinko EE, Nagey DA, Nanda J. Effects of physical activity on preterm birth. Am J Epidemiol. 1998;147(7):628–35. https://doi.org/10.1093/oxfordjournals.aje.a009503.
Mollart L. Single-blind trial addressing the differential effects of two reflexology techniques versus rest, on ankle and foot oedema in late pregnancy. Complement Ther Nurs Midwifery. 2003;9(4):203–8. https://doi.org/10.1016/S1353-6117(03)00054-4.
Montoya-Williams D, Lemas DJ, Spiryda L, Patel K, Carney OO, Neu J, Carson TL. The neonatal microbiome and its partial role in mediating the association between birth by cesarean section and adverse pediatric outcomes. Neonatology. 2018;114(2):103–11. https://doi.org/10.1159/000487102.
Mueller SM, Grunwald M. Taktile Körperstimulation (Massage) in der Pränatal- und Geburtsmedizin. Man Med. 2019;57(4):254–9. https://doi.org/10.1007/s00337-019-0536-4.
Mueller SM, Grunwald M. Effects, side effects and contraindications of relaxation massage during pregnancy: A systematic review of randomized controlled trials. J Clin Med. 2021;10(16):3485. https://doi.org/10.3390/jcm10163485.
Newnham JP, Moss TJ. Antenatal glucocorticoids and growth. Single versus multiple doses in animal and human studies. Semin Neonatol. 2001;6(4):285–92. https://doi.org/10.1053/siny.2001.0064.
Oberlander TF, Warburton W, Misri S, Aghajanian J, Hertzman C. Neonatal outcomes after prenatal exposure to selective serotonin reuptake inhibitor antidepressants and maternal depression using population-based linked health data. Arch Gen Psychiatry. 2006;63(8):898–906.
O'Connor TG, Heron J, Golding J, Beveridge M, Glover V. Maternal antenatal anxiety and children's behavioural/emotional problems at 4 years—report from the Avon longitudinal study of parents and children. Br J Psychiatry. 2002;180:502–8.
Offermann H, Gebauer C, Pulzer F, Bläser A, Thome U, Knüpfer M. Cesarean section increases the risk of respiratory adaptive disorders in healthy late preterm and two groups of mature newborns. Z Geburtshilfe Neonatol. 2015;219(6):259–65. https://doi.org/10.1055/s-0035-1545323.
Okhowat J, Murtinger M, Schuff M, Wogatzky J, Spitzer D, Vanderzwalmen P, et al. Massage therapy improves in vitro fertilization outcome in patients undergoing blastocyst transfer in a cryo-cycle. Altern Ther Health Med. 2015;21(2):16–22.
Paarlberg KM, Vingerhoets AJJMD, Passchier J, Dekker GA, van Geijn HP. Psychosocial factors and pregnancy outcome: a review with emphasis on methodological issues. J Psychosom Res. 1995;39(5):563–95. https://doi.org/10.1016/0022-3999(95)00018-6.
Plagemann A. Grundlagen perinataler Prägung und Programmierung. Monatsschr Kinderheilkd. 2016;164(2):91–8. https://doi.org/10.1007/s00112-015-3419-3.
Previti G, Pawlby S, Chowdhury S, Aguglia E, Pariante CM. Neurodevelopmental outcome for offspring of women treated for antenatal depression. A systematic review. Arch Womens Ment Health. 2014;17(6):471–83. https://doi.org/10.1007/s00737-014-0457-0.
Ruiz RJ, Fullerton J, Dudley DJ. The interrelationship of maternal stress, endocrine factors and inflammation on gestational length. Obstet Gynecol Surv. 2003;58(6):415–28.
Sandall J, Tribe RM, Avery L, Mola G, Visser GHA, Homer CSE, et al. Short-term and long-term effects of caesarean section on the health of women and children. Lancet. 2018;392(10155):1349–57. https://doi.org/10.1016/S0140-6736(18)31930-5.
Schlegel ML, Whalen JL, Williamsen PM. Integrative therapies for women with a high risk pregnancy during antepartum hospitalization. Am J Matern Child Nurs. 2016;41(6):356. https://doi.org/10.1097/NMC.0000000000000279.
Sevelsted A, Stokholm J, Bønnelykke K, Bisgaard H. Cesarean section and chronic immune disorders. Pediatrics. 2015;135(1):e92–8. https://doi.org/10.1542/peds.2014-0596.
Shobeiri F, Manoucheri B, Parsa P, Roshanaei G. Effects of counselling and sole reflexology on fatigue in pregnant women: a randomized clinical trial. J Clin Diagn Res. 2017;11(6):QC01–4. https://doi.org/10.7860/JCDR/2017/22681.9972.
Smith CA, Collins CT, Crowther CA, Levett KM. Acupuncture or acupressure for pain management in labour. Cochrane Database Syst Rev. 2011;7:CD009232. https://doi.org/10.1002/14651858.CD009232.
Smith CA, Levett KM, Collins CT, Armour M, Dahlen HG, Suganuma M. Relaxation techniques for pain management in labour. Cochrane Database Syst Rev. 2018a;3:CD009514. https://doi.org/10.1002/14651858.CD009514.pub2.

Smith CA, Levett KM, Collins CT, Dahlen HG, Ee CC, Suganuma M. Massage, reflexology and other manual methods for pain management in labour. Cochrane Database Syst Rev. 2018b;3:CD009290. https://doi.org/10.1002/14651858.CD009290.pub3.

Smorti M, Ponti L, Tani F. Maternal depressive symptomatology during pregnancy is a risk factor affecting newborn's health: a longitudinal study. J Reprod Infant Psychol. 2019;37(4):444–52. https://doi.org/10.1080/02646838.2019.1581919.

Sutham K, Na-Nan S, Paiboonsithiwong S, Chaksuwat P, Tongsong T. Leg massage during pregnancy with unrecognized deep vein thrombosis could be life threatening: a case report. BMC Pregnancy Childbirth. 2020;20(1):237. https://doi.org/10.1186/s12884-020-02924-w.

Talge NM, Neal C, Glover V, Early Stress, Translational Research and Prevention Science Network: Fetal and Neonatal Experience on Child and Adolescent Mental Health. Antenatal maternal stress and long-term effects on child neurodevelopment. How and why? J Child Psychol Psychiatry. 2007;48(3–4):245–61. https://doi.org/10.1111/j.1469-7610.2007.01714.x.

Torkzahrani S, Mahmoudikohani F, Saatchi K, Sefidkar R, Banaei M. The effect of acupressure on the initiation of labor: a randomized controlled trial. Women Birth. 2017;30(1):46–50. https://doi.org/10.1016/j.wombi.2016.07.002.

Ugboma HA, Akani CI. Abdominal massage: another cause of maternal mortality. Niger J Med. 2004;13(3):259–62.

van den Bergh BRH, Marcoen A. High antenatal maternal anxiety is related to ADHD symptoms, externalizing problems, and anxiety in 8- and 9-year-olds. Child Dev. 2004;75(4):1085–97. https://doi.org/10.1111/j.1467-8624.2004.00727.x.

Wadhwa PD, Porto M, Garite TJ, Chicz-DeMet A, Sandman CA. Maternal corticotropin-releasing hormone levels in the early third trimester predict length of gestation in human pregnancy. Am J Obstet Gynecol. 1998;179(4):1079–85.

Wampach L, Heintz-Buschart A, Fritz JV, Ramiro-Garcia J, Habier J, Herold M, et al. Birth mode is associated with earliest strain-conferred gut microbiome functions and immunostimulatory potential. Nat Commun. 2018;9(1):5091. https://doi.org/10.1038/s41467-018-07631-x.

World Health Organization. WHO recommendation on episiotomy policy. Hg. v. WHO Reproductive Health Library, Geneva; 2018. https://apps.who.int/iris/bitstream/handle/10665/272447/WHO-RHR-18.12-eng.pdf?ua=1. Accessed 12 May 2021.

Relevance of Touch for Early Childhood Development

7

Stephanie Margarete Mueller and Martin Grunwald

Contents

Human neonates are neurologically and behaviorally altricial. Like other altricial mammals (e.g., dogs and cats), humans cannot move independently and purposefully or eat solid food after birth. Therefore, adult care is essential for the good physical and mental development of infants and young children. In addition to personal hygiene, warmth, and a supply of food, adequate physical contact with infants and toddlers is crucial for healthy development (Cascio et al. 2019; Gliga et al. 2019; Bales et al. 2018; Montagu 1986). This is especially true for infants born prematurely. If adequate touch stimuli are missing or if the infant or toddler experiences touch stimuli only as violence or pain, then they usually develop severe and irreparable developmental disorders or die (Spitz 1945; Nelson et al. 2013, 2014; McGoron et al. 2012). In humans, as well as in other altricial mammals, adequate social touch is required by the infant for stress regulation, social bonding, neural and physical growth, and maturation processes.

S. M. Mueller (✉) · M. Grunwald
Haptic Research Lab, Paul-Flechsig-Institute for Brain Research, Leipzig University, Leipzig, Germany
e-mail: s.mueller@medizin.uni-leipzig.de; mgrun@medizin.uni-leipzig.de

S. M. Mueller et al., *Human Touch in Healthcare*, https://doi.org/10.1007/978-3-662-67860-2_7

7.1 Premature Infants

Typically, a fetus grows in its mother's womb for 40 weeks. If the fetus is born before 37 weeks of gestation, this is referred to as preterm or premature birth (Martius and Novotny 2006). Premature birth is not only associated with a low body weight of the infant but also maturational and developmental delays or serious diseases that require medical care in a neonatal unit. Worldwide, the number of premature births is increasing, and the WHO estimates that this now affects 1 in 10 births (Kassabian et al. 2020; Howson et al. 2013; Fig. 7.1).

Staying in a neonatal ward is a challenge for premature infants in several respects. If they are very premature, they receive medical care in an incubator, and many of the necessary treatments and examination procedures are unpleasant or even painful for the premature infant. Therefore, their growth and living environment is very different from that in the uterus. If they are not yet strong enough to suckle, premature infants must be fed artificially via a feeding tube. Additionally, until their respiratory system and lungs are fully mature, their breathing is supported by external oxygen supplementation. Premature infants cannot yet regulate their body temperature, and their immune system is still weak, so all the treatments must be carried out with careful hygiene and at a constant ambient temperature. All these measures severely limit the parents' physical contact with their newborn. The majority of touch experienced by preterm infants involves uncomfortable or painful medical procedures (Harrison 2001).

7.1.1 Premature Infants and Postnatal Physical Contact

Especially in premature infants, appropriate touch and movement interventions can have a significant positive impact on development processes. Since the early 1980s, the effects of kangaroo care have been systematically studied in premature infants. In **kangaroo care**, the premature infant is placed skin-to-skin on the chest of a primary caretaker or volunteer, who sits reclined and is covered with a blanket or fur. However, there is no mandatory rule to apply the method and hospitals may even restrict its use to medically stable preterm infants to prevent infections and complications. In contrast, kangaroo care can, in principle, also be performed with intubated preterm infants or infants in critical condition, and studies have demonstrated positive effects of kangaroo care in this context (Eichel 2001).

In addition to the kangaroo method, **preterm infant massages (PrM)** are increasingly being used on neonatal units to achieve various positive

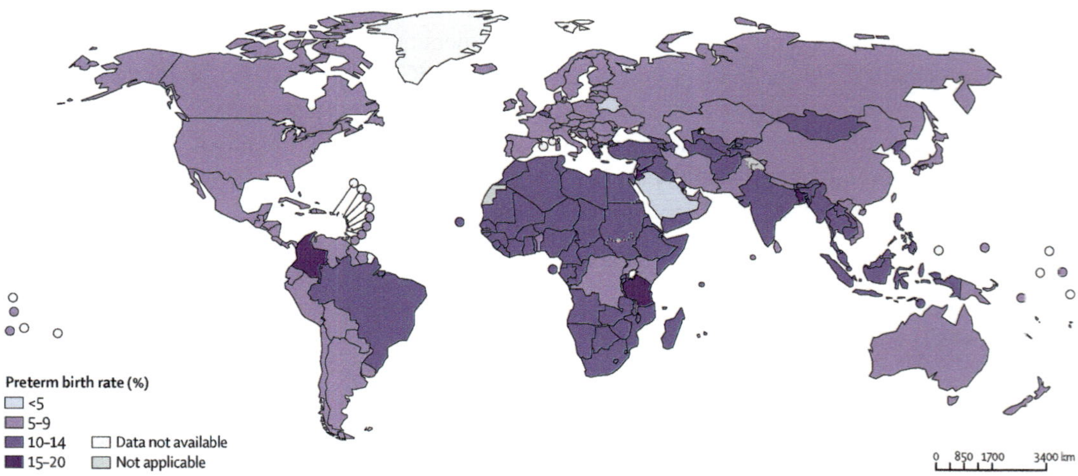

Fig. 7.1 Estimated percentage of preterm births worldwide. (Graphic: Chawanpaiboon et al. 2019)

physical and neurobiological effects (Rangey and Sheth 2014; Procianoy et al. 2010). These massages usually involve a combination of touch and movement stimulation of the premature infant. In most existing studies on preterm massages, the massages were performed three times daily for 5–10 consecutive days, and the developmental status at discharge was measured to determine the effects of the intervention.

Application Example:
Preterm infant massage. The premature infant first lies in the prone position and is gently but firmly stroked for 5 min with the warmed palm. Slow, rhythmic touch with moderate pressure is used on the infant's head, body, and limbs following this sequence: head to neck (six times), shoulder to hand (six times) left and right, neck to back to bottom (six times), and bottom to feet (six times) left and right. The premature infant is then carefully turned onto its back. The following movement stimulation consists of five 1 min sequences of passive limb movements. First, one arm, then the second arm, then each leg individually, and finally, both legs are slowly flexed and stretched. The child is then returned to the prone position, and the body and limbs are again stroked with moderate pressure for 5 min (Field et al. 1986; White and Labarba 1976). The infant should be calm and relaxed during the procedure; the touch and movement should be adjusted according to the infant's cues. If the infant shows signs of stress (like crying, mottled skin, hiccups, gagging, apnoea, or bradycardia) the massaging individual should pause and keep their hands still on the infant's body. ◄

Study results show that the positive effects of contact with preterm infants on both the parents and infants go far beyond bonding effects. Interestingly, the kangaroo method and premature infant massage act on similar dimensions and achieve comparable effect sizes (Rangey and Sheth 2014; Procianoy et al. 2010).The largest and most replicated effects of kangaroo care and preterm massage are **faster weight gain and earlier hospital discharge** than preterm infants who did not receive these treatments (Rangey and Sheth 2014; Procianoy et al. 2010).

In previous studies, over a 10-day intervention period, preterm infants treated with PrM were shown to gain, on average, between 13 and 47% more body weight daily than controls (Ferber et al. 2002; Field et al. 1986; Massaro et al. 2009; White and Labarba 1976). Some studies reported that the increased weight gain occurred despite the same number of feedings and caloric intake as the control group (Field et al. 1986). Furthermore, postnatal weight *loss* was more pronounced and lasted longer in the children in the control groups (White and Labarba 1976; Ferber et al. 2002) (Fig. 7.2).

In addition to health status and age, the infant's weight is associated with the length of its hospital stay. Consequently, it is not surprising that preterm infants treated with preterm massage tend to be discharged on average 3–6 days earlier than other infants (Field et al. 1986; deRoiste and Bushnell 1996; Gonzalez et al. 2009; Mendes and Procianoy 2008). Other studies have also found a trend toward earlier discharge following preterm massage, but their effects did not reach significance (Massaro et al. 2009; Procianoy et al. 2010; White and Labarba 1976).

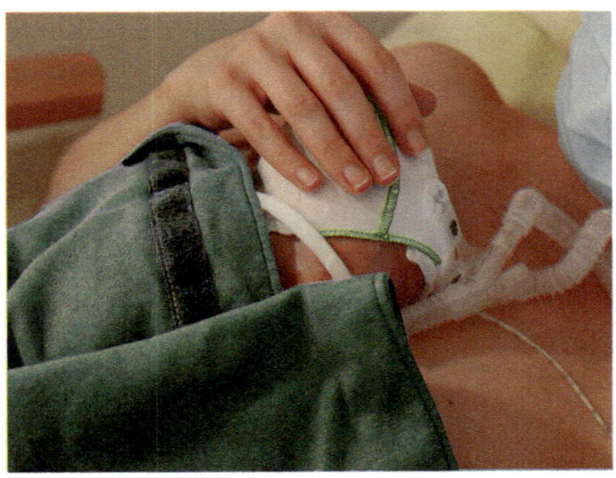

Fig. 7.2 Kangaroo method. Skin-to-skin contact in a semi-reclined position with a premature infant. (Photo: Haptic Research Lab, University of Leipzig)

Other positive outcomes of both kangaroo care and PrM include the following (Álvarez et al. 2017; Scafidi et al. 1986; Field et al. 1986; Yates et al. 2014; Niemi 2017; Mueller et al. 2022):

- Deeper sleep.
- Longer active/wakeful phases.
- Improved attention, habituation, and self-regulation.
- Stabilization of the heartbeat and breathing.
- Reduced stress responses/faster calming.
- Reduction in preterm apnea frequency.

In addition, a specific effect of kangaroo care is that mothers who perform direct skin-to-skin contact on their upper body tend to show an **increase in lactation** volume and duration (Furman et al. 2002).

Interestingly, premature infant massage may have additional effects compared to kangaroo care. In a long-term study on brain maturation processes, a group of extremely low birth weight (750–1500 g) preterm infants received 15 min of preterm massage four times per day in addition to regular kangaroo care. The group was compared to a control group treated with standard therapy and kangaroo care. In the group comparison, preterm infants who received PrM in addition to kangaroo care showed better **cognitive and psychomotor** development scores at 2 years of age (Procianoy et al. 2010; deRoiste and Bushnell 1996) despite the fact that both groups showed equal head circumference, weight, and height both at the time of discharge from the hospital and at the age of 2 years. The authors discussed the positive developmental effect of PrM + Kangaro as a possible consequence of a permanent change in the parent-child interactions (deRoiste and Bushnell 1996). Moreover, there was a tendency for patients in the PrM + Kangaroo group to be discharged 4 days earlier; however, the difference did not reach significance. In terms of hospital-related outcomes, the only significant difference was a lower incidence of late sepsis in the PrM + Kangaroo group. A **lower incidence of late sepsis** in preterm infants receiving PrM was also shown in another study (Mendes and Procianoy 2008).

Another specific effect of PrM is greater **bone mineralization** in the treated preterm infants. Preterm infants are at increased risk of deficient bone mineralization, and this increases the risk of fractures (e.g., femoral neck fracture) in early childhood. The effect of increased bone mineralization with PrM most likely results from the movement stimulation (passive limb movements) that is part of PrM treatment (Schulzke et al. 2007). Indeed, in previous studies, compared to preterm infants (birth weight: 1000–1500 g) who were only held and stroked but received no movement stimulation, the experimental groups with additional passive limb movements showed significantly increased bone mineral content and bone mineral density (Moyer-Mileur et al. 1995, 2000, 2008; Litmanovitz et al. 2003, 2007). Beyond that, both groups (PrM with and without passive limb movement) showed similar benefits in weight gain compared to standard therapy when controlling for birth weight, birth age, head circumference, and caloric intake.

► **Important** Both kangaroo care and preterm massage promote healthy physical and neural development of the infant. Kangaroo care also promotes the psychological bond between parents and children.

7.1.2 Biological Effect Model of Body Contact in Premature Infants

In a study investigating the mechanisms of weight gain in preterm infants, it was shown that PrM and passive limb movement acted through different metabolic pathways; in particular, while limb movement increased caloric intake, preterm massage caused an increase in vagus nerve activity (Diego et al. 2014), which, in turn, increased gastrointestinal motility (Diego et al. 2005); additionally, another study demonstrated an association between preterm massage and the levels of serum insulin and insulin-like growth factor 1 (IGF-1) (Field et al. 2008). Furthermore, another study reported that children treated with preterm infant massage showed increased weight

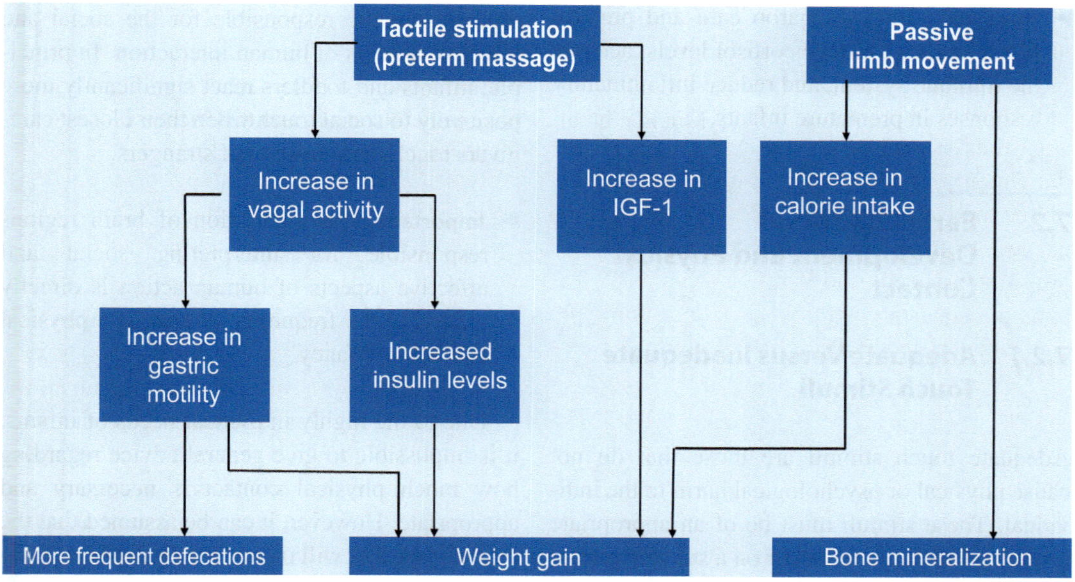

Fig. 7.3 Effects of preterm infant massage. (Fig. from: Mueller and Grunwald 2019. Path diagram based on Field et al. 2011, extended.)

gain despite the same caloric intake as children in the control groups (Scafidi et al. 1986). Meta-analytic path analyses suggest that the weight gain associated with preterm massage is caused by both insulin release triggered by vagus activity and increased gastrointestinal motility. Furthermore, the release of IGF-1 also contributes to weight gain, independent of vagus activation (Field et al. 2011) (Fig. 7.3).

Recent physiological evidence also highlights the central role of **vagus nerve activity** in immune regulation (Olofsson et al. 2012). Accordingly, stimulation of efferent parts of the vagus nerve leads to the release of acetylcholine, which, in turn, inhibits the synthesis and release of pro-inflammatory cytokines (cf. Sect. 2.4). This signal chain prevents an overshooting of inflammatory reactions and tissue damage (Borovikova et al. 2000). An increase in vagus activity in premature infants treated with PrM could, thus, support healing processes during infections and after operations. In addition, these vagus-mediated anti-inflammatory processes may contribute to the lower incidence of late sepsis in preterm infants treated with preterm infant massage (Mendes and Procianoy 2008; Procianoy et al. 2010).

Further evidence for the stress-reducing and immune-enhancing effect of both preterm infant massage and kangaroo care is related to the decreases in cortisol levels observed following these interventions. Indeed, some studies have shown lower **cortisol levels** in the intervention group up to 60 min after performing preterm massage (Acolet et al. 1993; Gitau et al. 2002). However, in some preterm infants, cortisol levels remained the same or increased during massage. One explanation for this opposite effect could be pain sensations triggered by excessive pressure or stretching forces during massage. In contrast, cortisol systematically decreased in the groups receiving kangaroo care. It should be noted that premature infants in the control groups (60 min rest) also showed a decrease in blood cortisol levels (Acolet et al. 1993; Mooncey et al. 1997). Nevertheless, painless physical stimulation can have additional stress-reducing effects that affect the immune system. For example, one recent study found an increase in the cytotoxicity of natural killer cells after preterm massage in stable premature infants (Ang et al. 2012). Further studies with good methodological standards are needed to substantiate the findings on immune effects.

▶ **Important** Both kangaroo care and preterm infant massage reduce cortisol levels, activate the immune system, and reduce inflammatory responses in premature infants.

7.2 Early Childhood Development and Physical Contact

7.2.1 Adequate Versus Inadequate Touch Stimuli

Adequate touch stimuli are those that do not cause physical or psychological harm to the individual. These stimuli must be of an appropriate intensity and duration, occur on a suitable part of the body, and occur at the right time. If social touch is performed too vigorously, for an inappropriate time period (too long or too short), at the wrong time, and to the wrong part of the body, then the positive biological effects of social touch are not elicited, or even harmful effects (e.g., stress and injuries) may occur. Numerous studies have shown that infants and toddlers register different stroking speeds and show a higher heart rate at unpleasant speeds (Aguirre et al. 2019; Gursul et al. 2018; Croy et al. 2016). Slow stroking movements of approximately 3 cm per second are perceived as pleasant by most infants and toddlers (Croy et al. 2019). This stroking speed is optimal for stimulating C-tactile nerve endings in the skin. When standardized stroking stimuli are applied to the upper arm of children aged 5–12 years old, the older children perceive these stimuli significantly more positively than younger children. In addition, girls evaluate these stroking stimuli as more pleasant than boys (Croy et al. 2019).

In addition, it has been demonstrated that in young children (5 years old), there is an association between the development of the right hemispheric insula and other brain areas and more pronounced body-communicative aspects of the parent–child relationship (Brauer et al. 2016). Specifically, more frequent adequate parent–child physical interaction is related to greater neural maturation processes in those brain regions that are responsible for the social and affective aspects of human interaction. In principle, infants and toddlers react significantly more positively to social touch when their closest caregivers touch them instead of strangers.

▶ **Important** The maturation of brain regions responsible for interpreting social and affective aspects of human action is directly related to the frequency of adequate physical contact in infancy.

Due to the highly individual needs of infants, it is impossible to give general advice regarding how much physical contact is necessary and appropriate. However, it can be assumed that the infant or toddler will indicate their need for physical contact and provide feedback on the adequate execution of physical contact using nonverbal signs and vocalizations.

▶ **Important** Other sensory cues may influence how touch stimuli are experienced in the context of body communication between an infant or toddler and their social environment. For example, coherent acoustic, visual, and olfactory stimuli (e.g., calm voice) during body communication promote the positive and stress-reducing effects of physical contact in infants and toddlers.

7.2.2 Growth Processes Through Social Touch

Touch stimuli activate various mechanoreceptors in the skin, hair follicles, tendons, muscles, and joints, depending on the body area, temperature, pressure intensity, and speed of the stimuli. The signals triggered by these stimuli reach various brain regions via nerve fibers. In children, the neural **activation leads to the maturation of these brain areas** (i.e., the insula, amygdala, and prefrontal cortex) (Tuulari et al. 2019; Jönsson et al. 2017; Feldman et al. 2014; Dunbar 2010). The neurochemical effects of various growth hormones are responsible for these maturation processes; indeed, these hormones both promote neuronal growth and influence the growth of body cells (cf. Sect. 7.1.2). Adequate touch stimuli during social physical interactions thus trigger complex **neural and physical growth processes** in infants and toddlers. The effects of physical contact cannot be replaced by other sensory channels. In this respect, socially mediated touch is indispensable "nourishment" for infants and toddlers (Grunwald 2017).

7.2.3 Stress Regulation Through Social Touch

Socially mediated adequate touch positively affects stress regulation in infants and young children (and even adults). Indeed, through touch, less of the stress hormone cortisol, which is produced in the adrenal cortex, is produced, thus resulting in a stress-reducing effect (Harrison et al. 2000; Feldman et al. 2010; van Oers et al. 1998; Walker 2010). Moreover, the decrease in stress associated with adequate touch is also indicated by the reduction in heart rate, the relaxation of the muscles, and the decrease in feelings of anxiety following this type of touch. The stress-reducing effects of adequate social touch are relevant throughout the life course (Murphy et al. 2018; Croy et al. 2019; cf. Sect. 2.4.3).

Maternal breastfeeding is commonly used for infant nourishment. However, the physical skin contact during this form of social touch also triggers several other physiological processes in both the infant and the mother, and the release of the hormone oxytocin is responsible for these processes. Specifically, oxytocin is released during mechanical stimulation of the nipples and other touch stimuli (cf. Sect. 2.4.1). In the mother, oxytocin triggers lactation in the mammary glands, as well as physiological relaxation in the body (Winberg 2005; Doan et al. 2007; Krol and Grossmann 2018; Tharner et al. 2012). The whole-body stimulation of the infant during breastfeeding also causes the release of oxytocin into the infant's body. The increased oxytocin levels in the infant's blood during breastfeeding and skin contact promote the relaxation response in the infant (Jonas and Woodside 2016). Similar stress-reducing effects have also been observed during **co-sleeping.** In this sleep situation, the infant sleeps close to the parents (not necessarily in the same bed) or a sibling. Sleep duration, sleep depth, as well as anxious behavior during the daytime are usually reduced by this form of social and physical proximity (Barry 2019; Iwata et al. 2013; Ward 2015). Incidentally, it should be remembered that an overwhelming majority of parents sleep in the same room with their partner, and concurrently, it is not uncommon for an infant or toddler to be expected to sleep alone in their bed and possibly even in a separate room.

7.2.4 Bonding and Social Attention Through Touch

The development of strong social and emotional bonds between people is tied to direct physical contact, and it is well known that oxytocin is a key biological factor in forming and maintaining social bonds. This hormone is released immediately after or during social touch and is sometimes referred to as the "love hormone." In addition to various physical phenomena influenced by oxytocin (lowering of the blood pressure, cortisol level inhibition, heart rate slowing, and skeletal muscle relaxation), oxytocin activates the neural networks responsible for processing social environmental cues (e.g., insula and superior temporal sulcus) (Feldman 2012; Carter 2014; Herpertz and Bertsch 2016; Peled et al. 2013). Additionally, oxytocin promotes the stability of social relationships, especially between infants and parents. Interestingly, it seems that oxytocin is released more strongly in females compared to males, although the cause and significance of these differences are still unclear. A significant increase in oxytocin levels has been shown in fathers who are intensively involved with their newborn infant (Feldman et al. 2010). However, studies suggest that touch stimuli are processed differently by men and women at the neuronal level. For example, using standardized stroking stimuli (a Robot arm moving a brush), an fMRI study demonstrated that a specific brain region crucial for social attention and social cognition processes (superior temporal sulcus) was activated in females from the age of 5 years old, but this specific activation pattern in response to gentle touch stimuli was not found in the male study participants (aged 5–35 years) (Björnsdotter et al. 2014).

> **Important** Social touch is crucial for the healthy growth of infants and young children. In addition, social touch promotes the development and maintenance of social relationships and contributes to stress regulation.

7.2.5 Maldevelopment and Pathologies Due to a Lack of Contact

Numerous studies have examined the effects of a lack of touch on mental and physical development in animal models and human infants. **Physical deprivation**, which refers to the complete absence of adequate physical stimuli, consistently leads to irreparable developmental damage or even death in infants. Developmental and maturational disorders caused by a lack of social touch affect both neural and physical development (Spitz 1945; Ardiel and Rankin 2010; Bick et al. 2015; Gupta and Schork 1995; Bos et al. 2009; Ghera et al. 2009; Humphreys et al. 2015). If the lack of touch is prolonged and extensive, the resulting developmental and maturational disorders are usually irreparable. The specific psychopathological consequences of a lack of touch include motor disorders, speech and articulation disorders, anxiety and memory disorders, and general cognitive impairment. Furthermore, on the behavioral level, severe social and communication disorders, as well as personality and body image disorders, may occur following a lack of contact (Levin et al. 2014, 2015; Nelson et al. 2013, 2014).

7.2.6 Language Development Through Socially Mediated Tactile Experiences

One of the greatest enigmas in social science is why humans can speak and how they acquire this ability in early infancy. One certainty in this process is that a child's language acquisition depends on the extent language is used to interact with the child. The biological ability for language acquisition seems to be genetically predetermined in our species; however, language acquisition is tied to social interactions (Tomasello 2009; Pleyer and Hartmann 2019). Accordingly, linguistic stimuli promote the infant's language development. If a child does not hear spoken language, they will not develop language skills. In addition, the processing of language-related tactile stimuli influences the development of a toddler's speech behavior, although this connection has only recently been investigated. In methodologically sophisticated studies, it has been demonstrated that the simultaneous presentation of speech stimuli and corresponding touch stimuli directed at the infant's body help to form the infant's first linguistic-bodily concepts (Abu-Zhaya et al. 2016; Seidl et al. 2015; Tincoff et al. 2019; Lew-Williams et al. 2019). The infant's language learning success regarding its own and foreign body parts is faster when clearer signals coupling between touch stimuli and language signals are used. The simultaneous transmission of linguistic stimuli and sensory body signals (e.g., the infant's head is touched when naming "head") also **promotes the infant's recognition of word meaning**. Studies have shown that the majority of parents intuitively use this coupling between speech and body touch in their everyday communication with infants and toddlers.

Similarly, the body touches that correspond to linguistic cues also promote object-related language development in toddlers (Nomikou and Rohlfing 2011; Kadlaskar et al. 2020). Language acquisition in infants and toddlers is tied to multimodal sensory impressions, which arise from physical interaction with one's own body, social others, or the external environment. In addition to tactile-haptic experiences, these impressions include visual, acoustic, gustatory, and olfactory sensory stimuli, which promote language acquisition in the context of individual and social actions. A child's immediate social environment (parents, close relatives) and their direct interactions with the child are the central driving force for language development (Tamis-LeMonda et al. 2014; Masur et al. 2005; Tincoff et al.

2019). Exclusively visual-acoustic stimulation, without social and physical interactions (such as in the context of computer-based simulations), cannot simulate the multisensory requirements for learning or replace the required social-linguistic role models.

References

Abu-Zhaya R, Seidl A, Cristia A. Multimodal infant-directed communication: how caregivers combine tactile and linguistic cues. J Child Lang. 2016;44:1088–116. https://doi.org/10.1017/S0305000916000416.

Acolet D, Modi N, Giannakoulopoulos X, Bond C, Weg W, Clow A, Glover V. Changes in plasma cortisol and catecholamine concentrations in response to massage in preterm infants. Arch Dis Childhood. 1993;68(1 Spec No):29–31.

Aguirre M, Couderc A, Epinat-Duclos J, Mascaro O. Infants discriminate the source of social touch at stroking speeds eliciting maximal firing rates in CT-fibers. Dev Cogn Neurosci. 2019;36:100639. https://doi.org/10.1016/j.dcn.2019.100639.

Álvarez MJ, Fernández D, Gómez-Salgado J, Rodríguez-González D, Rosón M, Lapeña S. The effects of massage therapy in hospitalized preterm neonates. A systematic review. Int J Nurs Stud. 2017;69:119–36. https://doi.org/10.1016/j.ijnurstu.2017.02.009.

Ang JY, Lua JL, Mathur A, Thomas R, Asmar BI, Savasan S, et al. A randomized placebo-controlled trial of massage therapy on the immune system of preterm infants. Pediatrics. 2012;130(6):E1549–58. https://doi.org/10.1542/peds.2012-0196.

Ardiel EL, Rankin CH. The importance of touch in development. Paediatr Child Health. 2010;15(3):153–6.

Bales KL, Witczak LR, Simmons TC, Savidge LE, Rothwell ES, Rogers FD, et al. Social touch during development: long-term effects on brain and behavior. Neurosci Biobehav Rev. 2018;95:202–19. https://doi.org/10.1016/j.neubiorev.2018.09.019.

Barry ES. Co-sleeping as a proximal context for infant development: the importance of physical touch. Infant Behav Dev. 2019;57:101385. https://doi.org/10.1016/j.infbeh.2019.101385.

Bick J, Fox N, Zeanah C, Nelson CA. Early deprivation, atypical brain development, and internalizing symptoms in late childhood. Neuroscience. 2015;342:140. https://doi.org/10.1016/j.neuroscience.2015.09.026.

Björnsdotter M, Gordon I, Pelphrey KA, Olausson H, Kaiser MD. Development of brain mechanisms for processing affective touch. Front Behav Neurosci. 2014;8:24. https://doi.org/10.3389/fnbeh.2014.00024.

Borovikova LV, Ivanova S, Zhang M, Yang H, Botchkina GI, Watkins LR, et al. Vagus nerve stimulation attenuates the systemic inflammatory response to endotoxin. Nature. 2000;405(6785):458–62. https://doi.org/10.1038/35013070.

Bos KJ, Fox N, Zeanah CH, Iii N, Charles A. Effects of early psychosocial deprivation on the development of memory and executive function. Front Behav Neurosci. 2009;3:16. https://doi.org/10.3389/neuro.08.016.2009.

Brauer J, Xiao Y, Poulain T, Friederici AD, Schirmer A. Frequency of maternal touch predicts resting activity and connectivity of the developing social brain. Cereb Cortex. 2016;26(8):3544–52. https://doi.org/10.1093/cercor/bhw137.

Carter CS. Oxytocin pathways and the evolution of human behavior. Annu Rev Psychol. 2014;65:17–39. https://doi.org/10.1146/annurev-psych-010213-115110.

Cascio CJ, Moore D, McGlone F. Social touch and human development. Dev Cogn Neurosci. 2019;35:5–11. https://doi.org/10.1016/j.dcn.2018.04.009.

Chawanpaiboon S, Vogel JP, Moller AB, Lumbiganon P, Petzold M, Hogan D, et al. Global, regional, and national estimates of levels of preterm birth in 2014: a systematic review and modeling analysis. Lancet Glob Health. 2019;7(1):e37–46.

Croy I, Luong A, Triscoli C, Hofmann E, Olausson H, Sailer U. Interpersonal stroking touch is targeted to C tactile afferent activation. Behav Brain Res. 2016;297:37–40. https://doi.org/10.1016/j.bbr.2015.09.038.

Croy I, Sehlstedt I, Wasling HB, Ackerley R, Olausson H. Gentle touch perception: from early childhood to adolescence. Dev Cogn Neurosci. 2019;35:81–6. https://doi.org/10.1016/j.dcn.2017.07.009.

deRoiste A, Bushnell IWR. Tactile stimulation. Short- and long-term benefits for pre-term infants. Br J Dev Psychol. 1996;14:41–53.

Diego MA, Field T, Hernandez-Reif M. Vagal activity, gastric motility, and weight gain in massaged preterm neonates. J Pediatr. 2005;147(1):50–5. https://doi.org/10.1016/j.jpeds.2005.02.023.

Diego MA, Field T, Hernandez-Reif M. Preterm infant weight gain is increased by massage therapy and exercise via different underlying mechanisms. Early Hum Dev. 2014;90(3):137–40. https://doi.org/10.1016/j.earlhumdev.2014.01.009.

Doan T, Gardiner A, Gay CL, Lee KA. Breast-feeding increases sleep duration of new parents. J Perinat Neonat Nurs. 2007;21(3):200–6. https://doi.org/10.1097/01.JPN.0000285809.36398.1b.

Dunbar RIM. The social role of touch in humans and primates: behavioural function and neurobiological mechanisms. Neurosci Biobehav Rev. 2010;34(2):260–8.

Eichel P. Kangaroo care: expanding our practice to critically ill neonates. Newborn Infant Nurs Rev. 2001;1(4):224–8.

Feldman R. Oxytocin and social affiliation in humans. Horm Behav. 2012;61(3):380–91.

Feldman R, Singer M, Zagoory O. Touch attenuates infants' physiological reactivity to stress. Dev Sci. 2010;13(2):271–8. https://doi.org/10.1111/j.1467-7687.2009.00890.x.

Feldman R, Rosenthal Z, Eidelman AI. Maternal-preterm skin-to-skin contact enhances child physiologic organization and cognitive control across the first 10 years

of life. Biol Psychiatry. 2014;75(1):56–64. https://doi.org/10.1016/j.biopsych.2013.08.012.
Ferber SG, Kuint J, Weller A, Feldman R, Dollberg S, Arbel E, Kohelet D. Massage therapy by mothers and trained professionals enhances weight gain in preterm infants. Early Hum Dev. 2002;67(1–2):37–45.
Field TM, Schanberg SM, Scafidi F, Bauer CR, Vega-Lahr N, Garcia R, et al. Tactile/kinesthetic stimulation effects on preterm neonates. Pediatrics. 1986;77(5):654–8.
Field T, Diego M, Hernandez-Reif M, Dieter JNI, Kumar AM, Schanberg S, Kuhn C. Insulin and insulin-like growth factor-1 increased in preterm neonates following massage therapy. J Dev Behav Pediatr. 2008;29(6):463–6. https://doi.org/10.1097/DBP.0b013e3181856d3b.
Field T, Diego M, Hernandez-Reif M. Potential underlying mechanisms for greater weight gain in massaged preterm infants. Infant Behav Dev. 2011;34(3):383–9. https://doi.org/10.1016/j.infbeh.2010.12.001.
Furman L, Minich N, Hack M. Correlates of lactation in mothers of very low birth weight infants. Pediatrics. 2002;109(4):e57.
Ghera MM, Marshall PJ, Fox NA, Zeanah CH, Nelson CA, Smyke AT, Guthrie D. The effects of foster care intervention on socially deprived institutionalized children's attention and positive affect: results from the BEIP study. J Child Psychol Psychiatry. 2009;50(3):246–53. https://doi.org/10.1111/j.1469-7610.2008.01954.x.
Gitau R, Modi N, Gianakoulopoulos X, Bond C, Glover V, Stevenson J. Acute effects of maternal skin-to-skin contact and massage on saliva cortisol in preterm babies. J Reprod Infant Psychol. 2002;20(2):83–8. https://doi.org/10.1080/02646830220134595.
Gliga T, Farroni T, Cascio CJ. Social touch: a new vista for developmental cognitive neuroscience? Dev Cogn Neurosci. 2019;35:1–4. https://doi.org/10.1016/j.dcn.2018.05.006.
Gonzalez AP, Vasquez-Mendoza G, García-Vela A, Guzmán-Ramirez A, Salazar-Torres M, Romero-Gutierrez G. Weight gain in preterm infants following parent-administered Vimala massage. A randomized controlled trial. Am J Perinatol. 2009;26(4):247–52. https://doi.org/10.1055/s-0028-1103151.
Grunwald M. Homo hapticus. Warum wir ohneTastsinn nicht leben können. DroemerKnaur; 2017. ISBN: 978-3-426-27706-5 .
Gupta MA, Schork NJ. Touch deprivation has an adverse effect on body image: some preliminary observations. Int J Eat Disord. 1995;17(2):185–9.
Gursul D, Goksan S, Hartley C, Mellado GS, Moultrie F, Hoskin A, et al. Stroking modulates noxious-evoked brain activity in human infants. Curr Biol. 2018;28(24):R1380–1. https://doi.org/10.1016/j.cub.2018.11.014.
Harrison LL. The use of comforting touch and massage to reduce stress for preterm infants in the neonatal intensive care unit. Newborn Infant Nurs Rev. 2001;1(4):235–41.
Harrison LL, Williams AK, Berbaum ML, Stem JT, Leeper J. Physiologic and behavioral effects of gentle human touch on preterm infants. Res Nurs Health. 2000;23(6):435–46. https://doi.org/10.1002/1098-240X(200012)23:6<435::AID-NUR3>3.0.CO;2-P.
Herpertz SC, Bertsch K. Oxytocin effects on brain functioning in humans. Biol Psychiatry. 2016;79(8):631–2. https://doi.org/10.1016/j.biopsych.2016.02.004.
Howson CP, Kinney MV, McDougall L, Lawn JE. Born too soon: preterm birth matters. Reprod Health. 2013;10 Suppl 1:S1. https://doi.org/10.1186/1742-4755-10-S1-S1.
Humphreys KL, Gleason MM, Drury SS, Miron D, Nelson CA 3rd, Fox NA, Zeanah CH. Effects of institutional rearing and foster care on psychopathology at age 12 years in Romania: follow-up of an open, randomised controlled trial. Lancet Psychiatry. 2015;2(7):625–34. https://doi.org/10.1016/S2215-0366(15)00095-4.
Iwata S, Iwata O, Matsuishi T. Sleep patterns of Japanese preschool children and their parents: implications for co-sleeping. Acta Paediatr. 2013;102(6):e257–62. https://doi.org/10.1111/apa.12203.
Jonas W, Woodside B. Physiological mechanisms, behavioral and psychological factors influencing the transfer of milk from mothers to their young. Horm Behav. 2016;77:167–81. https://doi.org/10.1016/j.yhbeh.2015.07.018.
Jönsson EH, Bendas J, Weidner K, Wessberg J, Olausson H, Wasling HB, Croy I. The relation between human hair follicle density and touch perception. Sci Rep. 2017;7(1):2499. https://doi.org/10.1038/s41598-017-02308-9.
Kadlaskar G, Waxman S, Seidl A. Does human touch facilitate object categorization in 6-to-9-month-old infants? Brain Sci. 2020;10(12):940. https://doi.org/10.3390/brainsci10120940.
Kassabian S, Fewer S, Yamey G, Brindis CD. Building a global policy agenda to prioritize preterm birth: A qualitative analysis on factors shaping global health policymaking. Gates Open Res. 2020;4:65. https://doi.org/10.12688/gatesopenres.13098.1.
Krol KM, Grossmann T. Psychologische Effekte des Stillens auf Kinder und Mütter. Bundesgesundheitsblatt Gesundheitsforschung Gesundheitsschutz. 2018;61(8):977–85. https://doi.org/10.1007/s00103-018-2769-0.
Levin AR, Zeanah CH Jr, Fox NA, Nelson CA. Motor outcomes in children exposed to early psychosocial deprivation. J Pediatr. 2014;164(1):S. 123. https://doi.org/10.1016/j.jpeds.2013.09.026.
Levin AR, Fox NA, Zeanah CH Jr, Nelson CA. Social communication difficulties and autism in previously institutionalized children. J Am Acad Child Adolesc Psychiatry. 2015;54(2):108. https://doi.org/10.1016/j.jaac.2014.11.011.
Lew-Williams C, Ferguson B, Abu-Zhaya R, Seidl A. Social touch interacts with infants' learning of auditory patterns. Dev Cogn Neurosci. 2019;35:66–74. https://doi.org/10.1016/j.dcn.2017.09.006.

Litmanovitz I, Dolfin T, Friedland O, Arnon S, Regev R, Shainkin-Kestenbaum R, et al. Early physical activity intervention prevents decrease of bone strength in very low birth weight infants. Pediatrics. 2003;112(1 Pt 1):15–9.

Litmanovitz I, Dolfin T, Arnon S, Regev RH, Nemet D, Eliakim A. Assisted exercise and bone strength in preterm infants. Calcif Tissue Int. 2007;80(1):39–43. https://doi.org/10.1007/s00223-006-0149-5.

Martius J, Novotny A. Gynäkologie, Geburtshilfe und Neonatologie. Lehrbuch für Pflegeberufe. 12th ed. Stuttgart: Kohlhammer Verlag; 2006.

Massaro AN, Hammad TA, Jazzo B, Aly H. Massage with kinesthetic stimulation improves weight gain in preterm infants. J Perinatol. 2009;29(5):352–7. https://doi.org/10.1038/jp.2008.230.

Masur EF, Flynn V, Eichorst DL. Maternal responsive and directive behaviours and utterances as predictors of children's lexical development. J Child Lang. 2005;32(1):63–91.

McGoron L, Gleason MM, Smyke AT, Drury SS, Nelson CA III, Gregas MC, et al. Recovering from early deprivation: attachment mediates effects of caregiving on psychopathology. J Am Acad Child Adolesc Psychiatry. 2012;51(7):683–93. https://doi.org/10.1016/j.jaac.2012.05.004.

Mendes EW, Procianoy RS. Massage therapy reduces hospital stay and occurrence of late-onset sepsis in very preterm neonates. J Perinatol. 2008;28(12):815–20. https://doi.org/10.1038/jp.2008.108.

Montagu A. Touching. The human significance of the skin. 3rd ed. New York: Harper & Row; 1986. Online verfügbar unter http://www.loc.gov/catdir/description/hc044/85045216.html.

Mooncey S, Giannakoulopoulos X, Glover V, Acolet D, Modi N. The effect of mother-infant skin-to-skin contact on plasma cortisol and beta-endorphin concentrations in preterm newborns. Infant Behav Dev. 1997;20(4):553–7.

Moyer-Mileur L, Luetkemeier M, Boomer L, Chan GM. Effect of physical activity on bone mineralization in premature infants. J Pediatr. 1995;127(4):620–5.

Moyer-Mileur LJ, Brunstetter V, McNaught TP, Gill G, Chan GM. Daily physical activity program increases bone mineralization and growth in preterm very low birth weight infants. Pediatrics. 2000;106(5):1088–92.

Moyer-Mileur LJ, Ball SD, Brunstetter VL, Chan GM. Maternal-administered physical activity enhances bone mineral acquisition in premature very low birth weight infants. J Perinatol. 2008;28(6):432–7. https://doi.org/10.1038/jp.2008.17.

Mueller SM, Ackermann BW, Martin S, Seifert K, Mohr A, Alali W, Thome UH, Grunwald M. Incidence of intermittent hypoxia increases during clinical care in extremely preterm infants. Neonatology. 2022;120(1):102–10. https://doi.org/10.1159/000527725.

Mueller SM, Grunwald M. Frühgeborenenmassage: taktile Körperstimulation in der Neonatalmedizin. Man Med. 2019;57(4):260–5. https://doi.org/10.1007/s00337-019-0546-2.

Murphy MLM, Janicki-Deverts D, Cohen S. Receiving a hug is associated with the attenuation of negative mood that occurs on days with interpersonal conflict. PLoS One. 2018;13(10):e0203522. https://doi.org/10.1371/journal.pone.0203522.

Nelson CA III, Fox NA, Zeanah CH Jr. Anguish of the abandoned child. Sci Am. 2013;308(4):62–7.

Nelson CA, Fox NA, Zeanah CH. Romania's abandoned children. Deprivation, brain development, and the struggle for recovery. Cambridge: Harvard University Press; 2014.

Niemi A-K. Review of randomized controlled trials of massage in preterm infants. Children. 2017;4(4):21. https://doi.org/10.3390/children4040021.

Nomikou I, Rohlfing KJ. Language does something: body action and language in maternal input to three-month-olds. IEEE Trans Auton Ment Dev. 2011;3(2):113–28. https://doi.org/10.1109/TAMD.2011.2140113.

van Oers HJ, de Kloet ER, Whelan T, Levine S. Maternal deprivation effect on the infant's neural stress markers is reversed by tactile stimulation and feeding but not by suppressing corticosterone. J Neurosci. 1998;18(23):10171–9.

Olofsson PS, Rosas-Ballina M, Levine YA, Tracey KJ. Rethinking inflammation. Neural circuits in the regulation of immunity. Immunol Rev. 2012;248(1):188–204. https://doi.org/10.1111/j.1600-065X.2012.01138.x.

Peled L, Wagner S, Perry A, Shamay-Tsoory SG. Get in touch: the role of oxytocin in social touch. J Mol Neurosci. 2013;51:S90.

Pleyer M, Hartmann S. Constructing a consensus on language evolution? Convergences and differences between biolinguistic and usage-based approaches. Front Psychol. 2019;10:2537. https://doi.org/10.3389/fpsyg.2019.02537.

Procianoy RS, Mendes EW, Silveira RC. Massage therapy improves neurodevelopment outcome at two years corrected age for very low birth weight infants. Early Hum Dev. 2010;86(1):7–11. https://doi.org/10.1016/j.earlhumdev.2009.12.001.

Rangey PS, Sheth M. Comparative effect of massage therapy versus kangaroo mother care on body weight and length of hospital stay in low birth weight preterm infants. Int J Pediatr. 2014;2014:434060. https://doi.org/10.1155/2014/434060.

Scafidi F, Field TM, Schanberg SM, Bauer CR, Vegalahr N, Garcia R, et al. Effects of tactile kinesthetic stimulation on the clinical course and sleep wake behavior of preterm neonates. Infant Behav Dev. 1986;9(1):91–105.

Schulzke SM, Trachsel D, Patole SK. Physical activity programs for promoting bone mineralization and growth in preterm infants. Cochrane Database Syst Rev. 2007;(2):CD005387. https://doi.org/10.1002/14651858.CD005387.pub2.

Seidl A, Tincoff R, Baker C, Cristia A. Why the body comes first: effects of experimenter touch on infants' word finding. Dev Sci. 2015;18(1):155–64. https://doi.org/10.1111/desc.12182.

Spitz RA. Hospitalism; an inquiry into the genesis of psychiatric conditions in early childhood. Psychoanal Study Child. 1945;1:53–74.

Tamis-LeMonda CS, Kuchirko Y, Song L. Why is infant language learning facilitated by parental responsiveness? Curr Dir Psychol Sci. 2014;23(2):121–6. https://doi.org/10.1177/0963721414522813.

Tharner A, Luijk MPCM, Raat H, Ijzendoorn MH, Bakermans-Kranenburg MJ, Moll HA, et al. Breastfeeding and its relation to maternal sensitivity and infant attachment. J Dev Behav Pediatr. 2012;33(5):396–404. https://doi.org/10.1097/DBP.0b013e318257fac3.

Tincoff R, Seidl A, Buckley L, Wojcik C, Cristia A. Feeling the way to words: parents' speech and touch cues highlight word-to-world mappings of body parts. Lang Learn Dev. 2019;15(2):103–25. https://doi.org/10.1080/15475441.2018.1533472.

Tomasello M. Constructing a language. A usage-based theory of language acquisition. Cambridge: Harvard University Press; 2009.

Tuulari JJ, Scheinin NM, Lehtola S, Merisaari H, Saunavaara J, Parkkola R, et al. Neural correlates of gentle skin stroking in early infancy. Dev Cogn Neurosci. 2019;35:36–41. https://doi.org/10.1016/j.dcn.2017.10.004.

Walker C-D. Maternal touch and feed as critical regulators of behavioral and stress responses in the offspring. Dev Psychobiol. 2010;52(7):638–50. https://doi.org/10.1002/dev.20492.

Ward TCS. Reasons for mother-infant bed-sharing: a systematic narrative synthesis of the literature and implications for future research. Matern Child Health J. 2015;19(3):675–90. https://doi.org/10.1007/s10995-014-1557-1.

White JL, Labarba RC. The effects of tactile and kinesthetic stimulation on neonatal development in the premature infant. Dev Psychobiol. 1976;9(6):569–77. https://doi.org/10.1002/dev.420090610.

Winberg J. Mother and newborn baby: mutual regulation of physiology and behavior--a selective review. Dev Psychobiol. 2005;47(3):217–29. https://doi.org/10.1002/dev.20094.

Yates CC, Mitchell AJ, Booth MY, Williams DK, Lowe LM, Whit Hall R. The effects of massage therapy to induce sleep in infants born preterm. Pediatr Phys Ther. 2014;26(4):405–10. https://doi.org/10.1097/PEP.0000000000000081.

Effects of Massages and Other Touch Interventions on Various Diseases

8

Stephanie Margarete Mueller

Contents

8.1 Interpersonal Touch as an Active Substance

A wide variety of physiological processes can be set in motion by interpersonal touch, which has already been mentioned in previous chapters (e.g., Sects. 2.4 and 5.5). The findings are largely consistent with the findings of psychoneuroimmunology and psychoneuroen-

S. M. Mueller (✉)
Haptic Research Lab, Paul-Flechsig-Institute for Brain Research, Leipzig University, Leipzig, Germany
e-mail: s.mueller@medizin.uni-leipzig.de

S. M. Mueller et al., *Human Touch in Healthcare*, https://doi.org/10.1007/978-3-662-67860-2_8

docrinology. It is known from these disciplines that psychological factors influence the nervous system and interact with both the immune system and the endocrine system. That is, changes in one of the systems can result in changes in all the other systems. These interactions can have both positive and negative consequences for the whole organism. For example, moments of relaxation or pleasure are associated with improved mood, reductions in stress hormones, and a strengthened immune system. In contrast, stress, pain, and negative psychological states cause physical tension, headaches, high blood pressure, indigestion, and increased blood glucose levels. Based on this knowledge, relaxation techniques such as progressive muscle relaxation (PMR), yoga, and autogenic training now belong to the basic concepts of health promotion, curation and palliation, and rehabilitation, especially medical and psychiatric. Paradoxically, however, relaxation massages occupy a subordinate position in medical thinking and are still devalued occasionally as "feel-good treatment." This is regrettable because massages can:

- Generate a comprehensive relaxation response, without much practice and in a short time
- Benefit even severely injured, mobility-impaired, and cognitively impaired patients or patients with otherwise low compliance (Mueller and Grunwald 2019)

The abundance of current research shows that any appropriate manual body stimulation leads to relevant physiological and psychological changes. These effects can also be demonstrated with massages. The following chapter presents the effects of several tactile relaxation interventions as complementary treatments for physical and mental conditions. Techniques of manual therapy, manual medicine, or osteopathy are not the subject of this chapter.

▶ **Important** Relaxation massage, reflexology, and acupressure are complementary measures that may be applied in support of other evidence-based medical interventions. In this regard, medical guidelines also provide orientation.

8.2 Methodological Critique

Since the 2000s, an increasing number of studies on the clinically relevant effects of massage have been conducted. However, there are big differences regarding the methodological quality of these studies. Some include only small samples (<30 persons) and are conducted without a control group. Other studies only use qualitative survey data, results are selectively reported, and control groups differ from the experimental group in their characteristics and pretest values. This makes the interpretation of results and the calculation of effect sizes difficult or even impossible. In addition, because of the multitude of techniques (including foot reflexology, light Thai massage, Swedish massage, hand massages, reiki/therapeutic touch, acupressure, and shiatsu) and the diversity of patient groups (type of disease, stage of disease, and treatment approach), the comparability of the results is limited because not every technique has been studied for every patient group. To counteract the methodological limitations and present results that are as robust as possible, only randomized controlled trials, reviews, and meta-analyses reporting experimental studies are cited in this chapter. If there is a deviation from this rule, it will be indicated at the relevant point.

8.3 Touch and Its Influence on Physical and Mental Disorders

8.3.1 Diabetes Mellitus

8.3.1.1 Reductions in Blood Glucose Levels

Recent research showed promising effects of relaxation massages in patients with diabetes mellitus type 1 as well as type 2. For example, more pronounced reductions in blood glucose levels were achieved in **children with type 1 diabetes** when massage was used in addition to standard therapy (insulin, physical activity, and diet). In this study, parents were instructed to massage their child for 15 min every night for 2 months before bedtime (Ghazavi et al. 2008). The hands, face, upper body, and upper and lower extremities were massaged by a parent. In contrast, children in the comparison group performed 15 min of PMR each evening. An audio recording guided PMR in the presence of the parents. The third group of children (the control group) received only standard therapy during the study. Before and after the 2-month intervention, the HbA1c level in the children's blood was determined. HbA1c provides information on the average blood glucose level over the last 8–12 weeks. After 2 months of intervention, 68% of the massaged children, 62.5% of the children who had performed PMR, and 50% of the children on standard therapy showed lower HbA1c levels than before the intervention.

In another study, children with type 1 diabetes received professional Swedish massage three times per week for 15 min on the whole body (Sajedi et al. 2011). Massage oil was used. The intervention was carried out for 3 months. Immediately after each massage, blood glucose levels were measured. In the massage group, the blood glucose level decreased continuously over the intervention period. Post-massage blood glucose decreased approximately 10 mg/dL per week, from 200.3 ± 61.7 mg/dL (equivalent to approximately 11.1 mmol/L) after the first week (3 massages) to 116.9 ± 28.8 mg/dL (equivalent to approximately 6.5 mmol/L) after the 12th week (36 massages). In the control group with standard treatment, blood glucose levels remained stable between 187.8 and 209.4 mg/dL throughout the test period.

> **Important** Regular relaxing massages, in addition to insulin therapy and an adapted diet, can significantly reduce blood glucose levels.

Stress-reducing effects are discussed as the underlying mechanism. During stress, the energy resources of the body are mobilized, which leads to an increase in blood glucose levels (cf. Sect. 2.4.3). Stress reduction should therefore have a regulating effect on blood glucose levels. Some results suggest that massage may also positively affect blood glucose levels in **patients with type 2 diabetes.** In one study, women with type 2 diabetes were massaged once a week for 30 min (Ghasemi Pour et al. 2013). After 10 weeks of intervention, significantly lower HbA1c levels were measured in the massaged women than in the control group. Similar effects were found in a study without a control group in the before and after comparison (Andersson et al. 2004). In contrast, other studies failed to show any change in HbA1c levels in patients with type 2 diabetes (Wändell et al. 2010). The authors discuss how different stress levels may explain the different results among the participants. Massage may help reduce stress-related high blood glucose levels in individuals with very high stress levels (Wändell et al. 2010). In addition, the frequency, type of massage, and pressure applied could play a role (Bayat et al. 2019). So far, it has not been conclusively clarified which characteristics a massage must have to be effective as a complementary treatment for diabetes mellitus. However, stress-reducing and relaxation-promoting effects are triggered primarily by stroking massages performed with medium pressure and without pain.

8.3.1.2 Symptom Reduction and an Increase in Quality of Life

In addition to the potential positive effects of relaxation massage on blood glucose levels, there is evidence of other beneficial effects. Massage-studies report **less neuropathic pain** (Gok Metin et al. 2017) and **improved blood flow to the skin** (Castro-Sánchez et al. 2011) in patients with type 2 diabetes. Repeatedly, positive effects on the **physical and emotional quality of life** have also been shown (Wändell et al. 2012; Gok Metin et al. 2017). These results are based on studies with moderate to good methodological quality. Nevertheless, the findings should be verified in future studies.

8.3.1.3 Specific Precautions for Massage in Diabetes

Patients injecting insulin should **not be massaged at the injection site** for at least 90 min after insulin administration. Some studies show that massage of the injection site may contribute to increased insulin bioavailability (Berger et al. 1982). Under experimental conditions, blood insulin levels of 56.4 ± 8.7 mU/L were measured after 30 min of massaging the injection site, as well as a six times faster reduction in blood glucose compared to the control group (Linde 1986). In the control group, blood insulin levels were only 19.7 ± 2.2 mU/L.

Other precautions involve the skin of patients with diabetes, especially that of the lower legs and feet (Ezzo et al. 2001). The skin of many patients with diabetes is very dry, making it prone to skin cracks. Accordingly, moisturizing massage lotions should always be used to allow better gliding of the hands on the skin during a massage. In addition, the applied pressure should be carefully adjusted, and no rough or edged tools should be used to prevent injuries. Due to the high prevalence of atherosclerosis in patients with diabetes, injuries heal very slowly, and the risk of infections caused by bacteria or fungi increases. Therefore, before each massage, the body parts to be massaged should be thoroughly inspected for wounds, swelling, or inflammation. If there are signs of diabetic foot syndrome or neuropathic symptoms, consultation with the attending physician is required (see Table 4.1 in Sect. 4.1.3 Risk factors for diabetic foot syndrome).

8.3.2 Cancer

8.3.2.1 Safety of Oncological Massages

Many cancer patients wish to improve their well-being and reduce symptoms through complementary methods. Since the turn of the millennium, there has been a pronounced increase in the number of studies in this field. In particular, the effects of body-oriented methods are increasingly studied. About 30 years ago, patients with cancer were advised not to undergo massage or lymphatic drainage out of concern that it would promote metastasis (Batavia 2004). Today, patients at all disease stages are included in research efforts. It is evident from numerous animal and human studies that massage does not generally worsen cancer or lead to other complications (Corbin 2005). Provided a few precautions are taken, relaxation massage, reflexology, acupressure treatments, and lymphatic drainage can be performed on patients with acute or metastatic cancer. Therapists who wish to use massage on such patients should consider the following conditions (Corbin 2005; Sagar et al. 2007):

- **Coagulation disorders:** Patients with cancer may have low platelet counts due to taking anticoagulant medications (e.g., warfarin and heparin), as a side effect of chemotherapy/radiotherapy, or due to the cancer itself (e.g., leukemia). There is, thus, an increased risk of bruising and internal bleeding. Therefore, to prevent injuries, massages should always be performed with low pressure and in coordination with what the patient perceives as pleasant and not painful. Deep-tissue massages should be avoided.
- **Bone metastases:** Patients with bone metastases are at increased risk for fractures. Therapists should be aware of the location of metastases and avoid placing pressure on these areas.
- **Open wounds/radiodermatitis:** Injured skin areas are at risk of triggering pain or infection through touch. As with all open wounds or inflamed body areas, it is important to avoid massages in such areas.
- **Tumor position:** Although metastasis by massage is unlikely (exception: osteosarcoma; see below), manipulation should not be performed directly over tumor positions to avoid pain and unpleasant sensations. Special care should be taken with skin carcinomas, as the skin at these sites is often unstable and prone to bleeding.

▶ Important *NOTE!* **Osteosarcoma**: Patients with osteosarcoma constitute an important exception and are a contraindication to massage. In animal models, massage directly over osteosarcoma resulted in worsening and greater spread of the carcinoma (Wang et al. 2014). In a study of 134 osteosarcoma patients, those who had been massaged at the site of the osteosarcoma *prior to* diagnosis showed worse progression of the disease and more frequent metastases (Wu et al. 2010). Whether massages at distant body sites from the osteosarcoma can have negative consequences for these patients has not yet been systematically investigated.

8.3.2.2 Full Body Massages and Therapeutic Touch

The care of patients with cancer should always be holistic, with consideration of the patient's bio-psychosocial needs. Such a diagnosis is often accompanied by psychological challenges, such as fears of disease progression or recurrence, fear of death, uncertainties about the diagnosis, social isolation, depression, and a negative body image due to surgery, weight loss, or other physical changes (Russell et al. 2008; Grunwald and Mueller 2017). (For more in-depth information on body image changes due to illness, see Sect. 1.5)

Light Thai massages, Swedish massages, and therapeutic touch (TT) have been shown in various studies to affect patients with cancer positively. Massages, as well as TT, can induce relaxation, which is characterized by **lowered blood pressure, a lower heart rate, and slowed breathing** (Post-White et al. 2003). The effects are not merely due to social support or social presence, as studies have shown that both massages and TT can reduce **anxiety, fatigue, and pain** in oncological patients, but the mere presence of another person has no such effect (Post-White et al. 2003).

In one study, patients received 4 weeks of 45-min sessions of each of the three conditions (Swedish massage with unscented oil, TT, and mere presence) in random order. TT (alternative labels: Healing touch or Reiki) was performed by placing the hands flat on various parts of the client's body or hovering directly above the body surface. Practitioners often refer to this technique as a biofield or energy treatment through which disturbed "energy fields" or "energy flows" can be restored. Such "energy field changes" have not yet been scientifically proven, and only a few studies on TT meet strict scientific criteria. However, based on the known physiological changes that can be triggered through social touch, relaxation processes, and placebo effects, standardized touch therapies are interesting procedures (cf. Sects 2.4 and 5.3). In the direct comparison of TT and massages, it was shown that massages reduce pain in oncological patients more successfully and improve mood more reliably (Post-White et al. 2003). Recent reviews that included patients with different types of cancer at different stages of treatment highlight the positive effects of massage on anxiety, fatigue, and pain (Shin et al. 2016; Calcagni et al. 2019). Accordingly, massage benefits patients at all stages of the disease, including those under palliative care (Jane et al. 2011; Khiewkhern et al. 2013). Additionally, massage can contribute to **improve sleep, general well-being, reduce anger, and reduce listlessness** (Jane et al. 2011; Listing et al. 2009). It is possible that the use of scented massage oils may enhance the positive effects (Shin et al. 2016). There is preliminary evidence that aromatic oils may lead to more robust and longer-lasting symptom reductions. However, it is not yet clear whether the oil (less friction) or the aroma (fragrance) is the relevant factor. A study in which one group of patients (blood cancer, isolation ward) was massaged with oil and a second group with aroma oil showed comparable positive effects with and without aroma (Stringer et al. 2008). Compared to the control group without intervention (rest), both oil-massage groups with and without aroma showed reduced cortisol levels, less negative, and more positive emotions.

It is not conclusively clear what causes contradictory results in different studies, e.g., pain-reducing effects in some studies but not in others. Different explanations are discussed. On the one hand, attitudes toward treatment and expectancy effects may influence the success of treatments (cf. Sect. 5.3 Placebo effects). On the other hand, different baseline levels of symptoms may play a role. For example, stress-, anxiety-, and pain-reducing effects are only measurable if patients show a minimum level of these symptoms in the pretest (Toth et al. 2013; Listing et al. 2010). In addition, methodological flaws in the study design can lead to contradictory results.

8.3.2.3 Hand and Foot Massages

Two recent reviews and one meta-analysis show that through reflexology as well as hand and foot effleurage, small to moderate positive **effects on pain** in cancer patients can be achieved (Unlu et al. 2018; Gholamzadeh et al. 2019; Najafpour and Shayanfard 2020). In addition, a number of studies show **improvements in anxiety, depression, sleep, and quality of life** in cancer patients (Unlu et al. 2018; Gholamzadeh et al. 2019; Lee et al. 2015).

Currently, however, there is no scientific evidence that specific points on the feet or hands are associated with specific organs or that tactile stimulation of specific points would affect diseases of specific organs (Ernst et al. 2011; Ernst 2009; Wang et al. 2008). This is true both when the treatment is performed by trained personnel and when it is performed by the patients themselves (Song et al. 2015). Accordingly, reflexology must not be used to diagnose or treat diseases! However, reflexology can trigger short-term relaxation effects. The effects resemble those that can be induced by effleurage of the hands, feet, or body (Lee et al. 2015).

The reported studies used variations of 20–40-min treatment sessions, once to twice per week.

> ▶ **Important** **Reductions in pain and anxiety** can be achieved through several massage techniques (light Thai massage, Swedish massage, and hand and foot massages), reflexology, acupressure, and TT in patients with different types of cancer. In addition, all types of interventions **reduced fatigue**, which in turn improved physical and psychological well-being.

8.3.2.4 Acupressure

To date, only a few studies with good methodological quality have investigated the effect of **acupressure** on patients with cancer (Calcagni et al. 2019). The existing studies show positive effects on similar dimensions as Swedish massage and reflexology: **anxiety, pain, and fatigue.** For example, in hospitalized patients with different types of cancer, 10 acupressure sessions were performed (one time per day) (Beikmoradi et al. 2015). Treatment lasted approximately 30 min, with acupressure points stimulated for 2 min each (bilateral: LI4, LI10, H7, and Hu9; unilateral: DU20, Ren6, Yin tang, and UB13). In the placebo acupressure group, points 2 cm adjacent to the actual acupressure points were stimulated. The control group received standard care only. A significant reduction in anxiety was measured in the acupressure group. A non-significant trend toward anxiety reduction was noted in the placebo group, and a trend toward anxiety *increase* was noted in the control group (non-significant).

Short-term positive effects of acupressure have also been shown for pain. For example, patients with cancer who received acupressure treatment during a bone marrow biopsy (2 min bilateral LI4 and H7) reported significantly lower pain scores after the procedure than patients in the control group (standard treatment) (Sharifi Rizi et al. 2017). Patients who received only placebo acupressure (points 2 cm next to the acupressure points were lightly touched) also reported significantly lower pain scores than the control group. However, pain reduction was more substantial in the acupressure group.

Similarly, patients with leukemia who participated in 12 outpatient acupressure appointments (three times per week; bilateral LIV3, ST36, LI11, and LI4) showed significantly lower pain scores immediately after each session than before the sessions (Sharif Nia et al. 2017). Participants reported pain on a 10-point visual analog scale (VAS). On average, pain scores improved from 8 to 5.5 immediately after the intervention. No change was observed in the control group.

Acupressure can also positively affect postoperative pain perception (Hsiung et al. 2015). In that study, patients with gastric cancer were treated with acupressure (P6 and ST36, bilateral, 3 min per point) for 3 consecutive days after partial gastric resection. In both the acupressure and control groups, pain intensity decreased continuously over the 3 days. On average, participants in the acupressure group showed faster remission of postoperative pain.

Acupressure effects on fatigue were shown in a study in which patients with breast cancer were treated with acupressure 3 days per week for 12 weeks (Zhang et al. 2017). Stimulated on both sides were LI4, ST36, and SP6 for 10 min each. After 6 and 12 weeks of treatment, the acupressure group reported significantly lower levels of physical and mental fatigue and higher levels of activity and motivation than the standard treatment group. After 12 weeks, the acupressure group also reported significantly lower scores on depression and anxiety scales and better sleep than the standard treatment group.

However, no reliable effects have been found on **chemotherapy-induced nausea and vomiting**. Review articles summarizing multiple studies of acupressure showed no effects for adults (Lee et al. 2008) or children (Khakpour et al. 2019). A meta-analysis suggests that there may be a small effect on the severity of nausea (both acute and delayed) but not on the frequency of vomiting (Miao et al. 2017).

As with all other complementary methods, acupressure must always be performed in addition to standard treatment.

> **Important** It remains unclear whether the various types of massage and touch interventions differ in effectiveness and whether patients with certain types of cancer respond better to massage than other patients. Further systematic studies are needed.

8.3.2.5 Effects on Immune Markers in Cancer Patients

Chemotherapy and radiotherapy can lead to a reduction in white blood cells. Measures to counteract this loss can help protect oncology patients from infections. In various studies, a beneficial effect of relaxation massages on immune markers has been shown (cf. Sect. 2.4.4). However, it is unclear whether these effects have a clinically relevant impact on the health status of patients and what dose would be required for this. Nevertheless, the results available so far are promising and will be briefly presented here:

For example, patients with colorectal cancer were treated with massage therapy between two cycles of chemotherapy (Khiewkhern et al. 2013). Within 1 week, they received three light Thai massages with aroma oil, each lasting 45 min. The head, face, neck, back, shoulders, arms, hands, lower legs, and feet were massaged. Blood samples were taken 5 min before the first massage and 1–2 days after the last massage. At the post-test, the increase in the number of lymphocytes was significantly higher (218 cells/μL) in the massage group than in the control group, a difference of 11%. In contrast, the number of other white blood cells (neutrophil granulocytes, CD4, and CD8) showed no difference between the groups. As secondary effects, the study also reported significant reductions in anxiety, fatigue, and pain but not nausea and depression.

This finding is consistent with a study involving women with breast cancer who had completed their last radio/chemotherapy cycle at least 3 months ago (Hernandez-Reif et al. 2005). The 58 participants were divided into a massage group, a PMR group, and a control group with no intervention. The massage group received three 30-min full-body massages per week for 5 weeks. The head, face, neck, back, shoulders, arms, hands, lower legs, and feet were massaged. The PMR group performed guided 30-min PMR three times per week for 5 weeks. Between the first and last days of the intervention, the massage group showed a significant increase in natural killer (NK) cells (12%) and lymphocytes (9%). However, the increase in killer cell toxicity (9%) was not significant. In contrast, in the PMR group, killer cell toxicity increased significantly (19%), but the increase in white blood cells (lymphocytes = 2%; NK = 7%) did not reach significance. No significant changes were observed in the control group (lymphocytes = 0%; NK = −7%; toxicity = 0%). In addition, significant increases in dopamine (59%) and serotonin (36%) were measured in the massage group but not in the PMR and control groups. Cortisol, epinephrine, or norepinephrine levels did not change in any of the three groups.

Other studies showed positive effects on immune markers immediately after massage (Billhult et al. 2009; Imanishi et al. 2009), but not in the long-term pre-post comparison after multiple massages (Imanishi et al. 2009; Billhult et al. 2008). Possible explanations for the lack of effects could be environmental conditions, the type and dose of massage, or the social support provided to the control group. The control group spent the same amount of time in the company of a nurse, which may have been perceived as social support and may have also elicited positive effects. In two of the studies, the massages were performed immediately following the outpatient radiotherapy session, directly in the oncology ward. The women were likely less able to relax in the oncology ward than in a neutral or pleasant environment. Supporting this hypothesis is the fact that no effects on cortisol, oxytocin, anxiety, depression, or quality of life were found in this study either (Billhult et al. 2008).

The results of another study suggest that attitudes toward massage may also have a relevant influence on immune effects. In this study, an increase in igA levels was found only in women who had a positive attitude toward massage (Fernández-Lao et al. 2012).

▶ **Important** A calm, relaxing, disturbance-free atmosphere and a pleasant room temperature are required to enable positive effects through oncological massages.

8.3.3 Asthma

Improvement of **asthmatic symptoms in children** is reported as a positive effect of massage in several review articles. Currently, however, only one randomized controlled trial exists, which can be viewed in full text (Field et al. 1998). Of four other publications that promise positive effects (Tian et al. 2014b,a; Fattah and Hamdy 2011; Goli and Shabestari 2017), only English abstracts are available but no full texts, so an assessment of the reliability of the findings is not possible. A review article with meta-analysis published in English also suggests positive effects but is based entirely on Asian studies for which full texts cannot be retrieved (Wu et al. 2017).

Because of the unreliable research base, only the results of the randomized controlled trial are briefly presented here to offer a cautious view of possible effects (Field et al. 1998). Thirty-two children participated in the study (16 between the ages of 4 and 8 years and 16 between the ages of 9 and 14 years). Children were randomly assigned to either the massage group or the PMR group (control group). Both interventions were delivered by the children's parents, who were previously trained in whole-body massage or PMR. The interventions were performed every evening before bedtime for 20 min for 30 consecutive days. Pulmonary function tests were performed before and at the end of the 30-day intervention. The study results showed that younger children, in particular, could benefit from massage. Children aged 6–8 years showed significant improvements in attitude toward asthma and improved lung functions. At follow-up, maximum expiratory flow (peak flow) increased from 2.6 to 3.7 L/s (42.3% increase) and forced expiratory vital capacity (lung volume) increased from 1.3 to 1.7 L (30.7% increase). In addition, forced expiratory volume in the first second of expiration (FEV1) increased from 1.1 to 1.5 L (36.4% increase), and FEF25-75 (forced expiratory flow) even showed an increase from 1.3 to 3.0 L/s (130.7%). In the older children, the massage group showed significant improvements in attitude toward asthma and FEF25-75 (from 1.7 to 3.5 L/s equals a 105.8% increase). In the PMR group, there were no significant changes in either the young or older children.

Whether or to what extent adults with asthma might benefit from massage has not been systematically studied.

▶ **Important** Massage can positively affect attitudes toward asthma and lung function in children with asthma.

Patients with **cystic fibrosis** could also potentially benefit from massage. In this rare metabolic disease, lung function and breathing are impaired. Currently, there is only one randomized controlled trial investigating the effect of relaxation massages. In this study, children were massaged for 20 min before bedtime by a parent (Hernandez-Reif et al. 1999). Participants in the control group were read to by a parent for 20 min each evening. At the end of the 30-day intervention, the maximum expiratory rate (peak flow) of the children in the massage group was significantly higher than before the intervention and in the control group. In addition, parental and child illness-related anxiety decreased in the massage group, and children's mood improved (less negative or depressed feelings).

8.3.4 Dialysis for Chronic Kidney Disease

Chronic kidney disease affects more than 10% of the general population worldwide (Kovesdy 2022). For patients with end-stage renal disease, hemodialysis is the most commonly used form of kidney replacement therapy. Patients who have to be treated regularly with dialysis often suffer from accompanying conditions. These include depression, anxiety, sleep disorders, sleep apnea, fatigue, and restless leg syndrome (Murtagh et al. 2007; Cukor et al. 2008). A growing number of studies suggest that massage can positively impact these accompanying conditions. Interestingly, the studies investigating the effect massage can have on these symptoms are very similar in their methodological approach. In most of these studies, patients are massaged on their feet during dialysis sessions, about an hour after dialysis begins. This approach has several advantages. First, it makes the studies relatively comparable. Second, patients receive a welcome change during the long dialysis sessions and do not have to attend additional appointments. With a minimum duration of 4 h per dialysis session and usually three sessions per week, additional appointments could have a negative impact on willingness to participate.

8.3.4.1 Fatigue, Mood, Sleep, and Quality of Life

Both as a consequence of the disease and due to dialysis treatments, many patients suffer from exhaustion (fatigue) and reduced quality of life. Therefore, various tactile interventions (Swedish massage, reflexology, and acupressure) have been investigated for their effectiveness in randomized controlled trials.

For example, in one study, patients were assigned to one of four groups and massaged on the feet using either almond oil (group 1), chamomile oil (group 2), or no oil (group 3) (Habibzadeh et al. 2020). The fourth group received no massage and served as a control group. Participants were massaged for 20 min (10 min per foot) three times a week for 2 months, 1 h after the start of dialysis. Before the Swedish massage began, the feet were washed and dried. All three massage groups showed significant improvements in **fatigue and quality of life** at follow-up. The two groups massaged with oil showed greater effects than the group massaged without oil. This effect was confirmed by another study in which massages were performed with or without aromatic oil (Mohammadpourhodki et al. 2021). The authors reported that at follow-up, patients who received aromatic oil massages rated their quality of life significantly more positively than patients who received massages without oil. Some authors suggest that the use of fragrances may increase positive effects. For example, one study compared the effects of aromatherapy (inhalation) and aromatic oil massage (Varaei et al. 2020). Participants were randomly assigned to one of the two groups or a control group. A piece of fleece wetted with a drop of aroma oil and pinned to the collar for 20 min was used for inhalation. The analysis showed that compared to the pretest, fatigue remained about the same in the inhalation group, decreased significantly in the massage group, and increased in the control group without intervention. At the two follow-up examinations, eight and 16 weeks after the end of the study, significantly lower fatigue values were still found in both intervention groups compared to the control group.

Other studies found positive effects on **sleep quality, depression, anxiety, stress, and fatigue** from foot reflexology, acupressure, and back massage (Unal and Balci Akpinar 2016; Hmwe et al. 2015; Shariati et al. 2012). Thereby, interventions on the feet and legs were more effective in improving sleep and fatigue than back massages. A possible explanation for this could be that foot massages reduce the incidence of uremic restless leg syndrome.

8.3.4.2 Uremic Restless Legs Syndrome

Restless legs syndrome (RLS) is a common problem in patients with chronic renal failure. Between 20 and 80% of dialysis patients suffer from RLS. The prevalence in the general population is only 2–15% (Rye and Trotti 2012; Winkelmann 2008). Because it is more pronounced during rest, it impairs sleep, contributes to fatigue, and reduces quality of life. Lifestyle changes (including sleep hygiene, less caffeine, and less alcohol) can positively impact RLS symptoms (Klingelhoefer et al. 2014). In addition, drug treatments are possible but may be associated with side effects (drowsiness, nausea, and blood pressure changes). Recent studies suggest that **foot and leg massages** can also positively affect RLS.

In all studies, symptom severity was measured using the International Restless Legs Syndrome Study Group Rating Scale (Walters et al. 2003). It consists of ten questions that can be scored between 0 and 4. Higher total scores indicate more severe RLS: 1–10 mild, 11–20 moderate, 21–30 severe, and 31–40 very severe symptoms.

Patients were massaged twice a week on the feet and lower legs using effleurage, for 3 consecutive weeks, during dialysis (Hashemi et al. 2015). Lavender oil was used. The massage lasted only 5 min per leg. At the end of the 3 weeks, the mean RLS score of the intervention group was significantly reduced (pre: $M = 22.4$; post: $M = 12.4$). Comparably large effects were seen with olive oil (Nasiri et al. 2019) or glycerin oil (Mirbagher Ajorpaz et al. 2020). In the control group, which received only the standard treatment, no changes in RLS severity occurred (pre: $M = 22.9$; post: $M = 23.2$).

A single case study suggests that improvement in RLS symptoms may last up to 2 weeks after the end of the intervention (Russell 2007). The patient received 45 min of effleurage of the feet and legs to the hips 2× per week for 3 weeks.

Currently, it is not known which mechanisms cause the effects. However, several hypotheses exist (Mitchell 2011):

- First, the release of dopamine might contribute to symptom reduction. This is supported by the fact that levodopa (a precursor of the endogenous substance dopamine) is used as a drug treatment for RLS and that increased urinary dopamine levels have been found in healthy persons after massages (cf. Sect. 2.4).
- Second, the increased blood flow caused by the massages might have a symptom-reducing effect by improving tissue oxygenation and stimulating cellular metabolism.
- Third, the sensory signals generated by massage might modulate neural activity in the thalamus. In patients with idiopathic RLS, it has been shown that activation in the thalamus is associated with paresthesia of the legs.

▶ **Important** Foot and leg massages during dialysis, of as little as 5 min per leg, can achieve significant and clinically relevant symptom reductions in restless leg syndrome. This improves sleep quality and reduces fatigue.

8.3.5 HIV/AIDS

The treatment of patients with HIV and AIDS aims to slow down the replication rate of the HIV viruses and prevent opportunistic infections. HIV drug treatment reduces viral replication and can positively affect the number of CD4 lymphocytes (T helper cells), resulting in a longer asymptomatic infection phase. During the course of HIV infection, the number of CD4 lymphocytes continuously decreases. Cell counts of less than 200/mm^3 indicate a severely advanced disease, usually with pronounced AIDS symptoms.

Opportunistic infections are associated with low numbers of NK cells. Consequently, the goal is to increase the number of NK cells to prevent infections. In addition, patients who remain asymptomatic despite advanced HIV infection and low CD4 cell counts appear to have higher NK cell activity (Solomon et al. 1993).

Various studies showed a significant **increase in the number of NK cells** in patients with HIV in connection with weekly relaxation massages over several weeks (Ironson et al. 1996; Diego et al. 2001). In other studies, however, such effects did not occur or occurred only in subgroups (Shor-Posner et al. 2006; Birk et al. 2000). The authors discuss how several 20-min massages per week could possibly achieve better effects than one longer massage per week. They argue that two to five short massages per week could achieve a greater cumulative relaxation effect because they may be less strenuous for patients than long massages. The relaxing and anxiety-reducing effects of massages are thought to be the key driver for an increase in NK cells. **Anxiety-reducing effects and positive effects on the quality of life** can be enhanced if, in addition to massages, other stress-regulating procedures (e.g., meditation and stress management training) are applied (Williams et al. 2005).

An influence of massages on CD4 lymphocytes has not been reliably proven so far.

> **Important** Massage can increase the number of NK cells in patients with HIV, especially if other stress-regulating techniques are also used.

8.3.6 Depression and Anxiety Disorders

When comparing studies on massage effects in different patient groups, it is noticeable that some effects (including improved sleep, improved mood, stress reduction, and pain reduction) are systematically reported (cf. Sect. 2.4 Physiological effects of touch). A comprehensive meta-analysis investigated which overarching effects could be achieved by relaxation massages, both in healthy individuals and in patients with diverse underlying diseases (Moyer et al. 2004). The authors found that regular massages over several weeks could **significantly reduce depression and anxiety**. Clinically relevant changes were measured for situational anxiety (state anxiety) and dispositional anxiety (trait anxiety). On average, 77% of participants in the massage groups experienced greater anxiety reduction than individuals in the control groups. Similarly, the reduction in depressive symptoms was more pronounced for 73% of those receiving massage than for those in the control groups. These effects are comparable to effect sizes reported in meta-analyses of psychotherapy efficacy. Accordingly, on average, 79% of patients treated with psychotherapy reached better outcome scores than untreated patients (Wampold 2009). That means massage therapy may be similarly effective as psychotherapy for treating secondary anxiety and depressive disorders. The findings were based on patient groups recruited for primary physical disorders (including HIV infection, back pain, hypertension, fibromyalgia, breast cancer, chronic fatigue syndrome, and multiple sclerosis). However, the cited meta-analysis does not include studies that examined whether patients with primary depression or anxiety disorders would benefit from massage therapy. The corresponding findings are summarized below.

> **Important** Massage therapy is similarly effective as psychotherapy in reducing anxiety and depression symptoms secondary to physical illnesses or disorders.

8.3.6.1 Primary Depression

Studies show that massage can significantly improve all levels of clinical depression, from mild to severe. Initial studies were conducted with depressed pregnant women. In this group of patients, the search for complementary and alternative treatments is particularly relevant, as many women fear that antidepressants may harm the child's development and discontinue the drugs during the course of pregnancy (Zoega et al. 2015). On the other hand, untreated depression during pregnancy is associated with pregnancy and birth complications as well as preterm birth and low birth weight (Gentile 2017). In one study, pregnant women were massaged twice a week for 16 weeks by their partner (Field et al. 2004). Professional massage therapists trained the partners to perform 20-min massages that were comfortable and safe for pregnant women (for more detail, see Sect. 6.1.3). The effects were compared with a group of women who performed PMR (audio recording) twice a week and a group that received standard gynecological care. In the massage group, significantly lower depression and anxiety scores (Current Mood Scale; General Depression Scale; State-Trait Anxiety Inventory [STAI]) were measured after a single massage and after 16 weeks, while no changes occurred in the PMR and standard care groups.

Comparable effects were reported for outpatients (men and women) with mild-to-moderate depressive disorders (Arnold et al. 2020). Participants received 45-min full-body oil massages plus 15 min of rest after the massage. The massages were performed by a professional massage therapist once a week for 4 weeks and included long strokes and soft kneading without any painful treatments. During the treatment, music or conversation were deliberately avoided. Some professionals refer to this particularly gentle and sensitive type of massage as "**psychoactive massage.**" Initial comparative experimental studies suggest that this type of massage may be particularly well suited to elicit anxiety-relieving and mood-lifting effects (Baumgart et al. 2020). Individuals in the comparison group performed 45 min of PMR once per week, which was guided by a coach in a relaxed environment. Approximately equal numbers of individuals in both groups received concomitant psychotherapy and psychotropic medication. At the end of intervention, both groups showed significant improvements; however, the people in the massage group reached significantly better scores on the Hamilton Depression Scale and the Bech-Rafaelsen Melancholia Scale (BRMS) than the people in the PMR group.

Patients undergoing acute psychiatric treatment are also likely to benefit from 'psychoactive' whole-body massages. In a study in which patients served as their own control group (intra-individual comparisons), in-patients with acute depression of the entire affective spectrum according to ICD-10 without comorbidity were examined (Müller-Oerlinghausen et al. 2004). The patients alternated between three massage appointments and two control appointments (relaxation and perception exercises) of 60 min each. Before and after each of the five sessions, participants were assessed on their symptoms using BRMS and STAI. On average, participants reported more positive changes after the massages than after the control appointments (massage: BRMS 20%, STAI 21%; control: BRMS 13%, STAI 14%).

In another study, children and adolescents (ages 8–18) in inpatient psychiatric treatment with adjustment disorder, conduct disorder, and depression showed significantly reduced anxiety (STAI) and depression scores after 5 days of massage therapy (Current Mood Scale; Field et al. 1992). In addition, their sleep improved significantly. The massages lasted 30 min and were limited to strokes with moderate pressure over the back and shoulders. The comparison group watched a movie with relaxing images and quiet music for 30 min daily. No changes in anxiety, depression, or sleep were observed in the film group at the end of the 5 days.

More in-depth studies are needed to determine the optimal frequency, type, and duration of massage applications as well as examine cumulative and long-term effects. In addition, systematic studies on the effectiveness of massage compared with psychotherapeutic and pharmacological interventions are required. Until reliable findings are available, massages can be used complementary to standard therapy.

▶ **Important** Preliminary findings suggest significant positive effects of 'psychoactive massage' in primary depression.

8.3.6.2 Anxiety Disorders

Anxiety disorders are among the most common mental health disorders, with a 12-month prevalence of about 15% (Jacobi et al. 2014; Thom et al. 2019), followed by affective disorders with a 12-month prevalence of about 9%. The most common forms of anxiety disorders are:

- Panic disorder with or without agoraphobia
- Generalized anxiety disorder
- Social anxiety disorder
- Specific phobias

The anxiety-reducing effects of massage have been repeatedly demonstrated for anxiety secondary to numerous physical diseases and conditions as well as generalized anxiety disorder (GAS; Rapaport et al. 2018). However, studies on massage effects on panic disorder, social anxiety, or specific phobias are not yet available.

In a longitudinal study, outpatients with generalized anxiety disorder were treated with Swedish massage (whole-body massage with effleurage and petrissage) twice a week for 45 min each (Rapaport et al. 2016). To take part in the study, participants had to be physically healthy and have generalized anxiety disorder as their primary psychiatric diagnosis (Structured Clinical Interview for DSM-IV; Hamilton Anxiety Scale [HAM-A] score > 14). The unique feature of the study is that massage was used as monotherapy. This means patients did not use psychotropic medication or participate in psychotherapy sessions during the 6-week study. A group of patients who received light touch treatments twice a week served as a control group. This consisted of gentle static touch to the limbs, trunk, and back over a period of 45 min. The results showed that after 6 weeks, both groups significantly improved in HAM-A scores. The effect was significantly greater in the massage group than in the light touch group. Some of the patients were treated for 6 additional weeks with massage therapy (Rapaport et al. 2021). On average, the HAM-A score decreased from on average 19.91 (SD = 2.17) to 10.00 (SD = 5.80) in the first 6 weeks and to 6.91 (SD = 3.11) in the following 6 weeks. These results suggest that the largest symptom-reducing effects occur during the first 6 weeks and that, for most patients, twice weekly massage therapy for 6 weeks is sufficient to reduce anxiety symptoms in a clinically relevant manner.

Another study showed that ten massage sessions spread over 12 weeks could also generate clinically relevant changes (Sherman et al. 2010). The effects of ten massages in 12 weeks were similar to those of 6 weeks of twice-weekly massage. However, in this study, 60% of participants also took antidepressant or antianxiety medications or attended psychotherapy. The massages lasted about 45 min and consisted of Myofascial Release and Swedish massage elements (Sherman et al. 2010). The goal of the massages was to relieve tension. Participants in the comparison groups received the same duration of thermotherapy (alternating hot and cold compresses) or quiet lying in a relaxation room. In this study, all three interventions resulted in comparable improvements in participants' HAM-A scores from, on average, 25 points before intervention to 15 points after intervention (range of change: 6.9–16.0). In addition, the study examined whether the effects persisted over the long term; the authors found that scores remained stable 12 weeks after the end of the intervention. The study did not include a control group without complementary treatments, so it cannot be assessed whether the effects would have occurred even without the treatments. However, comparisons with placebo-controlled drug trials suggest that placebo pills show smaller improvements in HAM-A scores, ranging from 2.3 to 10.2 points (Hidalgo et al. 2007). Therefore, in line with the 6-week study, it is likely that all three relaxation interventions reduce anxiety symptoms beyond medication and psychotherapy.

▶ **Important** For most patients with generalized anxiety disorder, twice-weekly massage therapy for 6 weeks is sufficient to reduce anxiety symptoms in a clinically relevant manner. The largest anxiety-reducing effects occur during the first 6 weeks of twice-weekly massage therapy.

8.3.7 Post-traumatic Stress Disorder

Post-traumatic stress disorder (PTSD) is a delayed response to a terrifying event or exceptionally threatening situation. Common symptoms include:

- Continued reliving of the event through intrusive thoughts, flashbacks, nightmares
- Social and emotional withdrawal, avoidance behavior, emotional numbness, apathy
- Arousal symptoms such as sleep disturbances, irritability, difficulty concentrating

Some patients also experience somatization, substance abuse, suicidality, or dissociative symptoms. Treatment of PTSD usually involves a combination of talking psychotherapy (e.g., cognitive behavioral therapy), confrontation therapy, and medication (antidepressants, anti-anxiety medications). More recently, EMDR (Eye Movement Desensitization and Reprocessing) has been increasingly used for treatment. It's efficacy is comparable or possibly superior to other confrontation therapies (Lewey et al. 2018; Cuijpers et al. 2020; Khan et al. 2018). In principle, a cautious and considered approach by trained trauma specialists and treatment based on guideline recommendations is indicated to prevent mental overload and further destabilization of the patient (Schaefer et al. 2019). In addition, complementary techniques can be used to support the treatment.

8.3.7.1 Massage Therapy

Some patients with PTSD seek complementary (body) therapies to counter feelings of tension, agitation, disembodiment, or pain. Depending on the nature of the trauma, patients may crave touch and yet suffer intrusive thoughts or panic attacks from touch; patients may also experience mistrust or fear of losing control. Treating traumatized individuals requires a high level of empathy, compassion, consideration, and patience from the professionals providing treatment. The most important conditions for massage treatments for PTSD are **safety, consent, and control**. Working with the patient, the therapist must create a safe environment in which the patient has a consensual say in which parts of the body are touched or when breaks are needed. Communication with the patient about how to proceed and responsiveness to the patient's needs are paramount. Highlighting the challenges posed by PTSD, we will briefly summarize study results on the effects of massage therapy. Although the findings suggest positive effects, no reliable statements can currently be made about the dose or contraindications for massages in PTSD.

In one of the first studies on the topic, children who showed **behavioral problems at school** were selected in the **aftermath of a severe natural disaster** (Hurricane Andrew 1992, Florida, USA; Field et al. 1996). Sixty children with moderate-to-high scores on the PTSD Scale (Frederick 1985) were randomly assigned to a massage group or a control group. Approximately 4 weeks had elapsed since the hurricane. The children had a mean age of 7.5 years and remained clothed during treatment. The massage group received 30 min of shoulder, neck, and back massage using long strokes with medium pressure twice a week for 4 weeks. The massages were performed by massage trainees. The control group spent the same amount of time and frequency watching cartoons with a massage trainee. Physical contact was maintained with the child by placing an arm around the child or having the child sit on the trainee's lap. Immediately after the massage, the children had lower state anxiety (STAI) and cortisol levels than before the massage. At the end of the 4-week intervention, the children's trait anxiety (Reynolds and Richmond 1985) and depressive symptoms (Center for Epidemiologic Studies Depression Scale) were significantly decreased. There were no changes in the control group (cartoons).

In a second study, 40 **war veterans** participated and were randomly assigned to a massage group or a waitlist control group (Field et al. 2020b). Participants had a mean age of 51 years and a mean of five military deployments, each lasting 6 months. No information was provided on how long ago the last deployment had occurred or how long the PTSD had been present. The patients completed two questionnaires on their current PTSD symptoms (including sleep, anxiety, depression, exhaustion, pain, and self-injurious intent) before the first and after the last massage (Forbes et al. 2001; Dewitt et al. 2018). Participants were massaged once a week for 30 min for 4 consecutive weeks on the head, neck, shoulders, and back, lying on their sides during the massage. After the intervention was terminated, both groups showed significant improvements in symptoms, which were slightly bigger in the massage group. However, the effects were extremely small. At 4 weeks of follow-up, almost all scores returned to baseline levels, except **self-injurious intentions**, which remained lower than before the intervention. Since improvements in symptoms were found in both the massage group and the control group, social support effects may have been generated by the repeated interviews, which also had a stabilizing effect in the control group.

Another study explored the effects of massage in combination with body-oriented mindfulness exercises on dissociative symptoms (Price 2007). The study involved 24 adult women who had been **victims of sexual abuse in** childhood. All participants had been receiving psychotherapeutic treatment for, on average, 6 years (range: 2–15 years), which continued concurrently with the study. The study had no control group. The intervention consisted of two sessions per week for 4 weeks. Each session lasted 60 min and consisted either entirely of massage applications or a combination of massage and mindfulness exercises. During the massages, the women were fully clothed. Massages were performed on the head, neck, back, legs, and arms, ranging from 10 to 60 min. The Dissociative Experiences Scale was used to evaluate symptomatology (Freyberger et al. 1998). During the intervention, **dissociative symptoms decreased significantly**. The process continued beyond the intervention: at the follow-up measurements, 1 and 3 months after the intervention, further reductions of dissociative symptoms were shown. The results suggest that body therapy interventions, complementary to psychotherapeutic treatments, can contribute to symptom reduction in PTSD.

8.3.7.2 ETF Tapping

One procedure that is increasingly receiving attention in the treatment of PTSD is called **tapping** (also known as Emotional Freedom Technique or EFT). This procedure also focuses on touch but does not use massage. Instead, the relevant touches are usually performed by the affected persons themselves while guided by a professional therapist.

It is a trauma-focused intervention with imaginal exposure in the form of trauma memories, stressful triggers in the present, and trauma-related anxiety about the future (Shapiro 2018; Schäfer et al. 2019). In the process, patients recall traumatic memories while performing tapping sequence. Consequently, it is not dissimilar to the EMDR (eye movement desensitization and reprocessing) approach. Hypotheses about the mechanisms of action of EMDR and tapping also match and are based on divided attention processes and conditioning processes. **Divided attention** is induced by eye movement (EMDR) or by touch (Tapping). During the retrieval of traumatic memories, the patient performs tapping on various areas of his or her body at a set sequence, speed, and frequency. Part of the patient's working memory resources are occupied and distracted by the attentional demand of this motor coordination task. Therefore, preoccupation with the traumatic memory is not possible. Accordingly, the distracting task has to be challenging enough so that it cannot be performed automatically. At the same time, however, the task must not bind the person's full attention and concentration, otherwise, recall and reappraisal of the traumatic memory would be prevented. Counterconditioning and extinction are thought to be the primary underlying mechanisms. The concept of **counterconditioning** is based on the assumption that opposing emotional states cannot occur simultaneously—for example, fear and relaxation. The goal is to link fear-inducing stimuli or thoughts with positive or neutral emotions. **Extinction** describes the attenuation of a conditioned response by repeatedly presenting the conditioned (initially neutral) stimulus without the expected consequence. In the case of tapping, trauma memories are retrieved simultaneously with a spatiotemporal working memory task, leaving few resources for emotional processes. A physiological state is created that is incompatible with the maladaptive conditioned reflexes of

PTSD (Feinstein and Church 2010; Landin-Romero et al. 2018). As a result, the intense negative emotionality of memories is reduced.

Tapping can significantly increase the speed and effectiveness of exposure therapy and cognitive behavioral therapy (Mollon 2007). For example, in a randomized controlled study, **war veterans with PTSD** were treated with six 1–h tapping sessions (Church et al. 2013). At completion, 90% of individuals in the intervention group no longer met the criteria for PTSD, while symptoms remained the same in the standard care control group. In addition, symptom improvements in the intervention group remained stable at follow-up measurements—3 and 6 months after treatment completion.

Tapping/exposure can also provide unusually rapid symptom relief for **adolescents with PTSD**, sometimes after only one session. Particularly striking effects were achieved with a group of 50 adolescents from Rwanda who were orphaned and traumatized 12 years earlier, during the genocide. After a single session, the symptom severity of all participants dropped below the diagnostic threshold for PTSD (Sakai et al. 2010). Interviews with the adolescents and their caregivers at the orphanage indicated substantial symptom reductions in flashbacks, nightmares, bedwetting, withdrawal, self-isolation, startle response, difficulty concentrating, aggression, and depression. At the follow-up examination 1 year after the intervention, symptom improvements remained stable. In another study, significant symptom improvements were also seen after just a single session in adolescents living in residential care due to physical or psychological **abuse experiences** (Church et al. 2012).

► **Important** Tapping in combination with exposure therapy should be performed by professional psychotherapists to avoid aggravation of PTSD symptoms.

A survey of 448 psychotherapists and psychological health practitioners confirms the high efficacy of tapping: 65% of therapists reported that 60–95% of patients were fully rehabilitated (Church et al. 2017). Ninety percent of therapists reported that less than 10% of patients did not respond or barely responded to treatment.

In a direct comparison of EMDR and tapping, comparable effects were obtained with both procedures (Karatzias et al. 2011).

Based on therapist experience reports, depending on the severity and complexity of PTSD symptomatology, an average of 6–10 tapping sessions of 1 h with exposure are recommended (Church et al. 2017). However, about one-third of patients may require more than ten sessions.

In addition to treating PTSD, tapping also shows large effects in individuals with **anxiety or panic disorders**, as a meta-analysis across 14 randomized controlled trials showed (Clond 2016).

8.3.8 ADHD and Autism

8.3.8.1 Massage Therapy for Attention Deficit Hyperactivity Disorder

Attention-deficit/hyperactivity disorder (ADHD) occurs with a prevalence of about 5% in childhood and adolescence and 2.5% in adulthood (Song et al. 2021). This makes it one of the most common mental disorders. The primary treatment approaches are psychotherapeutic procedures and pharmacological interventions (DGKJP et al. 2017). Both approaches are effective. However, pharmacological therapies improve symptoms for only a few hours and show no effects after the medication is discontinued. In addition, adverse effects may occur, including headache, sleep disturbance, gastrointestinal distress, depression, anxiety, irritability, loss of appetite, and dizziness (AHFS® Patient Medication Information 2023).

Various studies indicate that massages can have a positive effect on ADHD symptoms. Different massage techniques have already been investigated.

In one study, 7- to 18-year-old students ($M = 13$ years) received 20 min of **Swedish massage** twice a week (Khilnani et al. 2003). The students were massaged a total of nine times. A professional physical therapist performed all massages in a quiet room at the school. The head, neck, shoulders, arms, torso, legs, and back were massaged. The children remained fully clothed during the massage and lay on a portable massage table. Changes in behavior were determined using teacher interviews (Conners Rating Scale for Teachers) and compared to a waitlist control group. The results showed significant reductions in hyperactivity, anxiety, and daydreaming/inattention in the massage group; but not in the control group.

A meta-analysis of four studies using **Tuina Massage** also suggests positive effects (Chen et al. 2019). To perform Tuina massage (also known as TCM massage), regions over acupressure points and meridians are kneaded, stroked, shaken, and tapped. In the process, the person lies in underwear on a massage table and is treated on the whole body. In the studies, the treatments lasted about 30 min and were performed daily for at least 28 consecutive days. The meta-analysis found that Tuina massage produced, on average, 39% (range: 16–66%) more symptom reduction than methylphenidate.

In the most recent publication on the topic, an approach was taken that involved parents in the massage treatment (Asadi et al. 2020). In this study, a parent performed **foot massages** on the child 3 days per week, for 10 min each time. A total of 12 foot massages were performed over the course of 1 month. The massages were to be done at night about an hour before bedtime. Almond oil was used for the massages. The control group received no intervention. ADHD symptoms were assessed before and after the 1-month intervention using a parent-teacher questionnaire (Savari 2012). The questionnaire assessed five scales: memory and attention deficits, responsibility and organization, undirected movements, cooperation with others, and impulsivity. A total of 35–140 points could be obtained, with 35 points indicating mild ADHD symptomatology and 140 points indicating severe symptomatology. As a result, the massage group showed significantly lower symptoms at the end of the intervention than before (pre: $M = 80.3$ SD 10.92; post: $M = 69.79$ SD 10.63) and than the control group (pre: $M = 78.9$ SD 8.06; post: $M = 77.5$ SD 6.79). Specifically, the massage group showed highly significant improvements on three of the five ADHD symptom scales (memory and attention deficits, responsibility and organization, and cooperation with others). However, no improvement was recorded for impulsivity and undirected movements.

> **Important** Even short massages can reduce ADHD symptoms. In everyday life and during school requirements, hyperactivity, anxiety, daydreaming/inaccuracy, memory and attention deficits, responsibility and organization, and cooperation with others can be positively influenced.

8.3.8.2 Massage Technique for Autism Spectrum Disorders

Autism spectrum disorders (ASDs) are characterized by deficits in social interaction and communication, as well as stereotyped, repetitive behaviors, interests, and activities (DGKJP et al. 2016). The core symptoms manifest in early childhood and usually persist across the lifespan. In long-term studies, however, improvements in symptoms were observed in some of the children. The extent to which maturation processes, interventions, or other factors contribute to symptom improvement is currently under debate. Already known predictors for a decrease in symptoms are less pronounced symptoms at diagnosis, especially concerning social interaction, as well as higher intellectual abilities (DGKJP et al. 2016). For children who received minimal (<10 h per week) or no early intervention, three clusters of progression were determined (Lord et al. 2012; Kim et al. 2018): About one-third of patients with ASD improved 2 years after their initial diagnosis. Another third remained symptomatically stable. In the last third, symptoms worsened.

Recent studies suggest that intensive early intervention, particularly **applied behavior analysis (ABA),** can achieve moderate to large positive effects on cognitive, language, and social skills (e.g., Howard et al. 2005). Comparisons of different early intervention programs have found ABA to produce significant improvements in all measures of children's ability, whereas other intervention programs have produced less pronounced changes (Howard et al. 2005). The crucial factors for success are the intensity and duration of the support. High-intensity support of 25–40 h per week shows the largest improvements in IQ and behavioral measures (Eldevik et al. 2010; Howard et al. 2005). However, not only the intensity but also the duration of the interventions are relevant. Support programs of between 10 and 36 months show linearly increasing outcome measures of language, motor skills, and social skills (Linstead et al. 2017; Virués-Ortega 2010) (Fig. 8.1). Support programs lasting only a few weeks or a few months cannot achieve comparable effects, even at a very high intensity (Linstead et al. 2017). Support programs longer than 36 months are also unlikely to achieve additional effects (Virués-Ortega 2010).

Several studies suggest that **massage techniques** may also positively affect autism symptoms. The results from six experimental studies were recently summarized in a review article (Lee et al. 2010). According to the findings, children with ASD who received repeated massage showed better communication and social skills than children in the control groups, according to teacher and parent ratings. Massage interventions were conducted several times a week for 4 weeks to 24 months, typically lasted only 15 min, and featured stroking, tapping, or shaking touch. Children were fully clothed during the interventions, with only shoes removed. Two of the six studies used a technique that the authors referred to as "QiGong Sensory Training" or "Qigong Massage." The treatment consists of different **touch sequences, each performed three times** (videos for illustration can be viewed on YouTube under the keyword 'qigong sensory massage autism').

First, the child lies on the stomach and is lightly tapped three times from head to feet with

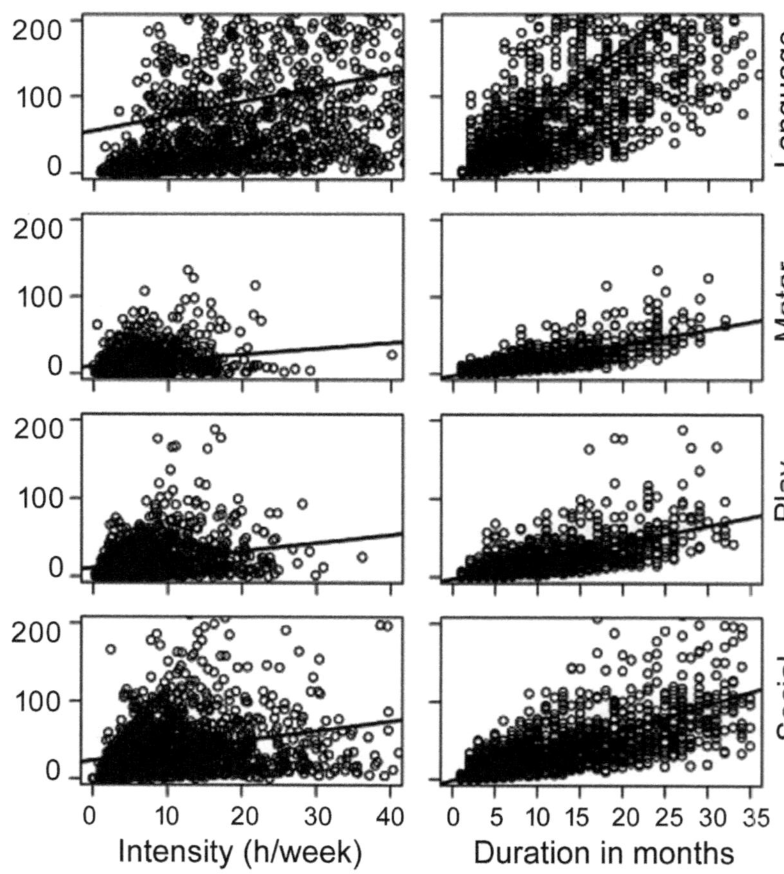

Fig. 8.1 Effects of intensive early intervention for autism spectrum disorders. Effects on motor, language, and social skills through ABA as a function of the duration and intensity of early intervention. (Translated from: Linstead et al. 2017)

one hand. Then the sequence is repeated three times with both hands. Then the sides of the body are tapped from head to feet. This is followed by tapping each arm and shaking the arms by loosely holding the hand and moving it back and forth. This is followed by briefly pressing each finger of the child between the thumb and index finger. The second part of the treatment is done in the supine position and includes stroking and gently pressing on the chest, tapping the front of the legs, stroking the calves (the leg is lifted), pressing the toes, and shaking the legs. The authors recommend adjusting the touches depending on the child's response and describe that if done regularly, touches become increasingly possible. It should be started with light, short 'patting' touches. Slow, stroking touches with gentle pressure should later be added.

A longitudinal study investigated the effects of QiGong Sensory Training on children with ASD over a 24-month period (Silva et al. 2016). The children were between 2 and 5 years old at the beginning of the study. Throughout the study, participants did *not* take psychotropic medications or receive intensive early intervention. No data were provided on the children's IQ, and there was no control group. The treatment protocol included daily 10–15-min QiGong massage sessions delivered by parents. Parents received professional training before the intervention began. During the first 5 months, the children were additionally treated once a week by a massage therapist who guided and encouraged the parents. During the second half of the first year, meetings with the therapist occurred only monthly. During the second year, the parents performed the treatments on their own.

At the end of the 24-month intervention, the following effects were evident: **Autism symptom severity** (CARS score according to Steinhausen, 1996) decreased highly significantly from a mean of 38.5 (SD = 8.1) to 32.8 (SD = 9.1); effect size $eta^2 = 0.559$. Overall, 25.8% of the children achieved a CARS score of 25.5 or lower, reaching neurotypical levels. Also, the scores obtained with the Autism Behavior Checklist (ABC; Krug et al. 2008) changed highly significantly from a mean of 81.1 (SD = 28.3) to 50.4 (SD = 29.2); the effect size was $eta^2 = 0.528$. Overall, 12.9% of the children achieved neurotypical ABC scores at the end of the 2 years.

Moreover, **unusual sensory reactions** to tactile stimuli declined significantly (Silva and Schalock 2012). They decreased from a mean of 29.8 (SD = 7.9) to 18.7 (SD = 8.8); $eta^2 = 0.634$. Almost one-third (32.3%) of the participating children no longer showed any defensive tactile responses at the end of the 2 years.

The results underline the relevance of sensory abnormalities for the diagnosis of early childhood developmental disorders (cf. Sect. 3.4.2). In the participating children, more severe sensory abnormalities were associated with more autistic behaviors and more pronounced autism symptomatology (Silva et al. 2016). Statistically, **all outcome measures improved significantly for both severe and mild symptom manifestations**. Children with lower baseline levels of sensory reactivity and autistic symptoms tended to benefit slightly more from the intervention than children with higher baseline levels (Fig. 8.2).

Long-term treatments with such or similar touch interventions could reduce overreactive sensory responses and contribute to linear positive effects on social, language, and behavioral aspects. Future studies should systematically compare the effects of touch treatment and ABA to make them comparable. If the effects of QiGong treatments are confirmed in randomized controlled trials, it would be necessary to evaluate whether children benefit to a similar extent from intensive ABA programs. The authors of the longitudinal QiGong study particularly emphasize the much smaller time commitment (QiGong: 15 min per day vs. ABA: 6–8 h per day) as a beneficial aspect (Silva et al. 2016). An additional gain lies in the **reduction of unusual sensory reactions** (cf. sensory processing disorders Sect. 3.4.2) due to the QiGong treatment. In addition, some participating parents reported **greater physical closeness and more loving affection** from their children. Also, one study suggests that oxytocin levels increase in the child and the massaging parent (Tsuji et al. 2015). In that study, the children were massaged by their mother for 3 months, 20 min a day. Oxytocin contributes to

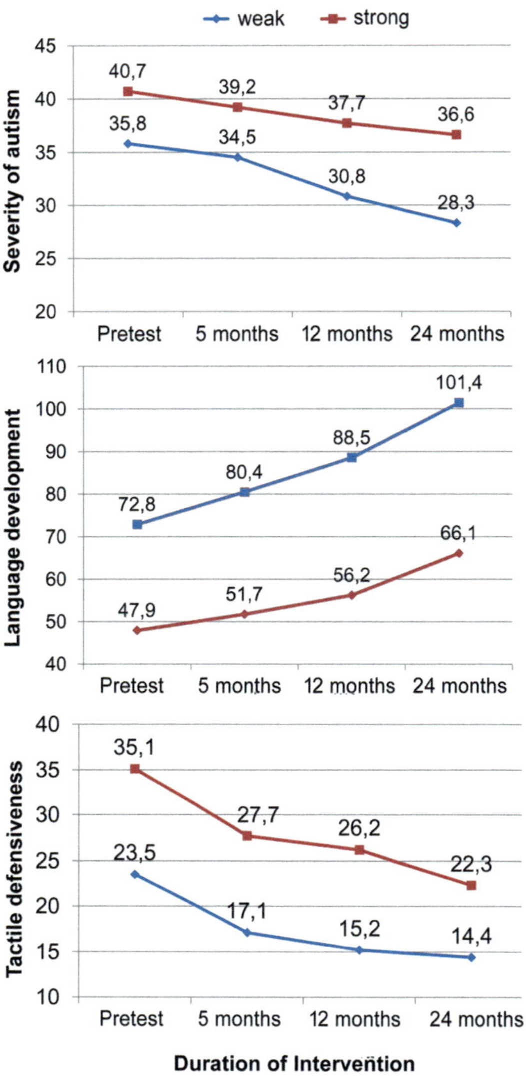

Fig. 8.2 Effects of daily QiGong massage. Developmental processes are grouped by the intensity of tactile defense at the pretest: low (blue) and strong (red). Children with weaker symptoms tended to benefit more from the intervention. (Translated from: Silva et al. 2016)

the pleasant experience of touch and to seeking physical contact with others. If these processes fail to occur due to low oxytocin levels, then less physical contact takes place, and a viscous cycle of less physical contact and less oxytocin occurs. Lack of physical contact makes social bonding more difficult, and situations in which social and communicative skills can be practiced occur less frequently (see Sect. 3.4.2).

8.3.9 Special Topic: Deep Pressure Stimulation/Weighted Vests and Blankets

Another method of applying pressure stimuli to the body is with weighted blankets, vests, or pillows. This method has been used in occupational and physical therapy for several years as a **calming and sleep-inducing tool**. Weighted blankets are an advancement of the "hug machine," developed in the 1960s by Temple Grandin (1992). Alternative ways to elicit pressure stimuli in children up to about 5 years of age include wrapping them in an exercise mat, piling athletic mats over the child, or resting them under a bean bag chair. These methods may be less effective with older children or adults because they are rejected as childish or because insufficient pressure can be applied. Grandin herself reports positive effects of the 'hug machine' in children with ASDs and children with ADHD in various observational studies and self-tests. According to this, calming effects can already be observed after 5-min applications. Recommended are 5–15-min applications of deep pressure stimulation. **Healthy adults (18–25-year-old college students**) also benefit from and report the relaxing, sleep-inducing effects of the 'hug machine' (Grandin 1992). However, no effect was found in approximately 40% of healthy adults.

By now, such devices are also commercially available under the product name squeeze machine.

The pressure on body tissues created by weighted blankets is much less than that of a 'hugging machine'. Suppliers of commercially available weighted blankets typically recommend a blanket weight of no more than 10% of body weight. This advice has been generalized from safety guidelines for backpacks to weighted blankets/vests (Mullen et al. 2008). Because weighted blankets, unlike weighted vests or backpacks, are intended for reclined or seated use and not for use while standing or moving, the safety guidelines may not transfer meaningfully. In one study, the safety of 30-pound (13.6 kg) weighted blankets was assessed using physiologic measures (blood pressure, heart rate, pulse oximetry, and skin conductance) (Mullen et al. 2008). Healthy adult participants between 18 and 58 years and body weights between 50.8 and 106.1 kg showed **no adverse physiological effects** when the blanket was **applied for 5 min**. The blankets' weight thus corresponded to between 12.8 and 26.8% of body weight. Of the participants, 81.3% found the weight of the blanket to be optimal and soothing; 15.6% of the participants would have preferred even heavier blankets. 3.1% of participants felt the blanket was too heavy. A correlation between body weight and preferred blanket weight was not shown. Participants were additionally asked about their well-being and answered the STAI before and after the blanket application. Sixty-three percent of participants reported **less anxiety/stress** on the STAI after the weighted blanket than after the control condition (no blanket), despite being a sample without anxiety symptomatology. A mixed sample of **psychiatric patients under acute inpatient care** showed no adverse physiological effects after 5 min of use (Champagne et al. 2015). Also, in this sample, 60% of patients reported a reduction in anxiety/tension (STAI and self-report) after applying the weighted blanket. In contrast, the remaining 40% of participants found the blanket uncomfortable and reported an increase in anxiety/tension in the STAI. No effects occurred in the control condition without a blanket.

Similarly, in one study, an inflatable vest was used to apply pressure to the upper body for 3 min, which reduced skin conductance, decreased arousal, and increased heart rate variability (Reynolds et al. 2015). These readings indicated a calming effect. However, in this study, the change in readings persisted only during the 3-min stimulation, not beyond. This may be due to the study setting, as a stress test followed a few minutes after the vest simulation. The anticipation of the approaching stress test likely reduced the relaxation response.

> **Important** For most individuals, deep pressure stimulation for 5–15 min, e.g., in the form of weighted blankets, has a calming and anxiety-reducing effect. For such short applications, blanket weights up to 27% of body weight have been tested for safety and shown to be safe. Some people find even stronger pressure stimuli pleasant. There is no correlation between body weight and preferred blanket weight. However, some people find deep-pressure stimuli unpleasant or oppressive and react negatively.

If weighted blankets are to be used for more extended periods of time, e.g., all night for sleeping, they should not be as heavy as for short interventions. Heavy blankets cause uncomfortable pressure sensations after some time, especially at joints. For **applications lasting longer than 15 min, blanket weights of up to 10% of body weight** have proven most comfortable. A recent review article concluded that weighted blankets are likely to produce **anxiety-relieving effects** but could not make any statement about their efficacy for sleep disorders (Eron et al. 2020). The main reason for this is the poor state of research due to studies without control groups and the use of subjective observational measures. However, a recent randomized controlled trial suggests **positive effects on sleep disturbance** (Ekholm et al. 2020). The study examined 120 outpatients with affective disorders (depression and anxiety) or ADHD and clinically relevant comorbid sleep disorders (Insomnia Severity Index; ISI > 14; Dieck et al. 2018). ISI scores > 14 indicate moderately severe sleep disorders; scores < 7 are considered not clinically relevant. Patients were grouped by matched diagnosis and randomly assigned to one of two groups: A) a weighted blanket weighing 6–8 kg (13–17 lbs), or B) a lighter blanket weighing 1.5 kg (3 lbs). After 4 weeks of use, the group that used the **heavy blanket showed significantly lower depression scores, anxiety scores, fatigue/exhaustion scores, and ISI scores** compared to before the intervention and compared to the group with the lighter blankets. The weighted blankets did not affect absolute sleep time, but patients reported sleeping better through the night. ISI scores decreased in all patient groups over the 4-week measurement period, while they remained the same or even increased in control persons. The most pronounced effects were observed in patients with generalized anxiety disorder. In the group with heavy blankets, ISI scores decreased from 16.3 after the first week to 6.2 after the fourth week. In comparison, in the group diagnosed with generalized anxiety disorder who used the light blanket, the ISI value *increased* from 16.9 to 20.0 during the same period. During a 12-month follow-up, the positive effects persisted with continued use of the weighted blanket.

▶ **Important** Daily use of weighted blankets during sleep can reduce sleep disturbances. Improved sleep positively affects depression and anxiety symptoms, as well as exhaustion and fatigue during the day. For applications lasting longer than 15 min, blanket weights of no more than 10% of body weight have proven effective.

In addition to calming and anxiety reduction, attempts have been made to use weighted blankets and vests to increase **attention and cognitive performance** in children with neurodevelopmental disorders (including ASD and ADHD) or disabilities. However, several review articles and meta-analyses conclude that there is **no evidence for such effects** (Morrison 2007; Stephenson and Carter 2009; Losinski et al. 2016). Consequently, no reliable evidence exists to date that wearing weight vests during school would improve attention or reduce impulsive, stereotypic, and disruptive behavior. It is possible that weighted vests may have a positive effect on attention in children with ADHD when the children perform still work alone in the room (Lin et al. 2014; Buckle et al. 2011). However, additional systematic studies are needed.

8.3.10 High Blood Pressure and Cardiovascular Diseases

Elevated blood pressure (hypertension) can cause cardiovascular disease, renal failure, heart attack, and stroke. Worldwide, approximately 10.5 million deaths are attributable to elevated blood pressure each year (Beaney et al. 2018). In about 90% of all high blood pressure cases, there is no identifiable organic cause; these are termed essential or primary hypertension. The main **risk factors for primary hypertension are an unhealthy diet, a lack of exercise, obesity, stress, and high salt and alcohol consumption** (Neuhauser et al. 2016). Hypertension is consequently closely related to lifestyle, making it the most important modifiable risk factor for disease and mortality. Cardiovascular disease causes at least 18 million deaths per year globally. It is the most common cause of death worldwide, accounting for an estimated 30% of all deaths (WHO 2022; Robert Koch Institute 2015).

The leading causes of death from cardiovascular disease are coronary heart disease (CHD, defined as myocardial infarction or angina pectoris) and stroke (Busch and Kuhnert 2017).

8.3.10.1 Essential (Primary) Hypertension

In a recent meta-analysis, data from 24 studies on massage for essential hypertension were pooled and analyzed (Xiong et al. 2015). It include only studies in which repeated massage treatments were performed and outcomes were compared with a control group. The meta-analysis suggests that **regular massage, in addition to antihypertensive medication**, may be more effective than antihypertensive medication alone. On average, systolic and diastolic blood pressure decreased more in people who had massage plus medication than in people who only took medication. The additional reduction with massage averaged 6.92 mmHg for systolic blood pressure (range: 3.80–10.05) and 3.63 mmHg for diastolic blood pressure (range: 1.09–6.18). It is known from epidemiological studies that reductions in systolic blood pressure by 10 mmHg and diastolic by 5 mmHg can reduce the likelihood of CHD by 22% and stroke by 41% (Law et al. 2009).

Whether regular massage positively affects blood pressure even without concomitant use of antihypertensive medication requires further investigation and the results of the meta-analysis are contradictory. On the one hand, *no* differences in changes in blood pressure were found when comparing massaged people and people who did not receive any blood pressure therapy.

On the other hand, the results of the meta-analysis suggest that massage may lower systolic blood pressure (but not diastolic blood pressure) more than antihypertensive medications. It is also known from studies on the effects of social support and physical contact that contact with close persons and pets can have a blood pressure-lowering effect and reduce cardiovascular reactivity to stress (for more details, see Sects. 5.5.3 and 5.5.4). In addition, lower blood pressure values were measured in various studies immediately after massage applications than before the massage (e.g., Arslan et al. 2021; Post-White et al. 2003). Compared to other complementary procedures (e.g., cupping, QiGong, ear acupuncture, listening to music, relaxation exercises, biofeedback, breathing exercises, yoga, and TaiChi), massages reduce blood pressure more reliably (Niu et al. 2019).

The inconsistent findings require more carefully designed randomized controlled trials to assess the effects of massage. The vast majority of studies in the above meta-analysis were from Chinese journals, making it difficult to verify the methodology and evaluate the results (Xiong et al. 2015). The studies included in the meta-analysis also varied widely in the frequency and duration of massage treatments. Some studies used 1 h of massage per week for 4 weeks, other studies conducted one massage per day for 6 months. At face validity, **massage several times a week** is more successful in reducing hypertension than once a week or less. This would be consistent with the underlying mechanisms discussed for the positive effects of massage on hypertension (Nelson 2015). Accordingly, more frequent massages reduce stress and increase positive mood more effectively (for more detail, see Sect. 2.4), and the massage-associated physiological and psychological processes have an **inhibitory effect on the sympathetic nervous system** and **reduce the activity of the HPA axis**, resulting in a decrease in blood pressure. Furthermore, relaxation processes and tissue manipulation lead to better blood flow, which could have additional positive effects on endothelial function.

▶ **Important** Regular massages may have a blood pressure-lowering effect. Complementary to blood pressure medication, massages can help prevent strokes and heart attacks.

8.3.10.2 Massage After Coronary Artery Bypass

Treatment of advanced CHD with high-grade coronary stenosis ultimately requires coronary bypass surgery. This surgical procedure is used when other procedures (e.g., stent placement) have been unsuccessful or are not an option. The standard approach to perform a coronary artery bypass is to open the chest using a median sternotomy (which is a longitudinal transection of the sternum) and perform open heart surgery. The postoperative period is characterized by severe pain. Many patients also experience psychological symptoms such as anxiety and depressed mood. Patients with marked symptoms of depression and anxiety after coronary bypass surgery have an increased risk of being rehospitalized after discharge from the hospital (Tully et al. 2008). Massage applications may be an effective way to **reduce pain and anxiety after cardiac surgery** and improve sleep.

In a recent meta-analysis, data from eight randomized controlled trials were pooled and compared (Miozzo et al. 2016). Patients received one to three massage sessions, each lasting 15–30 min, within the first 6 days after surgery. Hand massages, foot/leg massages, and back and shoulder massages were performed. Persons in the control groups received standard care or standard care with guided mental relaxation exercises. Pain and anxiety were assessed before and after each massage using VASs. The meta-analysis revealed highly significant and clinically relevant reductions in pain and anxiety in patients treated with massage therapy. Massaged patients rated pain on average 1.52 points (range: 0.84–2.20) lower on the VAS scale than patients in the control groups. In addition, the anxiety of the massaged patients was, on average, 1.48 points (range: 1.04–1.93) lower than that of the control people. Results from two other meta-analyses suggest similar effects on pain and anxiety (Boitor et al. 2017; Kukimoto et al. 2017). In addition, massaged patients reported **less fatigue and improved sleep** on the first 2 days after surgery (Priyasanthi et al. 2020). To date, however, it has not been investigated whether the anxiety- and pain-reducing massage effects after surgery allow for reduction in analgesic administration or reduce the likelihood of rehospitalization (Grafton-Clarke et al. 2019).

Summary
- To trigger relaxation (stress reduction) and psychological effects (reduce depression/anxiety), slow strokes and soft kneading whole-body massages (e.g., psychoactive massage; Slow Stroke® massage) are more suitable than trigger point treatment or treatment of densifications.
- Methods must be adapted to the needs of each patient and each disorder.
- The behavior of the person giving the massage and the environmental conditions are crucial for a comprehensive relaxation effect: a pleasantly warm environment; a quiet, protected environment; warmed hands and warmed oil; no conversations, interruptions, or disturbances; no pain.
- To date, there is no consensus on massage duration and frequency or whether there is a relationship between the type of massage (Swedish massage, psychoactive massage, foot reflexology) and the desired physiological effects.
- The stress-reducing effects of regular relaxation massages stay in effect for several days (Rapaport et al. 2012).
- Relaxation massages promote sleep, reduce fatigue, improve mood, and improve quality of life.
- Short-term reductions in acute pain can be achieved through various techniques (acupressure, foot reflexology, foot/hand massages, and back or full body massages).
- Positive effects on immune markers (e.g., in cancer or HIV) can be triggered by massages if deep relaxation (e.g., by psychoactive massage) is achieved.
- Regular massage can help reduce blood glucose levels in people with type I diabetes.
- Relaxation massages temporarily reduce blood pressure in healthy adults. In hypertension, relaxation massages can increase the effectiveness of antihypertensive drugs.
- In anxiety disorders, the loosening of body tissues through massage may be the primary mode of action to reduce symptoms. Significant effects in patients with generalized anxiety disorder were achieved by several weeks of Swedish massage therapy.
- Tension and anxiety can also be reduced in healthy persons, persons with affective disorders, or persons with neurodevelopmental disorders by deep pressure stimulation applied through massage or weighted blankets.
- EFT Tapping in combination with exposure therapy is comparable to EMDR in its effectiveness for PTSD.
- Even short foot and leg massages can reduce restless leg syndrome in dialysis patients, thereby improving sleep and fatigue.

8.4 Contraindications and Side Effects of Massage

8.4.1 Adverse Effects

Massages performed by trained clinical professionals are generally safe, as training curricula include detailed information on contraindications for manual therapy and Swedish massage. Nevertheless, the most important contraindications and precautions are briefly listed below. In addition to contraindications, the intensity and pressure used for massage are the most important causes of possible adverse effects. Techniques aiming to induce physiological relaxation and activation of the immune system **should be performed without pain**. Furthermore, some authors emphasize that medium pressure is superior to light stroking in inducing relaxation because light stroking can have an activating effect on the vegetative nervous system (Field et al. 2010), which would hinder relaxation. The amount of pressure that is perceived as pleasant and painless can differ substantially between patients and between body parts. Accordingly, it is vital to talk to the patient to find the optimal pressure intensity. Clinical studies of massage applied by professional therapists rarely report adverse side effects that go beyond transient tiredness and muscle soreness. However, case reports show that excessive force, exotic techniques, and insufficient anatomical or medical knowledge can lead to potentially life-threatening complications. These rare case reports include cervical fractures and dislocations of the spinal column (Poon et al. 2020; Abilash et al. 2017), compression injury of nerves in the arm and neck (Giese and Hentz 1998; Aksoy et al. 2009), internal bleeding and hepatic hematoma (Trotter 1999; Sun et al. 2015), as well as injuries to blood vessels in the neck leading to an aneurysm or even stroke (Patel et al. 2018; Dutta et al. 2018). Other complications include detachment of thromboses, which can lead to pulmonary or renal embolism (Behera et al. 2018; Mikhail et al. 1997), and dislodging of ureteral or venous stents (Haskal 2008; Kerr 1997). After manipulations of the cervical spine or trapezius muscle, tinnitus symptoms and even unilateral hearing loss have also been reported (Brügel and Schorn 1991; Medvedev 1994).

According to available studies, severe complications after massage are extremely rare. The complications presented in the case reports show a clear association with forceful and painful manipulations performed by lay persons or non-certified persons (Ernst 2003; Koren and Kalichman 2018).

More common but less harmful side effects of massage treatments include transient tiredness and an increase in tissue pain, swelling, superficial hematoma, and allergic reactions to oils or scents (Corbin 2005).

8.4.2 Contraindications

Contraindications can be divided into absolute contraindications for massage and those that must be decided on a case-by-case basis (relative contraindications). Absolute contraindications may be limited in time (e.g., postoperative) or refer only to a specific part of the body.

In the case of relative contraindications, the risk must be assessed by a physician or specialist staff, who decide, depending on the patient's condition, if only certain massage techniques should be used or if the intensity, force, and duration of the massages must be adjusted. **Relative contraindications exist for all conditions listed in Sect. 8.3** (which are completed by Table 8.1). Specific precautions for each disease are also reported in the respective subchapter (Sects 8.3.1–8.3.10). The massaging professional is urged to proceed with caution, pay special attention to any changes in the patient's symptoms, write responsible reports, and remain in communication with the physician.

As a general rule, massage of the abdomen should not be performed in pregnant women, as this may lead to miscarriage and rupture of the uterus (for further precautions for massage during pregnancy, see Sect. 6.1.7).

The list in Table 8.1 does not claim to be complete. In case of uncertainty, the manual therapist and the physician should coordinate possible care options.

Table 8.1 Absolute and relative contraindications of massage treatments

	Absolute contraindications (massages should not be performed)	Body area	Relative contraindications	Adaptations in case of relative contraindication
Fever or inflammation	In case of fever or acute inflammation	Global		
	Systemic inflammation, e.g., during an acute episode of rheumatism, arthritis, or systemic sclerosis	Global	During the non-acute phases of autoimmune diseases, massages may help with pain and fatigue	
	Disorientation or psychosis	Global		
Pregnancy	Complicated pregnancy with severe complications	Global		
	Healthy pregnancy	Local	Do not massage the abdomen; consider the increased risk of thrombosis; avoid supine position	(For further precautions for massage during pregnancy, see Sect. 6.1.7)
Skin	Acute inflammations, infections, and rashes (including decubitus, ulcer, and eczema)	Local	Observe trophic skin changes, e.g., in the context of diabetes or taking cortisone	Adapt massage technique (reduce pressure); do not massage in cases of severe changes
	Open wounds, fresh burns, scalds, and frostbite	Local	In chronic skin diseases (e.g., psoriasis and neurodermatitis), avoid massaging acute lesions and inflamed joints	Adapt the pressure and choose adequate massage oil
	Fresh scars (<4 weeks old)	Local		
	Contagious skin diseases (e.g., athlete's foot and jock itch)	Local		
	Contagious skin diseases (e.g., measles, rubella, chickenpox, and scabies)	Global		
	Skin tumors	Local		
Musculature, ligaments, and tendons	Acute inflammation	Local		
	Fresh injuries	Local		
	Ossifications	Local		
Bones and joints	Fresh fractures or conditions after surgery (e.g., knee prosthesis)	Local	Osteoporosis	Adjust the intensity and pressure of the massage
	Osteosarcoma	Local; in case of metastasis global		
	Acute inflammation of the bone, periosteum, one or more joints, bursae	Local		
	72 h after a sprain, strain, rupture, or dislocation	Local		

Table 8.1 (continued)

	Absolute contraindications (massages should not be performed)	Body area	Relative contraindications	Adaptations in case of relative contraindication
Vascular system	Large varices, deep vein thrombosis, and thrombophlebitis	No massage of the lower limbs until a medical assessment	Coagulation disorders	Adjust massage technique/reduce pressure
	Suspected embolism	All four limbs until medical clarification is obtained		
	Heart failure; myocardial infarction (less than 3 months ago).	Global		
	Unstable hypertension	Global		
Nervous system			Peripheral neuropathies	Adjust the intensity and pressure of the massage and observe skin changes or injuries
			Hyperesthesia; allodynia	Discontinue massage if it is uncomfortable or painful
Acute red flag symptoms	• Focal neurologic signs • Sudden deterioration of general condition	Global **Initiate first aid and contact emergency services**		

8.5 Looking Beyond the Horizon: Physical Activity as Medicine

▶ **Important** It should be emphasized that massages can only have a complementary effect on many diseases and are consequently not recommended as the sole treatment or as a substitute for medical assessment and therapy.

The health-promoting effects of massages can be enhanced by other body-oriented measures, such as sufficient physical exercise and a healthy diet. Recent research shows that a lack of exercise is one of the risk factors for several chronic diseases, such as CHD and type 2 diabetes (Lees and Booth 2004; Edwardson et al. 2012). This phenomenon is laconically referred to as **Sedentary Death Syndrome.** Overall, this summarizes the health risk of a sedentary lifestyle, the influence of physical inactivity on the development of chronic diseases, and the associated shortened lifespan.

The accurate functioning of virtually all processes in the body requires mechanical stimuli, which are triggered by movement as well as tensile and compressive forces. This principle applies to the molecular level (e.g., protein folding and opening of ion channels), the cellular level, and the organism as a whole. For example, mechanical forces are required to maintain healthy bones: muscular loading (strength training) can reduce the risk of osteoporosis, and chewing hard food helps to strengthen the jawbone as well as the gums, which can prevent tooth loss (see Sect. 1.2). In addition, muscle contractions trigger the release of several hundred different cytokines and other peptides (called **myokines**) that affect various organ functions. Receptors for these myokines have been found on cells of skeletal muscle, bone, adipose tissue, liver, pancreas, heart, immune, and brain cells (Pedersen and Febbraio 2012). Some myokines influence bone metabolism, improve vasodilator regulation of blood vessels, or have systemic effects on the immune system. Myokine circuits seem to be altered by a lack of physical activity and may be the relevant link between a lack of exercise and the development of chronic diseases (Pedersen and Febbraio 2012). Stretching and exercise also stimulate blood flow and lymphatic circulation in the tissues, which promote the removal of cellular waste products (cf. Sect. 2.3). Furthermore, regular physical activity can counteract stress and temporarily buffer the health consequences of social isolation and a lack of physical contact (Field et al. 2020a).

As an absolute minimum of physical activity, 30 min of moderate-intensity activity should be performed on 4–7 days per week (Berg and Halle 1999; Löllgen 2020; BZgA 2016; WHO 2019). Suitable moderate-intensity aerobic exercise includes, for example, brisk walking at 6 km/h (3.7 miles/h), or cycling at 15 km/h (9 miles/h) (Wolf et al. 2011). Epidemiological studies have shown that individuals who exercise more than this minimum have up to a 30% lower risk of CHD, stroke, diabetes mellitus, and certain cancers than inactive individuals (Hamer and Chida 2008; Hu et al. 1999, 2000; Schmid et al. 2014).

Furthermore, physical activity can not only prevent disease but also produce positive effects on disease progression and mortality in pre-existing conditions. For example, regular physical activity can reduce mortality in patients with CHD or type 2 diabetes by 30–40% (Khera et al. 2016; Sluik et al. 2012). Additionally, positive effects on well-being and organ function have been shown in patients with cardiac insufficiency, lung diseases, chronic kidney disease, some cancerous diseases, osteoporosis, degenerative spinal disorders, Parkinson's disease, and stroke (Löllgen 2020). Some physicians are therefore calling for a systematic study of the therapeutic possibilities of exercise so that specific recommendations can be made to patients (Löllgen et al. 2018). One possible implementation is "exercise on prescription" as a personalized secondary prevention in primary healthcare. The prescription specifies the type, intensity, and duration of exercise. Likewise, discontinuation criteria (including dizziness, shortness of breath, and an irregular pulse) and further rules of conduct (e.g., consult a physician) can be specified (Löllgen 2020).

References

Abilash K, Mohd Q, Ahmad ZAH, Towil B. Fracture-dislocation at C6-C7 level with quadriplegia after traditional massage in a patient with ankylosing spondylitis: a case report. Malays Orthop J. 2017;11(2):75.

AHFS® Patient Medication Information. Methylphenidate. 2023. https://medlineplus.gov/druginfo/meds/a682188.html#side-effects. Accessed 11 May 2023.

Aksoy IA, Schrader SL, Ali MS, Borovansky JA, Ross MA. Spinal accessory neuropathy associated with deep tissue massage: a case report. Arch Phys Med Rehabil. 2009;90(11):1969–72. https://doi.org/10.1016/j.apmr.2009.06.015.

Andersson K, Wändell P, Törnkvist L. Tactile massage improves glycaemic control in women with type 2 diabetes: a pilot study. Pract Diab Int. 2004;21(3):105–9. https://doi.org/10.1002/pdi.602.

Arnold MM, Müller-Oerlinghausen B, Hemrich N, Bönsch D. Effects of psychoactive massage in outpatients with depressive disorders: a randomized controlled mixed-methods study. Brain Sci. 2020;10(10):676. https://doi.org/10.3390/brainsci10100676.

Arslan G, Ceyhan Ö, Mollaoğlu M. The influence of foot and back massage on blood pressure and sleep quality in females with essential hypertension: a randomized controlled study. J Hum Hypertens. 2021;35:627. https://doi.org/10.1038/s41371-020-0371-z.

Asadi Z, Shakibaei F, Mazaheri M, Jafari-Mianaei S. The effect of foot massage by mother on the severity of attention-deficit hyperactivity disorder symptoms in children aged 6-12. Iran J Nurs Midwifery Res. 2020;25(3):189–94. https://doi.org/10.4103/ijnmr.IJNMR_78_19.

Batavia M. Contraindications for therapeutic massage: do sources agree? J Bodyw Mov Ther. 2004;8(1):48–57. https://doi.org/10.1016/S1360-8592(03)00084-6.

Baumgart SB, Baumbach-Kraft A, Lorenz J. Effect of psycho-regulatory massage therapy on pain and depression in women with chronic and/or somatoform back pain: a randomized controlled trial. Brain Sci. 2020;10(10):721. https://doi.org/10.3390/brainsci10100721.

Bayat D, Mohammadbeigi A, Parham M, Hashemi M, Asghari M. The effect of massage on diabetes and its complications: a systematic review. Crescent J Med Biol Sci. 2019;7(1):22–8.

Beaney T, Schutte AE, Tomaszewski M, Ariti C, Burrell LM, Castillo RR, et al. May measurement month 2017: an analysis of blood pressure screening results worldwide. Lancet Glob Health. 2018;6(7):e736–43. https://doi.org/10.1016/S2214-109X(18)30259-6.

Behera C, Devassy S, Mridha AR, Chauhan M, Gupta SK. Leg massage by mother resulting in fatal pulmonary thromboembolism. Med Legal J. 2018;86(3):146–50. https://doi.org/10.1177/0025817217706645.

Beikmoradi A, Najafi F, Roshanaei G, Pour Esmaeil Z, Khatibian M, Ahmadi A. Acupressure and anxiety in cancer patients. Iran Red Crescent Med J. 2015;17(3):e25919. https://doi.org/10.5812/ircmj.25919.

Berg A, Halle M. Korperliche Aktivitat und Kardiovaskulare Mortalitat: Von Der Epidemiologie zur Medizinischen Praxis. Med Welt. 1999;50(9):359–62.

Berger M, Cüppers HJ, Hegner H, Jörgens V, Berchtold P. Absorption kinetics and biologic effects of subcutaneously injected insulin preparations. Diabetes Care. 1982;5(2):77–91. https://doi.org/10.2337/diacare.5.2.77.

Billhult A, Lindholm C, Gunnarsson R, Stener-Victorin E. The effect of massage on cellular immunity, endocrine and psychological factors in women with breast cancer -- a randomized controlled clinical trial. Auton Neurosci. 2008;140(1–2):88–95. https://doi.org/10.1016/j.autneu.2008.03.006.

Billhult A, Lindholm C, Gunnarsson R, Stener-Victorin E. The effect of massage on immune function and stress in women with breast cancer--a randomized controlled trial. Auton Neurosci. 2009;150(1–2):111–5. https://doi.org/10.1016/j.autneu.2009.03.010.

Birk TJ, McGrady A, MacArthur RD, Khuder S. The effects of massage therapy alone and in combination with other complementary therapies on immune system measures and quality of life in human immunodeficiency virus. J Altern Complement Med. 2000;6(5):405–14. https://doi.org/10.1089/acm.2000.6.405.

Boitor M, Gélinas C, Richard-Lalonde M, Thombs BD. The effect of massage on acute postoperative pain in critically and acutely ill adults post-thoracic surgery: systematic review and meta-analysis of randomized controlled trials. Heart Lung. 2017;46(5):339–46. https://doi.org/10.1016/j.hrtlng.2017.05.005.

Brügel FJ, Schorn K. Zervikaler Tinnitus nach HWS-Behandlung. Laryngorhinootologie. 1991;70(6):321–5. https://doi.org/10.1055/s-2007-998046.

Buckle F, Franzsen D, Bester J. The effect of the wearing of weighted vests on the sensory behaviour of learners diagnosed with attention deficit hyperactivity disorder within a school context. S Afr J Occup Ther. 2011;41(3):37–41.

Busch MA, Kuhnert R. 12-Monats-Prävalenz einer koronaren Herzkrankheit in Deutschland. J Health Monit. 2017;2(1):64–9. https://doi.org/10.17886/RKI-GBE-2017-009.

BZgA. Nationale Empfehlungen für Bewegung und Bewegungsförderung. Sonderheft. 2016. Online verfügbar unter https://www.bundesgesundheitsministerium.de/fileadmin/Dateien/5_Publikationen/Praevention/Broschueren/Bewegungsempfehlungen_BZgA-Fachheft_3.pdf, zuletzt geprüft am 11.05.2021.

Calcagni N, Gana K, Quintard B. A systematic review of complementary and alternative medicine in oncology: Psychological and physical effects of manipulative and body-based practices. PLoS One. 2019;14(10):e0223564. https://doi.org/10.1371/journal.pone.0223564.

Castro-Sánchez AM, Moreno-Lorenzo C, Matarán-Peñarrocha GA, Feriche-Fernández-Castanys B, Granados-Gámez G, Quesada-Rubio JM. Connective tissue reflex massage for type 2 diabetic patients with peripheral arterial disease: randomized controlled trial. Evid Based Complement Alternat Med. 2011;2011:1–12. https://doi.org/10.1093/ecam/nep171.

Champagne T, Mullen B, Dickson D, Krishnamurty S. Evaluating the safety and effectiveness of the weighted blanket with adults during an inpatient mental health hospitalization. Occup Ther Ment Health. 2015;31(3):211–33. https://doi.org/10.1080/0164212X.2015.1066220.

Chen S-C, Yu BY-M, Suen LK-P, Yu J, Ho FY-Y, Yang J-J, Yeung W-F. Massage therapy for the treatment of attention deficit/hyperactivity disorder (ADHD) in children and adolescents: a systematic review and meta-analysis. Complement Ther Med. 2019;42:389–99. https://doi.org/10.1016/j.ctim.2018.12.011.

Church D, Piña O, Reategui C, Brooks A. Single-session reduction of the intensity of traumatic memories in abused adolescents after EFT: a randomized controlled pilot study. Traumatology. 2012;18(3):73–9.

Church D, Hawk C, Brooks AJ, Toukolehto O, Wren M, Dinter I, Stein P. Psychological trauma symptom improvement in veterans using emotional freedom techniques: a randomized controlled trial. J Nerv Ment Dis. 2013;201(2):153–60. https://doi.org/10.1097/NMD.0b013e31827f6351.

Church D, Stern S, Boath E, Stewart T, Feinstein D, Palmer-Hoffman J, Clond M. Using emotional freedom techniques (EFT) to treat PTSD in veterans: a review of the evidence, survey of practitioners, and proposed clinical guidelines. Perm J. 2017;21(2):16–23.

Clond M. Emotional freedom techniques for anxiety: a systematic review with meta-analysis. J Nerv Ment Dis. 2016;204(5):388–95. https://doi.org/10.1097/NMD.0000000000000483.

Corbin L. Safety and efficacy of massage therapy for patients with cancer. Cancer Control. 2005;12(3):158–64. https://doi.org/10.1177/107327480501200303.

Cuijpers P, van Veen SC, Sijbrandij M, Yoder W, Cristea IA. Eye movement desensitization and reprocessing for mental health problems: a systematic review and meta-analysis. Cogn Behav Ther. 2020;49(3):165–80. https://doi.org/10.1080/16506073.2019.1703801.

Cukor D, Coplan J, Brown C, Peterson RA, Kimmel PL. Course of depression and anxiety diagnosis in patients treated with hemodialysis: a 16-month fol-

low-up. Clin J Am Soc Nephrol. 2008;3(6):1752–8. https://doi.org/10.2215/CJN.01120308.
Dewitt B, Feeny D, Fischhoff B, Cella D, Hays RD, Hess R, et al. Estimation of a preference-based summary score for the patient-reported outcomes measurement information system: The PROMIS®-Preference (PROPr) Scoring System. Med Decis Making. 2018;38(6):683–98. https://doi.org/10.1177/0272989X18776637.
DGKJP, et al. Interdisziplinäre S3-Leitlinie Autismus-Spektrum-Störungen im Kindes-, Jugend- und Erwachsenenalter Teil 1: Diagnostik. 2016. Online verfügbar unter https://www.awmf.org/uploads/tx_szleitlinien/028-018l_S3_Autismus-Spektrum-Stoerungen_ASS-Diagnostik_2016-05_abgelaufen.pdf, zuletzt geprüft am 11.05.2021.
DGKJP, et al. Langfassung der S3 Leitlinie ADHS bei Kindern, Jugendlichen und Erwachsenen. 2017. Online verfügbar unter https://www.awmf.org/uploads/tx_szleitlinien/028-045l_S3_ADHS_2018-06.pdf, zuletzt geprüft am 11.05.2021.
Dieck A, Morin CM, Backhaus J. A German version of the Insomnia Severity Index. Somnologie. 2018;22(1):27–35. https://doi.org/10.1007/s11818-017-0147-z.
Diego MA, Field T, Hernandez-Reif M, Shaw K, Friedman L, Ironson G. HIV adolescents show improved immune function following massage therapy. Int J Neurosci. 2001;106(1–2):35–45. https://doi.org/10.3109/00207450109149736.
Dutta G, Jagetia A, Srivastava AK, Singh D, Singh H, Saran RK. "Crick" in neck followed by massage led to stroke: uncommon case of vertebral artery dissection. World Neurosurg. 2018;115:41–3. https://doi.org/10.1016/j.wneu.2018.04.008.
Edwardson CL, Gorely T, Davies MJ, Gray LJ, Khunti K, Wilmot EG, et al. Association of sedentary behaviour with metabolic syndrome: a meta-analysis. PLoS One. 2012;7(4):e34916. https://doi.org/10.1371/journal.pone.0034916.
Ekholm B, Spulber S, Adler M. A randomized controlled study of weighted chain blankets for insomnia in psychiatric disorders. J Clin Sleep Med. 2020;16(9):1567–77. https://doi.org/10.5664/jcsm.8636.
Eldevik S, Hastings RP, Hughes JC, Jahr E, Eikeseth S, Cross S. Using participant data to extend the evidence base for intensive behavioral intervention for children with autism. Am J Intellect Dev Disabil. 2010;115(5):381–405. https://doi.org/10.1352/1944-7558-115.5.381.
Ernst E. The safety of massage therapy. Rheumatology. 2003;42(9):1101–6.
Ernst E. Is reflexology an effective intervention? A systematic review of randomised controlled trials. Med J Aust. 2009;191(5):263–6. https://doi.org/10.5694/j.1326-5377.2009.tb02780.x.
Ernst E, Posadzki P, Lee MS. Reflexology: an update of a systematic review of randomised clinical trials. Maturitas. 2011;68(2):116–20. https://doi.org/10.1016/j.maturitas.2010.10.011.
Eron K, Kohnert L, Watters A, Logan C, Weisner-Rose M, Mehler PS. Weighted blanket use: a systematic review. Am J Occup Ther. 2020;74(2):7402205010p1–7402205010p14. https://doi.org/10.5014/ajot.2020.037358.
Ezzo J, Donner T, Nickols D, Cox M. Is massage useful in the management of diabetes? A systematic review. Diabetes Spectr. 2001;14(4):218–24. https://doi.org/10.2337/diaspect.14.4.218.
Fattah MA, Hamdy B. Pulmonary functions of children with asthma improve following massage therapy. J Altern Complement Med. 2011;17(11):1065–8. https://doi.org/10.1089/acm.2010.0758.
Feinstein D, Church D. Modulating gene expression through psychotherapy: the contribution of non-invasive somatic interventions. Rev Gen Psychol. 2010;14(4):283–95. https://doi.org/10.1037/a0021252.
Fernández-Lao C, Cantarero-Villanueva I, Díaz-Rodríguez L, Fernández-de-las-Peñas C, Sánchez-Salado C, Arroyo-Morales M. The influence of patient attitude toward massage on pressure pain sensitivity and immune system after application of myofascial release in breast cancer survivors: a randomized, controlled crossover study. J Manipulative Physiol Ther. 2012;35(2):94–100. https://doi.org/10.1016/j.jmpt.2011.09.011.
Field T, Morrow C, Valdeon C, Larson S, Kuhn C, Schanberg S. Massage reduces anxiety in child and adolescent psychiatric patients. J Am Acad Child Adolesc Psychiatry. 1992;31(1):125–31. https://doi.org/10.1097/00004583-199201000-00019.
Field T, Seligman S, Scafidi F, Schanberg S. Alleviating posttraumatic stress in children following hurricane Andrew. J Appl Dev Psychol. 1996;17(1):37–50. https://doi.org/10.1016/S0193-3973(96)90004-0.
Field T, Henteleff T, Hernandez-Reif M, Martinez E, Mavunda K, Kuhn C, Schanberg S. Children with asthma have improved pulmonary functions after massage therapy. J Pediatr. 1998;132(5):854–8. https://doi.org/10.1016/S0022-3476(98)70317-8.
Field T, Diego MA, Hernandez-Reif M, Schanberg S, Kuhn C. Massage therapy effects on depressed pregnant women. J Psychosom Obstet Gynaecol. 2004;25(2):115–22. https://doi.org/10.1080/01674820412331282231.
Field T, Diego M, Hernandez-Reif M. Moderate pressure is essential for massage therapy effects. Int J Neurosci. 2010;120(5):381–5. https://doi.org/10.3109/00207450903579475.
Field T, Poling S, Mines S, Bendell D, Veazey C. Touch deprivation and exercise during the COVID-19 lockdown April 2020. Mes Res Arch. 2020a;8(8). https://doi.org/10.18103/mra.v8i8.2204.
Field T, Sauvageau N, Gonzalez G, Diego M. Veterans with post-traumatic stress disorder are less stressed following massage therapy. Curr Res Complement Altern Med. 2020b;4(141). https://doi.org/10.29011/2577-2201.100041.

Forbes D, Creamer M, Biddle D. The validity of the PTSD checklist as a measure of symptomatic change in combat-related PTSD. Behav Res Ther. 2001;39(8):977–86. https://doi.org/10.1016/S0005-7967(00)00084-X.

Frederick CJ. Children traumatized by catastrophic situations. In: Eth S, Pynoos RS, editors. Post-traumatic stress disorder in children. Washington, DC: American Psychiatric Press; 1985. p. 73–97.

Freyberger HJ, Spitzer C, Stieglitz R-D, Kuhn G, Magdeburg N, Bernstein-Carlson E. Fragebogen zu dissoziativen Symptomen (FDS). Deutsche Adaptation, Reliabilität und Validität der amerikanischen Dissociative Experience Scale (DES). PPmP: Psychotherapie Psychosomatik Medizinische Pschologie. 1998;48(6):223–9.

Gentile S. Untreated depression during pregnancy: short- and long-term effects in offspring. A systematic review. Neuroscience. 2017;342:154–66. https://doi.org/10.1016/j.neuroscience.2015.09.001.

Ghasemi Pour M, Abdoli S, Valiani M, Feizi A. The effect of massage therapy on glycemic control (FBS, HBA1C) in women with diabetes type 2 [nur Abstract]. J Res Dev Nurs Midwifery. 2013;10:81–9.

Ghazavi Z, Talakoob S, Attari A, Joazi M. Effects of massage therapy and muscle relaxation on glycosylated hemoglobin in diabetic children. Shiraz E-Med J. 2008;9(1):11–6.

Gholamzadeh H, Ilkhani M, Ameri A, Shakeri N. Effect of reflexology on the side effects of chemotherapy in cancer patients: an integrative review. Evid Based Care. 2019;8(4):7–13. https://doi.org/10.22038/ebcj.2018.34389.1874.

Giese S, Hentz VR. Posterior interosseous syndrome resulting from deep tissue massage. Plast Reconstr Surg. 1998;102(5):1778–9.

Gok Metin Z, Arikan Donmez A, Izgu N, Ozdemir L, Arslan IE. Aromatherapy massage for neuropathic pain and quality of life in diabetic patients. J Nurs Scholsh. 2017;49(4):379–88. https://doi.org/10.1111/jnu.12300.

Goli H, Shabestari MS. Effectiveness of massage therapy in improving symptom in children with allergic asthma: a randomized clinical trial. BMJ Open. 2017;7(Suppl 1):bmjopen-2016. In: International Society for Evidence-Based Healthcare Congress, Kish Island, Iran 5 (52).

Grafton-Clarke C, Grace L, Roberts N, Harky A. Can postoperative massage therapy reduce pain and anxiety in cardiac surgery patients? Interact Cardiovasc Thorac Surg. 2019;28(5):716–21. https://doi.org/10.1093/icvts/ivy310.

Grandin T. Calming effects of deep touch pressure in patients with autistic disorder, college students, and animals. J Child Adolesc Psychopharmacol. 1992;2(1):63–72. https://doi.org/10.1089/cap.1992.2.63.

Grunwald M, Mueller SM. Wissenschaftliche Grundlagen der Palpation. In: Johannes Mayer CS, Jean-Pierre B, editors. Lehrbuch Osteopathische Medizin. 1.; 2017. Auflage, 251–65.

Habibzadeh H, Wosoi Dalavan O, Alilu L, Wardle J, Khalkhali H, Nozad A. Effects of foot massage on severity of fatigue and quality of life in hemodialysis patients: a randomized controlled trial. Int J Community Based Nurs Midwifery. 2020;8(2):92–102. https://doi.org/10.30476/IJCBNM.2020.81662.0.

Hamer M, Chida Y. Walking and primary prevention: a meta-analysis of prospective cohort studies. Br J Sports Med. 2008;42(4):238–43. https://doi.org/10.1136/bjsm.2007.039974.

Hashemi SH, Hajbagheri A, Aghajani M. The effect of massage with lavender oil on restless leg syndrome in hemodialysis patients: a randomized controlled trial. Nurs Midwifery Stud. 2015;4(4):e29617. https://doi.org/10.17795/nmsjournal29617.

Haskal ZJ. Massage-induced delayed venous stent migration. J Vasc Interv Radiol. 2008;19(6):945–9.

Hernandez-Reif M, Field T, Krasnegor J, Martinez E, Schwartzman M, Mavunda K. Children with cystic fibrosis benefit from massage therapy. J Pediatr Psychol. 1999;24(2):175–81. https://doi.org/10.1093/jpepsy/24.2.175.

Hernandez-Reif M, Field T, Ironson G, Beutler J, Vera Y, Hurley J, et al. Natural killer cells and lymphocytes increase in women with breast cancer following massage therapy. Int J Neurosci. 2005;115(4):495–510. https://doi.org/10.1080/00207450590523080.

Hidalgo RB, Tupler LA, Davidson JRT. An effect-size analysis of pharmacologic treatments for generalized anxiety disorder. J Psychopharmacol. 2007;21(8):864–72. https://doi.org/10.1177/0269881107076996.

Hmwe NTT, Subramanian P, Tan LP, Chong WK. The effects of acupressure on depression, anxiety and stress in patients with hemodialysis: a randomized controlled trial. Int J Nurs Stud. 2015;52(2):509–18. https://doi.org/10.1016/j.ijnurstu.2014.11.002.

Howard JS, Sparkman CR, Cohen HG, Green G, Stanislaw H. A comparison of intensive behavior analytic and eclectic treatments for young children with autism. Res Dev Disabil. 2005;26(4):359–83. https://doi.org/10.1016/j.ridd.2004.09.005.

Hsiung W-T, Chang Y-C, Yeh M-L, Chang Y-H. Acupressure improves the postoperative comfort of gastric cancer patients: a randomised controlled trial. Complement Ther Med. 2015;23(3):339–46. https://doi.org/10.1016/j.ctim.2015.03.010.

Hu FB, Sigal RJ, Rich-Edwards JW, Colditz GA, Solomon CG, Willett WC, et al. Walking compared with vigorous physical activity and risk of type 2 diabetes in women: a prospective study. JAMA. 1999;282(15):1433–9.

Hu FB, Stampfer MJ, Colditz GA, Ascherio A, Rexrode KM, Willett WC, Manson JAE. Physical activity and risk of stroke in women. JAMA. 2000;283(22):2961–7.

Imanishi J, Kuriyama H, Shigemori I, Watanabe S, Aihara Y, Kita M, et al. Anxiolytic effect of aromatherapy massage in patients with breast cancer. Evid Based

Complement Alternat Med. 2009;6(1):123–8. https://doi.org/10.1093/ecam/nem073.

Ironson G, Field T, Scafidi F, Hashimoto M, Kumar M, Kumar A, et al. Massage therapy is associated with enhancement of the immune system's cytotoxic capacity. Int J Neurosci. 1996;84(1-4):205–17. https://doi.org/10.3109/00207459608987266.

Jacobi F, Höfler M, Strehle J, Mack S, Gerschler A, Scholl L, et al. Psychische Störungen in der Allgemeinbevölkerung: Studie zur Gesundheit Erwachsener in Deutschland und ihr Zusatzmodul Psychische Gesundheit (DEGS1-MH). Nervenarzt. 2014;85(1):77–87. https://doi.org/10.1007/s00115-013-3961-y.

Jane S-W, Chen S-L, Wilkie DJ, Lin Y-C, Foreman S, Wang; Beaton, Randal D., et al. Effects of massage on pain, mood status, relaxation, and sleep in Taiwanese patients with metastatic bone pain: a randomized clinical trial. Pain. 2011;152(10):2432–42. https://doi.org/10.1016/j.pain.2011.06.021.

Karatzias T, Power K, Brown K, McGoldrick T, Begum M, Young J, et al. A controlled comparison of the effectiveness and efficiency of two psychological therapies for posttraumatic stress disorder: eye movement desensitization and reprocessing vs. emotional freedom techniques. J Nerv Ment Dis. 2011;199(6):372–8. https://doi.org/10.1097/NMD.0b013e31821cd262.

Kerr HD. Ureteral stent displacement associated with deep massage. WMJ. 1997;96(12):57–8.

Khakpour M, Dabbaghi B, Noorkhomami S, Javid A, Sezavar M, Ghazanfarpour M. Efficacy of acupressure on nausea and vomiting in children undergoing chemotherapy: a systematic review. Int J Pediatr. 2019;7(6). https://doi.org/10.22038/ijp.2019.39206.3338.

Khan AM, Dar S, Ahmed R, Bachu R, Adnan M, Kotapati VP. Cognitive behavioral therapy versus eye movement desensitization and reprocessing in patients with post-traumatic stress disorder: systematic review and meta-analysis of randomized clinical trials. Cureus. 2018;10(9):e3250. https://doi.org/10.7759/cureus.3250.

Khera AV, Emdin CA, Drake I, Natarajan P, Bick AG, Cook NR, et al. Genetic risk, adherence to a healthy lifestyle, and coronary disease. N Engl J Med. 2016;375(24):2349–58.

Khiewkhern S, Promthet S, Sukprasert A, Eunhpinitpong W, Bradshaw P. Effectiveness of aromatherapy with light thai massage for cellular immunity improvement in colorectal cancer patients receiving chemotherapy. Asian Pac J Cancer Prev. 2013;14(6):3903–7. https://doi.org/10.7314/apjcp.2013.14.6.3903.

Khilnani S, Field T, Hernandez-Reif M, Schanberg S. Massage therapy improves mood and behavior of students with attentiondeficit/hyperactivity disorder. Adolescence. 2003;38(152):623–38.

Kim SH, Bal VH, Benrey N, Choi YB, Guthrie W, Colombi C, Lord C. Variability in autism symptom trajectories using repeated observations from 14 to 36 months of age. J Am Acad Child Adolesc Psychiatry. 2018;57(11):837–848.e2. https://doi.org/10.1016/j.jaac.2018.05.026.

Klingelhoefer L, Cova I, Gupta S, Chaudhuri KR. A review of current treatment strategies for restless legs syndrome (Willis-Ekbom disease). Clin Med. 2014;14(5):520–4. https://doi.org/10.7861/clinmedicine.14-5-520.

Koren Y, Kalichman L. Deep tissue massage: what are we talking about? J Bodyw Mov Ther. 2018;22(2):247–51.

Kovesdy CP. Epidemiology of chronic kidney disease: an update 2022. Kidney Int Suppl. 2022;12(1):7–11.

Krug D, Arick J, Almond P. Autism screening instrument for educational planning. 3rd ed. Austin: Pro-Ed; 2008.

Kukimoto Y, Ooe N, Ideguchi N. The effects of massage therapy on pain and anxiety after surgery: a systematic review and meta-analysis. Pain Manage Nurs. 2017;18(6):378–90. https://doi.org/10.1016/j.pmn.2017.09.001.

Landin-Romero R, Moreno-Alcazar A, Pagani M, Amann BL. How does eye movement desensitization and reprocessing therapy work? A systematic review on suggested mechanisms of action. Front Psychol. 2018;9:1395. https://doi.org/10.3389/fpsyg.2018.01395.

Law MR, Morris JK, Wald NJ. Use of blood pressure lowering drugs in the prevention of cardiovascular disease: meta-analysis of 147 randomised trials in the context of expectations from prospective epidemiological studies. BMJ. 2009;338:b1665. https://doi.org/10.1136/bmj.b1665.

Lee J, Dodd M, Dibble S, Abrams D. Review of acupressure studies for chemotherapy-induced nausea and vomiting control. J Pain Symptom Manage. 2008;36(5):529–44. https://doi.org/10.1016/j.jpainsymman.2007.10.019.

Lee MS, Kim J-I, Ernst E. Massage therapy for children with autism spectrum disorders: a systematic review. J Clin Psychiatry. 2010;72(3):406–11. https://doi.org/10.4088/JCP.09r05848whi.

Lee S-H, Kim J-Y, Yeo S, Kim S-H, Lim S. Meta-analysis of massage therapy on cancer pain. Integr Cancer Ther. 2015;14(4):297–304. https://doi.org/10.1177/1534735415572885.

Lees SJ, Booth FW. Sedentary death syndrome. Can J Appl Physiol. 2004;29(4):447–60; discussion 444–6. https://doi.org/10.1139/h04-029.

Lewey JH, Smith CL, Burcham B, Saunders NL, Elfallal D, O'Toole SK. Comparing the effectiveness of EMDR and TF-CBT for children and adolescents: a meta-analysis. J Child Adolesc Trauma. 2018;11(4):457–72. https://doi.org/10.1007/s40653-018-0212-1.

Lin H-Y, Lee P, Chang W-D, Hong F-Y. Effects of weighted vests on attention, impulse control, and on-task behavior in children with attention deficit hyperactivity disorder. Am J Occup Ther. 2014;68(2):149–58. https://doi.org/10.5014/ajot.2014.009365.

Linde B. Dissociation of insulin absorption and blood flow during massage of a subcutaneous injection site. Diabetes Care. 1986;9(6):570–4. https://doi.org/10.2337/diacare.9.6.570.

Linstead E, Dixon DR, Hong E, Burns CO, French R, Novack MN, Granpeesheh D. An evaluation of the effects of intensity and duration on outcomes across treatment domains for children with autism spectrum disorder. Transl Psychiatry. 2017;7(9):e1234. https://doi.org/10.1038/tp.2017.207.

Listing M, Reisshauer A, Krohn M, Voigt B, Tjahono G, Becker J, et al. Massage therapy reduces physical discomfort and improves mood disturbances in women with breast cancer. Psychooncology. 2009;18(12):1290–9. https://doi.org/10.1002/pon.1508.

Listing M, Krohn M, Liezmann C, Kim I, Reisshauer A, Peters E, et al. The efficacy of classical massage on stress perception and cortisol following primary treatment of breast cancer. Arch Womens Ment Health. 2010;13(2):165–73. https://doi.org/10.1007/s00737-009-0143-9.

Löllgen H. Refresher: Körperliche Aktivität als Medikament. Zeitschrift für Komplementärmedizin. 2020;12(1):54–9. https://doi.org/10.1055/a-1070-8052.

Löllgen H, Wismach J, Bachl N. Körperliche Aktivität als Medikament. AVP. 2018;45(3):126–34.

Lord C, Luyster R, Guthrie W, Pickles A. Patterns of developmental trajectories in toddlers with autism spectrum disorder. J Consult Clin Psychol. 2012;80(3):477–89. https://doi.org/10.1037/a0027214.

Losinski M, Sanders SA, Wiseman NM. Examining the use of deep touch pressure to improve the educational performance of students with disabilities. Res Pract Persons Severe Disabil. 2016;41(1):3–18. https://doi.org/10.1177/1540796915624889.

Medvedev EA. Case of acute unilateral neurosensory hearing loss caused by massage of the trapezius muscle. Vestn Otorinolaringol. 1994;3:38–9.

Miao J, Liu X, Wu C, Kong H, Xie W, Liu K. Effects of acupressure on chemotherapy-induced nausea and vomiting-a systematic review with meta-analyses and trial sequential analysis of randomized controlled trials. Int J Nurs Stud. 2017;70:27–37. https://doi.org/10.1016/j.ijnurstu.2017.02.014.

Mikhail A, Reidy JF, Taylor PR, Scoble JE. Renal artery embolization after back massage in a patient with aortic occlusion. Nephrol Dial Transplant. 1997;12(4):797–8.

Miozzo AP, Stein C, Bozzetto CB, Plentz D, Méa R. Massage therapy reduces pain and anxiety after cardiac surgery: a systematic review and meta-analysis of randomized clinical trials. Clin Trials Regul Sci Cardiol. 2016;23–24:1–8. https://doi.org/10.1016/j.ctrsc.2016.11.003.

Mirbagher Ajorpaz N, Rahemi Z, Aghajani M, Hashemi SH. Effects of glycerin oil and lavender oil massages on hemodialysis patients' restless legs syndrome. J Bodyw Mov Ther. 2020;24(1):88–92. https://doi.org/10.1016/j.jbmt.2019.06.012.

Mitchell UH. Nondrug-related aspect of treating Ekbom disease, formerly known as restless legs syndrome. Neuropsychiatr Dis Treat. 2011;7:251–7. https://doi.org/10.2147/NDT.S19177.

Mohammadpourhodki R, Sadeghnezhad H, Ebrahimi H, Basirinezhad MH, Maleki M, Bossola M. The effect of aromatherapy massage with lavender and citrus aurantium essential oil on quality of life of patients on chronic hemodialysis: a parallel randomized clinical trial study. J Pain Symptom Manage. 2021;61(3):456–463.e1. https://doi.org/10.1016/j.jpainsymman.2020.08.032.

Mollon P. Thought field therapy and its derivatives: rapid relief of mental health problems through tapping on the body. Prim Care Commun Psychiatry. 2007;12(3/4):123.

Morrison EE. A review of research on the use of weighted vests with children on the autism spectrum. Education. 2007;127(3):323–8.

Moyer CA, Rounds J, Hannum JW. A meta-analysis of massage therapy research. Psychol Bull. 2004;130(1):3–18. https://doi.org/10.1037/0033-2909.130.1.3.

Mueller SM, Grunwald M. Taktile Körperstimulation (Massage) in der Pränatal- und Geburtsmedizin. Manuelle Medizin. 2019;57(4):254–9. https://doi.org/10.1007/s00337-019-0536-4.

Mullen B, Champagne T, Krishnamurty S, Dickson D, Gao RX. Exploring the safety and therapeutic effects of deep pressure stimulation using a weighted blanket. Occup Ther Ment Health. 2008;24(1):65–89. https://doi.org/10.1300/J004v24n01_05.

Müller-Oerlinghausen B, Berg C, Scherer P, Mackert A, Moestl H-P, Wolf J. Wirkungen einer "Slow Stroke"-Massage als komplementäre Therapie bei stationären depressiven Patienten. Ergebnisse einer kontrollierten Studie (SeSeTra)1. Deutsche medizinische Wochenschrift (1946). 2004;129(24):1363–8. https://doi.org/10.1055/s-2004-826874.

Murtagh FEM, Addington-Hall J, Higginson IJ. The prevalence of symptoms in end-stage renal disease: a systematic review. Adv Chronic Kidney Dis. 2007;14(1):82–99. https://doi.org/10.1053/j.ackd.2006.10.001.

Najafpour Z, Shayanfard K. Effect of reflexology in treating cancer pain: a meta-analysis. Int J Cancer Manag. 2020;13(7):e102195. https://doi.org/10.5812/ijcm.102195.

Nasiri M, Abbasi M, Khosroabadi ZY, Saghafi H, Hamzeei F, Amiri MH, Yusefi H. Short-term effects of massage with olive oil on the severity of uremic restless legs syndrome: A double-blind placebo-controlled trial. Complement Ther Med. 2019;44:261–8. https://doi.org/10.1016/j.ctim.2019.05.009.

Nelson NL. Massage therapy: understanding the mechanisms of action on blood pressure. A scoping review. J Am Soc Hypertens. 2015;9(10):785–93. https://doi.org/10.1016/j.jash.2015.07.009.

Neuhauser H, Diederichs C, Boeing H, Felix SB, Jünger C, Lorbeer R, et al. Bluthochdruck in Deutschland. Daten aus sieben bevölkerungsbasierten epidemiologischen Studien (1994–2012). Deutsches Ärzteblatt. 2016;113(48):809–15. https://doi.org/10.25646/2436.

Niu J-F, Zhao X-F, Hu H-T, Wang J-J, Liu Y-L, Lu D-H. Should acupuncture, biofeedback, massage, Qi gong, relaxation therapy, device-guided breathing, yoga and tai chi be used to reduce blood pressure?: Recommendations based on high-quality systematic reviews. Complement Ther Med. 2019;42:322–31. https://doi.org/10.1016/j.ctim.2018.10.017.

Patel SM, Ojha S, Das S, Krishnan P. Extracranial vertebral artery aneurysm: an unpleasant consequence of neck massage. J Neurosci Rural Pract. 2018;9(4):655.

Pedersen BK, Febbraio MA. Muscles, exercise and obesity: skeletal muscle as a secretory organ. Nat Rev Endocrinol. 2012;8(8):457–65. https://doi.org/10.1038/nrendo.2012.49.

Poon GM, Wong KL, Chen H, Saggi SS, Lai M, Wong MK, Chan D. Cervical spine fracture after a bone cracking traditional (Tui Na) massage. Ann Acad Med Singapore. 2020;49(11):915–8. https://doi.org/10.47102/annals-acadmedsg.2020149.

Post-White J, Kinney ME, Savik K, Gau JB, Wilcox C, Lerner I. Therapeutic massage and healing touch improve symptoms in cancer. Integr Cancer Ther. 2003;2(4):332–44. https://doi.org/10.1177/1534735403259064.

Price C. Dissociation reduction in body therapy during sexual abuse recovery. Complement Ther Clin Pract. 2007;13(2):116–28. https://doi.org/10.1016/j.ctcp.2006.08.004.

Priyasanthi Y, Deepa M, Sudha R. Effectiveness of back massage on pain, fatigue and quality of sleep among post CABG patients. TNNMC J Med Surg Nurs. 2020;8(1):19–23.

Rapaport MH, Schettler P, Bresee C. A preliminary study of the effects of repeated massage on hypothalamic–pituitary–adrenal and immune function in healthy individuals: a study of mechanisms of action and dosage. J Altern Complement Med. 2012;18(8):789–97.

Rapaport MH, Schettler P, Larson ER, Edwards SA, Dunlop BW, Rakofsky JJ, Kinkead B. A preliminary study of the efficacy and biology of Swedish massage vs. light touch. J Clin Psychiatry. 2016;77(7):883–91.

Rapaport MH, Schettler PJ, Larson ER, Carroll D, Sharenko M, Nettles J, Kinkead B. Massage therapy for psychiatric disorders. Focus. 2018;16(1):24–31. https://doi.org/10.1176/appi.focus.20170043.

Rapaport MH, Schettler PJ, Larson ER, Dunlop BW, Rakofsky JJ, Kinkead B. Six versus twelve weeks of Swedish massage therapy for generalized anxiety disorder: preliminary findings. Complement Ther Med. 2021;56:102593. https://doi.org/10.1016/j.ctim.2020.102593.

Reynolds CR, Richmond BO. Revised Children's Manifest Anxiety Scale. RCMAS manual. Los Angeles: Western Psychological Services; 1985.

Reynolds S, Lane SJ, Mullen B. Effects of deep pressure stimulation on physiological arousal. Am J Occup Ther. 2015;69(3):6903350010p1-5. https://doi.org/10.5014/ajot.2015.015560.

Robert Koch-Institut. Gesundheit in Deutschland. Gesundheitsberichterstattung des Bundes. Gemeinsam getragen von RKI und Destatis. 2015. Online verfügbar unter https://www.rki.de/DE/Content/Gesundheitsmonitoring/Gesundheitsberichterstattung/GBEDownloadsGiD/2015/02_gesundheit_in_deutschland.pdf?__blob=publicationFile, zuletzt geprüft am 11.05.2021.

Russell M. Massage therapy and restless legs syndrome. J Bodyw Mov Ther. 2007;11(2):146–50. https://doi.org/10.1016/j.jbmt.2006.12.001.

Russell NC, Sumler S-S, Beinhorn CM, Frenkel MA. Role of massage therapy in cancer care. J Altern Complement Med. 2008;14(2):209–14. https://doi.org/10.1089/acm.2007.7176.

Rye DB, Trotti LM. Restless legs syndrome and periodic leg movements of sleep. Neurol Clin. 2012;30(4):1137–66. https://doi.org/10.1016/j.ncl.2012.08.004.

Sagar SM, Dryden T, Wong RK. Massage therapy for cancer patients: a reciprocal relationship between body and mind. Curr Oncol. 2007;14(2):45–56. https://doi.org/10.3747/co.2007.105.

Sajedi F, Kashaninia Z, Hoseinzadeh S, Abedinipoor A. How effective is Swedish massage on blood glucose level in children with diabetes mellitus? Acta Med Iran. 2011;49(9):592–7.

Sakai CE, Connolly SM, Oas P. Treatment of PTSD in Rwandan child genocide survivors using thought field therapy. Int J Emerg Ment Health. 2010;12(1):41–50.

Savari K. Construction and validation of questionnaires used for the diagnosis of attention deficit hyperactivity. Q Educ Meas. 2012;3(9):65–80. Online verfügbar unter https://jem.atu.ac.ir/article_5647_b3ae7b2f950d57701d69892c91251ba0.pdf.

Schäfer I, Gast U, Hofmann A, Knaevelsrud C, Lampe A, Liebermann P, et al. Posttraumatische Belastungsstörung: S3 Leitlinie der Deutschsprachigen Gesellschaft für Psychotraumatologie (DeGPT). Hg. v. Berlin: Springer; 2019. Online verfügbar unter https://www.awmf.org/uploads/tx_szleitlinien/155-001l_S3_Posttraumatische_Belastungsstoerung_2020-02_1.pdf, zuletzt geprüft am 11.05.2021.

Schmid D, Steindorf K, Leitzmann MF. Epidemiologic studies of physical activity and primary prevention of cancer. German J Sports Med. 2014;65(1):5.

Shapiro F. Eye movement desensitization and reprocessing (EMDR) therapy. Basic principles, protocols, and procedures. 3rd ed. New York: Guilford Publications; 2018. Online verfügbar unter https://ebookcentral.proquest.com/lib/gbv/detail.action?docID=5153824.

Shariati A, Jahani S, Hooshmand M, Khalili N. The effect of acupressure on sleep quality in hemodialysis patients. Complement Ther Med. 2012;20(6):417–23. https://doi.org/10.1016/j.ctim.2012.08.001.

Sharif Nia H, Pahlevan Sharif S, Yaghoobzadeh A, Yeoh KK, Goudarzian AH, Soleimani MA, Jamali S. Effect of acupressure on pain in Iranian leukemia patients: a randomized controlled trial study. Int J Nurs Pract. 2017;23(2). https://doi.org/10.1111/ijn.12513.

Sharifi Rizi M, Shamsalinia A, Ghaffari F, Keyhanian S, Naderi Nabi B. The effect of acupressure on pain, anxiety, and the physiological indexes of patients with cancer undergoing bone marrow biopsy. Complement Ther Clin Pract. 2017;29:136–41. https://doi.org/10.1016/j.ctcp.2017.09.002.

Sherman KJ, Ludman EJ, Cook AJ, Hawkes RJ, Roy-Byrne PP, Bentley S, et al. Effectiveness of therapeutic massage for generalized anxiety disorder: a randomized controlled trial. Depress Anxiety. 2010;27(5):441–50. https://doi.org/10.1002/da.20671.

Shin E-S, Seo K-H, Lee S-H, Jang J-E, Jung Y-M, Kim M-J, Yeon J-Y. Massage with or without aromatherapy for symptom relief in people with cancer. Cochrane Database Syst Rev. 2016;6:CD009873. https://doi.org/10.1002/14651858.CD009873.pub3.

Shor-Posner G, Hernandez-Reif M, Miguez M-J, Fletcher M, Quintero N, Baez J, et al. Impact of a massage therapy clinical trial on immune status in young Dominican children infected with HIV-1. J Altern Complement Med. 2006;12(6):511–6. https://doi.org/10.1089/acm.2006.12.511.

Silva LMT, Schalock M. Sense and self-regulation checklist, a measure of comorbid autism symptoms: initial psychometric evidence. Am J Occup Ther. 2012;66(2):177–86. https://doi.org/10.5014/ajot.2012.001578.

Silva LMT, Schalock M, Gabrielsen KR, Gretchen HD. One- and two-year outcomes of treating preschool children with autism with a Qigong massage protocol: an observational follow-along study. Altern Integr Med. 2016;5(2):1–10. https://doi.org/10.4172/2327-5162.1000216.

Sluik D, Buijsse B, Muckelbauer R, Kaaks R, Teucher B, Tj A, et al. Physical activity and mortality in individuals with diabetes mellitus: a prospective study and meta-analysis. Arch Intern Med. 2012;172(17):1285–95.

Solomon GF, Benton D, Harker JO, Bonavida B, Fletcher MA. Prolonged asymptomatic states in HIV-Seropositive persons with CD4 + T-Cells/mm': preliminary psychoimmunologic findings. J Acquir Immunodefic Syndr. 1993;6(10):1172.

Song HJ, Son H, Seo H-J, Lee H, Choi SM, Lee S. Effect of self-administered foot reflexology for symptom management in healthy persons: a systematic review and meta-analysis. Complement Ther Med. 2015;23(1):79–89. https://doi.org/10.1016/j.ctim.2014.11.005.

Song P, Zha M, Yang Q, Zhang Y, Li X, Rudan I. The prevalence of adult attention-deficit hyperactivity disorder: a global systematic review and meta-analysis. J Glob Health. 2021;11:04009.

Steinhausen H-C. Psychische Störungen bei Kindern und Jugendlichen. Lehrbuch der Kinder- und Jugendpsychiatrie. 4. Aufl. München: Urban und Schwarzenberg; 1996.

Stephenson J, Carter M. The use of weighted vests with children with autism spectrum disorders and other disabilities. J Autism Dev Disord. 2009;39(1):105–14. https://doi.org/10.1007/s10803-008-0605-3.

Stringer J, Swindell R, Dennis M. Massage in patients undergoing intensive chemotherapy reduces serum cortisol and prolactin. Psychooncology. 2008;17(10):1024–31. https://doi.org/10.1002/pon.1331.

Sun F, Yuan Q-L, Zhang Y-G. Large buttocks hematoma caused by deep tissue massage therapy. Pain Med. 2015;16(7):1445–7.

Thom J, Bretschneider J, Kraus N, Handerer J, Jacobi F. Versorgungsepidemiologie psychischer Störungen: Warum sinken die Prävalenzen trotz vermehrter Versorgungsangebote nicht ab? Bundesgesundheitsblatt Gesundheitsforschung Gesundheitsschutz. 2019;62(2):128–39. https://doi.org/10.1007/s00103-018-2867-z.

Tian F-L, Li Q, Cui J-M. Effect of massage on change of TLRs expressions in inflammatory cells of children with asthma during chronic remission phase. Matern Child Health Care China. 2014a;29(21):3512–4.

Tian F-L, Li Q, Cui J-M. Effect of massage on histamine, histamine receptor and leukotrienes levels in peripheral blood of children with asthma. Matern Child Health Care China. 2014b;29(24):3987–9.

Toth M, Marcantonio ER, Davis RB, Walton T, Kahn JR, Phillips RS. Massage therapy for patients with metastatic cancer: a pilot randomized controlled trial. J Altern Complement Med. 2013;19(7):650–6. https://doi.org/10.1089/acm.2012.0466.

Trotter JF. Hepatic hematoma after deep tissue massage. N Engl J Med. 1999;341(26):2019–20.

Tsuji S, Yuhi T, Furuhara K, Ohta S, Shimizu Y, Higashida H. Salivary oxytocin concentrations in seven boys with autism spectrum disorder received massage from their mothers: a pilot study. Front Psychiatry. 2015;6:58. https://doi.org/10.3389/fpsyt.2015.00058.

Tully PJ, Baker RA, Turnbull D, Winefield H. The role of depression and anxiety symptoms in hospital readmissions after cardiac surgery. J Behav Med. 2008;31(4):281–90. https://doi.org/10.1007/s10865-008-9153-8.

Unal KS, Balci Akpinar R. The effect of foot reflexology and back massage on hemodialysis patients' fatigue and sleep quality. Complement Ther Clin Pract. 2016;24:139–44. https://doi.org/10.1016/j.ctcp.2016.06.004.

Unlu A, Kirca O, Ozdogan M. Reflexology and cancer. J Oncol Sci. 2018;4(2):96–101. https://doi.org/10.1016/j.jons.2018.01.001.

Varaei S, Jalalian Z, Yekani Nejad MS, Shamsizadeh M. Comparison the effects of inhalation and massage aromatherapy with lavender and sweet orange on fatigue in hemodialysis patients: a randomized clinical trial. J Complement Integr Med. 2020;18(1):193–200. https://doi.org/10.1515/jcim-2018-0137.

Virués-Ortega J. Applied behavior analytic intervention for autism in early childhood: meta-analysis, meta-regression and dose-response meta-analysis of multiple outcomes. Clin Psychol Rev. 2010;30(4):387–99. https://doi.org/10.1016/j.cpr.2010.01.008.

Walters AS, LeBrocq C, Dhar A, Hening W, Rosen R, Allen RP, et al. Validation of the International Restless Legs Syndrome Study Group rating scale for restless legs syndrome. Sleep Med. 2003;4(2):121–32. https://doi.org/10.1016/s1389-9457(02)00258-7.

Wampold BE. The great psychotherapy debate. Models, methods, and findings. Transferred to digital printing. New York: Routledge; 2009.

Wändell PE, Carlsson AC, Andersson K, Gafvels C, Tornkvist L. Tactile massage or relaxation exercises do not improve the metabolic control of type 2 diabetics. Open Diabetes J. 2010;3(1):6–10. https://doi.org/10.2174/1876524601003010006.

Wändell PE, Carlsson AC, Gåfvels C, Andersson K, Törnkvist L. Measuring possible effect on health-related quality of life by tactile massage or relaxation in patients with type 2 diabetes. Complement Ther Med. 2012;20(1–2):8–15. https://doi.org/10.1016/j.ctim.2011.09.007.

Wang M-Y, Tsai P-S, Lee P-H, Chang W-Y, Yang C-M. The efficacy of reflexology: systematic review. J Adv Nurs. 2008;62(5):512–20. https://doi.org/10.1111/j.1365-2648.2008.04606.x.

Wang J-Y, Wu P-K, Chen PC-H, Yen C-C, Hung G-Y, Chen C-F, et al. Manipulation therapy prior to diagnosis induced primary osteosarcoma metastasis--from clinical to basic research. PLoS One. 2014;9(5):e96571. https://doi.org/10.1371/journal.pone.0096571.

WHO. Global action plan on physical activity 2018-2030. More active people for a healthier world. Geneva: World Health Organization; 2019.

WHO. Cardiovascular diseases. 2022. https://www.who.int/health-topics/cardiovascular-diseases. Accessed 15 May 2023.

Williams A-L, Selwyn PA, Liberti L, Molde S, Njike VY, McCorkle R, et al. A randomized controlled trial of meditation and massage effects on quality of life in people with late-stage disease: a pilot study. J Palliat Med. 2005;8(5):939–52. https://doi.org/10.1089/jpm.2005.8.939.

Winkelmann J. Genetics of restless legs syndrome. Curr Neurol Neurosci Rep. 2008;8(3):211–6. https://doi.org/10.1007/s11910-008-0033-y.

Wolf R, Baumbach C, Habel F, Heiermann M, Sinn R. Körperliche Aktivität als kardiovaskuläre Therapie Wie viel ist gut und sicher? Sportmed Präventivmed. 2011;41(4):10–4. https://doi.org/10.1007/s12534-011-0209-0.

Wu P-K, Chen W-M, Lee OK, Chen C-F, Huang C-K, Chen T-H. The prognosis for patients with osteosarcoma who have received prior manipulative therapy. J Bone Joint Surg Br. 2010;92(11):1580–5. https://doi.org/10.1302/0301-620X.92B11.24706.

Wu J, Yang X-W, Zhang M. Massage therapy in children with asthma: a systematic review and meta-analysis. eCAM. 2017;2017:5620568. https://doi.org/10.1155/2017/5620568.

Xiong XJ, Li SJ, Zhang YQ. Massage therapy for essential hypertension: a systematic review. J Hum Hypertens. 2015;29(3):143–51. https://doi.org/10.1038/jhh.2014.52.

Zhang B, Dong J-N, Sun P, Feng C, Liu Y-C. Effect of therapeutic care for treating fatigue in patients with breast cancer receiving chemotherapy. Medicine. 2017;96(33):e7750. https://doi.org/10.1097/MD.0000000000007750.

Zoega H, Kieler H, Nørgaard M, Furu K, Valdimarsdottir U, Brandt L, Haglund B. Use of SSRI and SNRI antidepressants during pregnancy: a population-based study from Denmark, Iceland, Norway and Sweden. PLoS One. 2015;10(12):e0144474. https://doi.org/10.1371/journal.pone.0144474.

Index

S. M. Mueller et al., *Human Touch in Healthcare*, https://doi.org/10.1007/978-3-662-67860-2

GPSR Compliance

The European Union's (EU) General Product Safety Regulation (GPSR) is a set of rules that requires consumer products to be safe and our obligations to ensure this.

If you have any concerns about our products, you can contact us on ProductSafety@springernature.com

In case Publisher is established outside the EU, the EU authorized representative is:

Springer Nature Customer Service Center GmbH
Europaplatz 3
69115 Heidelberg, Germany

Batch number: 10732801

Printed by Printforce, the Netherlands